PHYSICAL THERAPY CASE FILES®
Neurological Rehabilitation

Annie Burke-Doe PT, MPT, PhD
Associate Professor
University of St. Augustine for Health Sciences
San Marcos, California

Series Editor: Erin E. Jobst, PT, PhD
Associate Professor
School of Physical Therapy
College of Health Professions
Pacific University
Hillsboro, Oregon

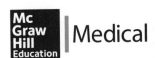

Medical

New York   Chicago   San Francisco   Athens   London   Madrid
Mexico City   Milan   New Delhi   Singapore   Sydney   Toronto

Physical Therapy Case Files®: Neurological Rehabilitation

1 2 3 4 5 6 7 8 9 0   DOC/DOC   18 17 16 15 14 13

ISBN 978-0-07-176378-3
MHID 0-07-176378-3

This book was set in Goudy by Cenveo® Publisher Services.
The editors were Catherine A. Johnson and Christina M. Thomas.
The production supervisor was Catherine H. Saggese.
Project management was provided by Yashmita Hota, Cenveo Publisher Services.
The cover designer was Thomas De Pierro.
RR Donnelley was the printer and binder.

Library of Congress Cataloging-in-Publication Data

Burke-Doe, Annie, author.
   Physical therapy case files. Neurological rehabilitation / Annie Burke-Doe.
      p. ; cm.
   Neurological rehabilitation
   Includes bibliographical references and index.
   ISBN-13: 978-0-07-176378-3 (pbk.)
   ISBN-10: 0-07-176378-3 (pbk.)
   I. Title.   II. Title: Neurological rehabilitation.
   [DNLM: 1. Nervous System Diseases—rehabilitation—Case Reports.   2. Physical Therapy Modalities—Case Reports.   WL 140]
   RC350.4
   616.8′043—dc23
                                                                        2013008991

CONTENTS

Kristen Barta, PT, DPT, NCS
Instructor
University of St. Augustine for Health Sciences
Austin, Texas

Annie Burke-Doe, PT, MPT, PhD
Associate Professor
University of St. Augustine for Health Sciences
San Marcos, California

Heather Scott David, PT, EdD(c), MPT, NCS
Adjunct Faculty
University of St. Augustine for Health Sciences
San Marcos, California

Michael Furtado, PT, DPT, NCS
Assistant Professor
University of Texas Medical Branch
School of Health Professions
Department of Physical Therapy
Galveston, Texas

Sharon L. Gorman, PT, DPTSc, GCS
Associate Professor
Department of Physical Therapy
Samuel Merritt University
Oakland, California

Timothy Harvey, PT, DPT
Samuel Merritt University
Oakland, California

Elizabeth A. Holt, PT, DPT
San Francisco, California

Christopher J. Ivey, PT, MPT, OCS, SCS, ATC, MS
Assistant Professor
University of St. Augustine for Health Sciences
San Marcos, California

Kristen M. Johnson, PT, EdD(c), MS, NCS
Assistant Professor
University of St. Augustine for Health Sciences
San Marcos, California

Jennifer Junkin, PT, DPT, MTC
Benchmark Physical Therapy
Conyers, Georgia

Aimie F. Kachingwe, PT, DPT, EdD, OCS, FAAOMPT
Associate Professor
Department of Physical Therapy
California State University Northridge
Northridge, California

Rolando T. Lazaro, PT, PhD, DPT, GCS
Associate Professor
Samuel Merritt University
Oakland, California

Cornelia Lieb-Lundell, PT, DPT, MA, PCS
Adjunct Faculty
University of St. Augustine for Health Sciences
San Marcos, California

Sheryl A. Low, PT, DPT, DSc, MPH, PCS
Chair and Associate Professor
Department of Physical Therapy
California State University Northridge
Northridge, California

Lisa Marie Luis, PT, DPT
Mount Shasta, California

Helen Luong, PT, DPT
El Camino Hospital Los Gatos Rehabilitation Center
Los Gatos, California

Terrence M. Nordstrom, PT, EdD
Assistant Academic Vice President and Associate Professor
Samuel Merritt University
Oakland, California

Anthony R. Novello, PT, DPT
Kaiser Permanente San Jose—Rehabilitation Services
San Jose, California

Beth Phillips, PT, DPA
Associate Professor
Department of Physical Therapy
California State University Northridge
Northridge, California

Delisa Rideout, DPT
Samuel Merritt University
Oakland, California

Jon Warren, MHSc, PGD Sports Med, Dip MT, MNZCP
Assistant Professor
University of St. Augustine for Health Sciences
San Marcos, California

Margaret A. Wicinski, PT, DPT, MTC, PCC, FAAOMPT
Assistant Professor
University of St. Augustine for Health Sciences
St. Augustine, Florida

Gail L. Widener, PT, PhD
Associate Professor
Department of Physical Therapy
Samuel Merritt University
Oakland, California

Wendy Wood, PT, DPT, GCS
Adjunct Faculty
University of St. Augustine for Health Sciences
San Marcos, California

ACKNOWLEDGMENTS

This *Physical Therapy Case Files: Neurological Rehabilitation* textbook is the culmination of the invaluable assistance and input from numerous talented people who have contributed in many ways toward its completion. First and foremost, I would like to offer thanks to all of the contributing authors for their commitment to this textbook. I am indebted to these individuals for their expertise and tireless work. Each contributor is acknowledged in the Contributor List; their names lend authority to this book, for which I am grateful.

I would also like to express gratitude and thanks to Erin Jobst, who has been a strong and consistent supporter for the *Physical Therapy Case Files* series. Without her help, it is unlikely that this book would have become a reality. I am also indebted to Joe Morita, the original editor from McGraw-Hill for introducing me to Erin Jobst and her never-ending talent and to the staff at McGraw-Hill for their help and support. Finally, efforts of this magnitude take a heavy toll on families of the authors; I would like to thank my husband Dan for the greatest love the world has known.

Annie Burke-Doe, PT, MPT, PhD

As the physical therapy profession continues to evolve and advance as a doctoring profession, so does the rigor of entry-level physical therapist education. Students must master fundamental foundation courses while integrating an understanding of new research in all areas of physical therapy. Evidence-based practice is the use of current best evidence in conjunction with the expertise of the clinician and the specific values and circumstances of the patient in making decisions regarding assessment and treatment. Evidence-based practice is a major emphasis in physical therapy education and in clinical practice. However, the most challenging task for students is making the transition from didactic classroom-based knowledge to its application in developing a physical therapy diagnosis and implementing appropriate evidence-based interventions. Ideally, instructors who are experienced and knowledgeable in every diagnosis and treatment approach could guide students at the "bedside" and students would supplement this training by self-directed independent reading. While there is certainly no substitute for clinical education, it is rare for clinical rotations to cover the scope of each physical therapy setting. In addition, it is not always possible for clinical instructors to be able to take the time necessary to guide students through the application of evidence-based tests and measures and interventions. Perhaps an effective alternative approach is teaching by using clinical case studies designed with a structured clinical approach to diagnosis and treatment. At the time of writing the *Physical Therapy Case Files* series, there were no physical therapy textbooks that contain case studies that utilize and reference current literature to support an illustrated examination or treatment. In my own teaching, I have designed case scenarios based on personal patient care experiences, those experiences shared with me by my colleagues, and searches through dozens of textbooks and websites to find a case study illustrating a particular concept. There are two problems with this approach. First, neither my own nor my colleagues' experiences cover the vast diversity of patient diagnoses, examinations, and interventions. Second, designing a case scenario that is not based on personal patient care experience or expertise takes an overwhelming amount of time. In my experience, detailed case studies that incorporate application of the best evidence are difficult to design "on the fly" in the classroom. The two-fold goal of the *Physical Therapy Case Files* series is to provide resources that contain multiple real-life case studies within an individual physical therapy practice area that will minimize the need for physical therapy educators to create their own scenarios and maximize the students' ability to implement evidence into the care of individual patients.

The cases within each book in the *Physical Therapy Case Files* series are organized for the reader to either read the book from "front to back" or to randomly select scenarios based on current interest. A list of cases by case number and by alphabetical listing by health condition is included in Section III to enable the reader to review his or her knowledge in a specific area. Sometimes a case scenario may include a more abbreviated explanation of a specific health condition or clinical test than was provided in another case. In this situation, the reader will be referred to the case with the more thorough explanation.

Every case follows an organized and well thought-out format using familiar language from both the World Health Organization's International Classification of Functioning, Disability, and Health (ICF) framework[1] and the American Physical Therapy Association's *Guide to Physical Therapist Practice*.[2] To limit redundancy and length of each case, we intentionally did not present the ICF framework or the *Guide's* Preferred Practice Patterns within each case. However, the section titles and the language used throughout each case were chosen to guide the reader through the evaluation, goal-setting, and intervention process and how clinical reasoning can be used to enhance an individual's activities and participation.

The front page of each case begins with a patient encounter followed by a series of open-ended questions. The discussion following the case is organized into *seven* sections:

1. **Key Definitions** provide terminology pertinent to the reader's understanding of the case. **Objectives** list the instructional and/or terminal behavioral objectives that summarize the knowledge, skills, or attitudes the reader should be able to demonstrate after reading the case. **PT considerations** provide a summary of the physical therapy plan of care, goals, interventions, precautions, and potential complications for the physical therapy management of the individual presented in the case.

2. **Understanding the Health Condition** presents an abbreviated explanation of the medical diagnosis. The intent of this section is *not* to be comprehensive. The etiology, pathogenesis, risk factors, epidemiology, and medical management of the condition are presented in enough detail to provide background and context for the reader.

3. **Physical Therapy Patient/Client Management** provides a summary of the role of the physical therapist in the patient's care. This section may elaborate on how the physical therapist's role augments and/or overlaps with those of other healthcare practitioners involved in the patient's care, as well as any referrals to additional healthcare practitioners that the physical therapist should provide.

4. **Examination, Evaluation, Diagnosis** guides the reader how to: organize and interpret information gathered from the chart review (in inpatient cases), appreciate adverse drug reactions that may affect patient presentation, and structure the subjective evaluation and physical examination. Not every assessment tool and special test that could possibly be done with the patient is included. For each outcome measure or special test presented, available reliability, validity, sensitivity, and specificity are discussed. When available, a minimal clinically important difference (MCID) for an outcome measure is presented because it helps the clinician to determine "the minimal level of change required in response to an intervention before the outcome would be considered worthwhile in terms of a patient/client's function or quality of life."[3]

5. **Plan of Care and Interventions** elaborates on a few physical therapy interventions for the patient's condition. The advantage of this section and the previous section is that each case does *not* exhaustively present every outcome measure, special test, or therapeutic intervention that *could be* performed. Rather, only selected outcome measures or examination techniques and interventions

are chosen. This is done to simulate a real-life patient interaction in which the physical therapist uses his or her clinical reasoning to determine the *most appropriate* tests and interventions to utilize with that patient during that episode of care. For each intervention that is chosen, the evidence to support its use with individuals with the same diagnosis (or similar diagnosis, if no evidence exists to support its use in that particular patient population) is presented. To reduce redundancy, standard guidelines for aerobic and resistance exercise have not been included. Instead, the reader is referred to guidelines published by the American College of Sports Medicine,[4] Goodman and Fuller,[5] and Paz and West.[6] For particular case scenarios in which standard guidelines are deviated from, specific guidelines are included.

6. **Evidence-Based Clinical Recommendations** includes a minimum of three clinical recommendations for diagnostic tools and/or treatment interventions for the patient's condition. To improve the quality of each recommendation beyond the personal clinical experience of the contributing author, each recommendation is graded using the Strength of Recommendation Taxonomy (SORT).[7] There are over one hundred evidence-grading systems used to rate the quality of individual studies and the strength of recommendations based on a body of evidence.[8] The SORT system has been used by several medical journals including *American Family Physician, Journal of the American Board of Family Practice, Journal of Family Practice,* and *Sports Health.* The SORT system has been chosen for two reasons: it is simple and its rankings are based on patient-oriented outcomes. The SORT system has only three levels of evidence: A, B, and C. Grade A recommendations are based on consistent, good-quality patient-oriented evidence (*e.g.,* systematic reviews, meta-analysis of high-quality studies, high-quality randomized controlled trials, high-quality diagnostic cohort studies). Grade B recommendations are based on inconsistent or limited-quality patient-oriented evidence (*e.g.,* systematic review or meta-analysis of lower-quality studies or studies with inconsistent findings). Grade C recommendations are based on consensus, disease-oriented evidence, usual practice, expert opinion, or case series (*e.g.,* consensus guidelines, disease-oriented evidence using only intermediate or physiologic outcomes). The contributing author of each case provided a grade based on the SORT guidelines for each recommendation or conclusion. The grade for each statement was reviewed and sometimes altered by the editors. Key phrases from each clinical recommendation are bolded within the case to enable the reader to easily locate where the cited evidence was presented.

7. **Comprehension Questions and Answers** include two to four multiple-choice questions that reinforce the content or elaborate and introduce new, but related concepts to the patient's case. When appropriate, detailed explanations about why alternative choices would not be the best choice are also provided.

My hope is that these real-life case studies will be a new resource to facilitate the incorporation of evidence into everyday physical therapy practice in various settings and patient populations. With the persistent push for evidence-based healthcare to promote quality and effectiveness[9] and the advent of evidence-based reimbursement guidelines, case scenarios with evidence-based recommendations will be an added benefit as physical therapists continually face the threat of decreased reimbursement rates for their services and will need to demonstrate evidence supporting their services. I hope physical therapy educators, entry-level physical therapy students, practicing physical therapists, and professionals preparing for Board Certification in clinical specialty areas will find these books helpful to translate classroom-based knowledge to evidence-based assessments and interventions.

Erin E. Jobst, PT, PhD

1. World Health Organization. International Classification of Functioning, Disability and Health (ICF). http://www.who.int/classifications/icf/en/. Accessed August 7, 2012.

2. American Physical Therapy Association. *Guide to Physical Therapist Practice (Guide)*. Alexandria, VA: APTA; 1999.

3. Jewell DV. *Guide to Evidence-based Physical Therapy Practice*. Sudbury, MA: Jones and Barlett; 2008.

4. American College of Sports Medicine. *ACSM's Guidelines for Exercise Testing and Prescription*. 8th ed. Philadelphia, PA: Wolters Kluwer/Lippincott Williams & Wilkins; 2010.

5. Goodman CC, Fuller KS. *Pathology: Implications for the Physical Therapist*. 3rd ed. Philadelphia, PA: W.B. Saunders Company; 2009.

6. Paz JC, West MP. *Acute Care Handbook for Physical Therapists*. 3rd ed. St. Louis, MO: Saunders Elsevier; 2009.

7. Ebell MH, Siwek J, Weiss BD, et al. Strength of Recommendation Taxonomy (SORT): a patient-centered approach to grading evidence in the medical literature. *Am Fam Physician*. 2004;69:548-556.

8. Systems to rate the strength of scientific evidence. Summary, evidence report/technology assessment: number 47. AHRQ publication no. 02-E015, March 2002. http://www.ahrq.gov/clinic/epcsums/strengthsum.htm. Accessed August 7, 2012.

9. Agency for Healthcare Research and Quality. www.ahrq.gov/clinic/epc/. Accessed August 7, 2012.

Introduction

The study of neurologic disease in physical therapy is exciting and dynamic because it is ever changing and always requires a framework related to the individual, his or her health condition, and contextual factors involved with recovery. While students are excited by the implications of returning patients to higher levels of function, they are also challenged by the exceedingly detailed requirements of learning the pathologies, treatments, and interventions. When confronted by the crushing memorization that is often required, the student has little time to step back and gain appreciation for the unique presentation of each individual and the art of the clinician providing care as determined by the most recent evidence.

This book provides a different approach to assist both the students and the faculty. Instead of making the mastery of diseases and interventions the main goal and then searching for applications of this knowledge, each clinical case can be used as a guide for integrating the best available evidence and as an example of a real-life case illustrating a practitioner's expertise in clinical decision-making. This text presents 31 cases representing individuals with a variety of neurologic conditions, ages, acuity levels, and practice areas. Each case incorporates and explains the use of evidence-based tests and measures and interventions, ending with graded clinical recommendations. Three cases present a unique opportunity for the reader to follow a patient with a complete spinal cord injury at the C7 neurological level as she moves from the intensive care unit (Case 14) to an inpatient rehabilitation facility (Case 15) and finally to an outpatient physical therapy clinic (Case 16). Through publication of *Physical Therapy Case Files: Neurological Rehabilitation*, I hope that students and faculty at many institutions will find this to be an enjoyable and effective way to learn neurologic physical therapy and its evidence-based real world applications.

Thirty-One Case Scenarios

Alzheimer's Disease

Annie Burke-Doe

CASE 1

At the request of her family, an 85-year-old female was evaluated for short-term memory loss by a neurologist. She recently had been found wandering in her neighborhood, looking for her way home. Her daughter described that her mother has had difficulty with cognitive function since the death of her husband 2 years earlier and that the family attributed the difficulty to grieving and depression. Her daughter also reported that her mother had fallen a number of times in the last 3 months and appeared more fatigued with activities. On cognitive examination, the patient was not oriented to date or month, but she could identify the day of the week and the season. She was able to name the state, county, and city, but not the clinic where she was being evaluated. She could recall three words immediately after they were spoken to her, but could not recall any after 5 minutes of distraction. She correctly spelled the first three letters of "world" backward. She could name a watch, a pen, and a sweater, but could not name a button, sleeve, or cuff. She correctly drew a clock, but could not set the hands to 9:15. The general neurologic examination was unrevealing, except for diminished light touch and vibration in the distal lower extremities and mildly unsteady gait. The patient was referred for physical therapy evaluation and treatment.

▶ Based on her health condition, what do you anticipate will be the contributors to activity limitations?
▶ What are the examination priorities?
▶ What is her rehabilitation prognosis?
▶ What are the most appropriate outcome measures for cognitive dysfunction?
▶ What are possible complications interfering with physical therapy?

KEY DEFINITIONS

ANOMIA: Inability to name objects

APRAXIA: Inability to execute or carry out learned purposeful movements, despite having the physical ability to perform the movements

CIRCUMLOCUTION: Roundabout or indirect way of speaking; the use of more words than necessary to express an idea

DEMENTIA: Decline in intellectual function severe enough to interfere with a person's relationships and ability to carry out daily activities

SUNDOWNING: State of confusion at the end of the day and into the night

Objectives

1. Describe Alzheimer's disease.
2. Identify key stages and changes in function with progression of Alzheimer's disease.
3. Identify reliable and valid outcome tools to measure cognitive decline.
4. Discuss appropriate components of the physical therapy examination for the individual with Alzheimer's disease.

Physical Therapy Considerations

PT considerations during management of the individual with dementia, history of falls, general motor and balance difficulties, and decreased endurance due to Alzheimer's disease:

▶ **General physical therapy plan of care/goals:** Assess cognition as well as noncognitive function including changes in affect, personality, and behavior; increase (or at least minimize declines in) strength, range of motion, and balance; promote functional movement; decrease fall risk

▶ **Physical therapy interventions:** Functional mobility training, balance training, gait training, facilitation of normal movement, therapeutic exercises, endurance training, patient/family/caregiver education

▶ **Precautions during physical therapy:** Falls

▶ **Complications interfering with physical therapy:** Presence of comorbidities, secondary impairments, progressively decreasing cognitive status, behaviors such as agitation and sundowning

Understanding the Health Condition

Alzheimer's disease is the most frequent cause of dementia, affecting an estimated 5 million people in the United States and 17 million worldwide.[1] As the Baby Boom generation ages, the number is projected to rise to 7.7 million by 2030, and between

11 and 16 million by 2050.[2] The principal risk factor is increased age,[3] with other factors including family history and genetic mutations.[1] Factor analysis of 663 patients with probable Alzheimer's disease reveals that memory, language, and praxis are the main cognitive deficits in Alzheimer's disease.[4] The disease onset is insidious; manifestations evolve over years from mildly impaired memory to severe cognitive loss.[1] In 2011, the National Institute on Aging-Alzheimer's Association workgroup developed a framework on the diagnostic guidelines for Alzheimer's disease. The workgroup suggested a hypothetical model for the trajectory of Alzheimer's disease in three stages. **The clinical stages include: (1) preclinical Alzheimer's disease, which precedes (2) mild cognitive impairment (MCI), followed by (3) a definitive diagnosis of Alzheimer's disease dementia.**[5-7] The long "preclinical" stage is currently being researched to determine the biomarkers and epidemiological and neuropsychological factors that best predict the risk of progression from asymptomatic to MCI to Alzheimer's disease.[8] Mild cognitive impairment is classified in two subtypes (amnestic and nonamnestic).[9] In amnestic MCI, the patients and their families are aware of increasing forgetfulness and the memory loss is more prominent than the subtle forgetfulness that occurs with normal aging.[10] Nonamnestic MCI is characterized by a subtle decline in functions not related to memory, but rather affecting attention, use of language, or visuospatial skills.[10]

The most frequent pathological features in the brains of patients with Alzheimer's disease include *extracellular* beta amyloid protein in diffuse plaques and beta amyloid protein in plaques containing elements of degenerating neurons, termed neuritic plaques.[11] *Intracellular* changes in pyramidal neurons include deposits of hyperphosphorylated and aggregated tau protein in the form of neurofibrillary tangles.[1,3,12] Amyloid plaques and intracellular tangles first appear in the hippocampus and then become widespread. Over time, there is widespread loss of neurons and synapses.[1]

Memory dysfunction in Alzheimer's disease involves impairment of learning new information, which is often characterized as short-term memory loss. In the early and moderate stages of the disease, recall of remote, well-learned material appears to be preserved, but the ability to retain recently acquired information is impaired. Closely associated with the loss of learning is progressive disorientation in time and place. In the later stages, frank failure of recall for previously well-remembered information is also observed.[13]

Impairments in language and executive function (*e.g.*, the ability to perform sequential tasks) are also a key component of Alzheimer's disease.[1,13] Verbal memory decline is often first manifested as difficulty in finding words in spontaneous speech and eventually results in reduced vocabulary, circumlocution, and word-finding pauses.[13] Anomia on confrontational naming tests is most notable for parts of an object (*e.g.*, a button) rather than the whole object (sweater). Problems with abstract thinking, organizing, planning, and problem solving become apparent as new behaviors such as socially inappropriate behavior, disinhibition, and poor task initiation or persistence emerge.[14] Executive dysfunction is present in the majority of individuals with Alzheimer's disease, even those with relatively mild dementia.[15]

Nearly all individuals with Alzheimer's disease eventually develop apraxia as the illness progresses. The most common type is ideomotor apraxia—the difficulty in translating an idea into a proper action.[13] Deficits in complex visual function such as agnosia are present, as well as spatial disorientation, acalculia, and left to right disorientation. Breakdown of elemental visual processing also occurs, leading to deficits in contrast and spatial frequency, motion detection, and figure-ground discrimination, which may influence driving[1] and other complex activities of daily living.

Noncognitive or behavioral symptoms associated with Alzheimer's disease often account for a larger proportion of caregiver burden or stress than the cognitive dysfunction. Personality changes are common, with passivity and apathy appearing more frequently than agitation in the early phases. One retrospective review suggested that social withdrawal, mood changes, or depression were present in more than 70% of cases, with a mean duration of more than 2 years *prior* to diagnosis of Alzheimer's disease.[16] Sundowning or "sundowning syndrome" is the occurrence or exacerbation of behavioral symptoms in the afternoon or evening.[17] Associated symptoms can include aggression, agitation, delusion, increased disorientation, and wandering.[18] Sundowning may be related to circadian rhythm disturbances and hormonal factors; it is often treated with bright light during the day and/or melatonin in the evening.[17]

Depression was observed in over 36% of 2354 individuals with Alzheimer's disease (with a mean Mini-Mental State Examination score of 17.8).[1,19] Anxiety has also been observed in about 37% of patients with Alzheimer's disease.[1,19] Catastrophic reactions (intense emotional outbursts of short duration characterized by tearfulness, aggressive behavior, and contrary behaviors) are associated with increased anxiety in individuals with Alzheimer's disease.[13] Psychosis and agitation can occur later in the disease course and are associated with more rapid decline.[1]

Another common problem with Alzheimer's disease is the individual's unawareness of the illness.[13] It is characterized by a lack of recognition of the full extent and implications of one's cognitive or functional disability. Prevalence of lack of insight into illness ranges from 30% to 50% in the mild and moderate stages of Alzheimer's disease.[20]

Throughout most of the disease course, Alzheimer's disease does not adversely affect the physical neurologic examination. In later stages, extrapyramidal signs (*e.g.*, rigidity) and gait disturbances may become prominent. Currently, there are only two treatments approved by the Food and Drug Administration for Alzheimer's disease: cholinesterase inhibitors (donepezil, rivastigmine, and galantamine) and the N-methyl-D-aspartate receptor antagonist memantine.[8] These drugs do not stop or limit disease progression. At best, they may provide symptomatic treatment that helps patients remain independent for longer periods and can assist with decreasing the caregiver burden. There is no cure for Alzheimer's disease.

Physical Therapy Patient/Client Management

A patient with Alzheimer's disease may present to the physical therapist at any stage of the disease continuum. More commonly, the individual presents in the intermediate stage of MCI and when the definitive diagnosis of Alzheimer's disease dementia has been made. At this stage, she may present with generalized weakness, loss of functional movement, and an increased risk of falling. In patients with dementia, cognitive deficits affect daily functioning to the extent that there is loss of independence in the community.[10] The physical therapist is an important part of the medical management of Alzheimer's disease as it relates to teaching the patient and the caregivers strategies to improve quality of life. All treatment planning should occur as part of a team effort in which the patient, family or significant others, physicians, nurses, social worker, and occupational therapist collaborate so that a consistent treatment plan and orientation are followed.[21] To enhance their effectiveness, therapists working with patients with cognitive impairment may benefit from advanced training in assessment of communication skills, neurologic functioning, and gerontology.[21]

Neuropsychological testing is used in the evaluation of Alzheimer's disease to understand the nature and extent of an individual's cognitive impairment. These tests are often conducted by a neuropsychologist, but can be performed by healthcare professionals trained in their use. A brief mental status examination, such as the Mini-Mental State Examination (MMSE), is often insensitive to early cognitive impairment. More useful measures include the Short Test of Mental Status (STMS) and the Montreal Cognitive Assessment (MoCA).[22-24] The STMS takes roughly 5 minutes to administer. It tests an individual's orientation, attention, immediate recall, arithmetic, abstraction, construction, information, and delayed recall (of approximately 3 minutes). In one study using the STMS, dementia was diagnosed with a sensitivity of 92% and specificity of 91% with cut-off scores ≤ 29.[24] Another study found that the sensitivity of the STMS in identifying dementia was 86.4%, with a specificity of 93.5% compared to other well-recognized and longer standardized tests of cognitive function.[25] The MoCA is another brief cognitive screening tool. It is a single page 30-point test that takes approximately 10 minutes to administer; it assesses different types of cognitive abilities, including orientation, short-term memory, executive function, language abilities, and visuospatial ability. In 277 adults, the sensitivity and specificity of the MoCA for detecting MCI were 90% and 87%, respectively, compared to 18% and 100%, respectively, for the MMSE.[23] In the same study, the sensitivity and specificity of the MoCA for detecting early Alzheimer's disease were 100% and 87% respectively, compared with 78% and 100%, respectively, for the MMSE. In individuals with Alzheimer's disease, dementia has a gradual onset over months to years. It is characterized by a history of worsening cognition and impairments in learning and recall of recently learned information. A diagnosis of dementia can be supported by the use of instruments such as the **Functional Activities Questionnaire (FAQ)**, which characterizes functional impairment that is within the range of dementia.[26,27] The FAQ provides performance ratings on 10 complex, higher-order activities. Used alone as a diagnostic tool, the FAQ was more sensitive than the Instrumental Activities of Daily Living Scale (85% vs. 57%) and almost as specific (81% vs. 92%) in distinguishing between normal and demented individuals.

Physical therapists are often consulted in the treatment of patients with Alzheimer's disease because of the gait, postural control, and mobility abnormalities that occur in Alzheimer's disease. These impairments are often among the first signs in individuals with central nervous system disorders.[28] The annual incidence of falls in persons with dementia is 40% to 60%, which is double the rate in cognitively intact elderly.[29] Even simple dual-task activities (*e.g.,* walking while performing a cognitive task) substantially decrease postural stability due to attention-related deficits in cognitively impaired geriatric patients with a history of falls.[30] It is estimated that 89% of long-term residents with dementia experience at least some degree of mobility impairment.[31]

Examination, Evaluation, and Diagnosis

During the examination, the physical therapist identifies impairments that can be causing functional problems, specific disabilities, and the stage of the disease in order to determine prognosis of the impairment and to determine what additional functional testing should be performed.[28] Key elements of the examination include patient history and a systems review to target areas requiring further assessment. Tests and measures may include posture, range of motion, muscle performance, gait, balance, and postural control. Observing performance of functional activities during the assessment is critical because these patients often have difficulty following commands. For a patient who has difficulty processing verbal and written stimuli, it may be beneficial to spread the interactions over an 8-hour work day in order to maximize the patient's performance and reduce fatigue or examination-induced stressors.[21] For example, instead of one 45-minute therapy session, the patient may be able to participate better in short 10-minute interactions. Patients with Alzheimer's disease may have specific problems integrating sensory input and may benefit from assessment of specific sensory systems. Patients with Alzheimer's disease frequently have changes in affect, personality, and behavior. Particular attention should be given to how the patient is responding to communication efforts. Determining activities she is familiar with and her daily rituals can assist the therapist and caregivers in developing alternative strategies to redirect an agitated patient. The therapist should also assess the need for or the current use of assistive devices, environmental barriers, and a home evaluation. Caregivers should be educated regarding the functional changes that may occur in the near future and ways to compensate for current functional losses.

Plan of Care and Interventions

The primary goal of physical therapy is to *maximize* functional independence, balance in sitting or standing with or without an assistive device, and safety awareness with all mobility, while *minimizing* secondary impairments. In the early stages, this patient population may appear physically healthy, but they are susceptible to falls and other accidents resulting in orthopaedic and other types of injuries.[32] Interventions are based on the individual's needs with a focus on maintaining the ability to function in the environment. Physical interventions may include walking, performance of activities of daily living, dancing, gardening,[32] aerobic exercise, involvement in intellectually stimulating activities, and participation in social activities.[9] Cognitive decline may be addressed through comprehensive cognitive stimulation that enhances neuroplasticity, reduces cognitive loss, and helps the patient to stretch functional independence through better cognitive performance.[33,34]

Due to greater loss in cognitive abilities and physical function, patients in the middle stage of Alzheimer's disease (like the patient described in the current case) will require more caregiver assistance. Patients who have sensory and perceptual changes can benefit from environment modifications including effective lighting, verbal orientation, physical escorts, consistent furniture placement, clear hallways, systematic storage systems for clothes and toiletry articles, and the use of contrasting colors to identify doors, windows, baseboards, and corners.[21] As a patient's cognitive status deteriorates, staff, family, and caregivers must be trained in nonverbal, positional, and manual cues as well as emotional communication techniques.[27] **Calming techniques** such as rocking,[32] the use of music,[35] and therapeutic touch including massage[36] have been shown to have some benefits in working with patients with dementia. Therapists can also train caregivers to ease the difficulties associated with unwanted behaviors such as agitation and sundowning. Some suggestions include: providing calm and repetitive tasks (*e.g.*, winding a ball of yard), exercising early in the day, keeping rooms well-lit during the day, reducing outside stimuli (*e.g.*, noise from television), controlling specific triggers, and keeping a behavioral log.[14] Current research suggests that **caregivers who received formal instruction** regarding techniques in custodial care, management of behavioral problems, and recommendations for simple home modifications need less assistance within the home[37] and report fewer negative appraisals of behavioral problems.[37-39]

The ability to maintain the patient's *safety* is a key factor in enabling her to stay at home rather than placing her in a long-term care facility. Wandering and getting lost is one of the most serious problems for patients with moderate to severe dementia.[13] The Safe Return Program is a nationwide service sponsored by the Alzheimer's Association to help police and private citizens identify, locate, and return people with dementia. Safe Return provides an identification item (wallet card, jewelry, or clothing label) for the registered person and a national toll-free telephone number to assist finding and returning the patient to home.

In the management of Alzheimer's disease, physical exercise and social activity are as important as nutrition and health maintenance. The physical therapist can assist the team in planning daily activities to provide structure, meaning, and accomplishment in a safe environment. As physical and cognitive functions are lost, adapting activities and routines will be essential to maintain patient participation. Therapy interventions, problem solving, and modifications need to be coordinated with all the team members.

Evidence-Based Clinical Recommendations

SORT: Strength of Recommendation Taxonomy

A: Consistent, good-quality patient-oriented evidence

B: Inconsistent or limited-quality patient-oriented evidence

C: Consensus, disease-oriented evidence, usual practice, expert opinion, or case series

1. An individual's stage of disease should be considered in determining expected cognitive function involvement and prognosis in Alzheimer's disease. **Grade A**

2. Physical therapists can use the Functional Activities Questionnaire (FAQ) to characterize functional impairments in individuals with dementia. **Grade A**

3. Emotional nonverbal communication and calming techniques such as massage, rocking, and music provide some benefits in working with patients with Alzheimer's disease. **Grade C**

4. When instruction regarding techniques in custodial care, management of behavioral problems, and recommendations for home modifications is provided to caregivers of individuals with Alzheimer's disease, they report fewer behavioral problems and need less assistance at home. **Grade A**

COMPREHENSION QUESTIONS

1.1 The most frequent pathological features in patients with Alzheimer's disease include which of the following?

A. Extracellular tau protein, neuritic plaques, and neurofibrillary tangles

B. Extracellular alpha amyloid protein, neuritic plaques, and neurofibrillary tangles

C. Intracellular beta amyloid protein, neuritic plaques, and neurofibrillary tangles

D. Extracellular beta amyloid protein, neuritic plaques, and neurofibrillary tangles

1.2 A physical therapist is working with a patient who demonstrates a subtle decline in cognitive function that is not related to memory as well as deficits in attentiveness and use of language. Which stage of Alzheimer's disease does this represent?

A. Preclinical Alzheimer's disease

B. Amnestic mild cognitive impairment

C. Nonamnestic mild cognitive impairment

D. Alzheimer's disease

ANSWERS

1.1 **D.** The most frequent pathological features in the brains of patients with Alzheimer's disease include extracellular beta amyloid protein in diffuse plaques and in plaques containing elements of degenerating neurons, termed neuritic plaques.[11] Intracellular changes in pyramidal neurons include deposits of hyperphosphorylated and aggregated tau protein in the form of neurofibrillary tangles.[1,3,12]

1.2 **C.** Nonamnestic mild cognitive impairment is characterized by a subtle decline in functions not related to memory. Deficits are noted in attentiveness, use of language, or visuospatial skills.

REFERENCES

1. Mayeux R. Early Alzheimer's disease. *N Engl J Med.* 2010;362:2194-2201.

2. Okie S. Confronting Alzheimer's disease. *N Engl J Med.* 2011;365:1069-1072.

3. Querfurth HW, LaFerla FM. Alzheimer's disease. *N Engl J Med.* 2010;362:329-344.

4. Talwalker S, Overall JE, Srirama MK, Gracon SI. Cardinal features of cognitive dysfunction in Alzheimer's disease: a factor-analytic study of the Alzheimer's Disease Assessment Scale. *J Geriatr Psychiatry Neurol.* 1996;9:39-46.

5. McKhann GM, Knopman DS, Chertkow H, et al. The diagnosis of dementia due to Alzheimer's disease: recommendations from the National Institute on Aging-Alzheimer's Association workgroups on diagnostic guidelines for Alzheimer's disease. *Alzheimers Dement.* 2011;7:263-269.

6. Albert MS, DeKosky ST, Dickson D, et al. The diagnosis of mild cognitive impairment due to Alzheimer's disease: recommendations from the National Institute on Aging-Alzheimer's Association workgroups on diagnostic guidelines for Alzheimer's disease. *Alzheimers Dement.* 2011;7:270-279.

7. Sperling RA, Aisen PS, Beckett LA, et al. Toward defining the preclinical stages of Alzheimer's disease: recommendations from the National Institute on Aging-Alzheimer's Association workgroups on diagnostic guidelines for Alzheimer's disease. *Alzheimers Dement.* 2011;7:280-292.

8. Farlow MR, Cummings JL. Effective pharmacologic management of Alzheimer's disease. The *Am J Med.* 2007;120:388-397.

9. Petersen RC. Mild cognitive impairment as a diagnostic entity. *J Intern Med.* 2004;256:183-194.

10. Petersen RC. Clinical practice. Mild cognitive impairment. *N Engl J Med.* 2011;364:2227-2234.

11. Duyckaerts C, Delatour B, Potier MC. Classification and basic pathology of Alzheimer disease. *Acta Neuropathol.* 2009;118:5-36.

12. Lee VM, Goedert M, Trojanowski JQ. Neurodegenerative tauopathies. *Annu Rev Neurosci.* 2001;24:1121-1159.

13. Geldmacher DS, Farlow M. Alzheimer disease. In: Gilman S, ed. *MedLink Neurolog.* San Diego, CA: MedLink Corporation; 2010.

14. American Psychiatric Association. *Diagnostic and Statistical Manual of Mental Disorders.* 4th ed. Washington DC: American Psychiatric Association; 1994.

15. Stokholm J, Vogel A, Gade A, Waldemar G. Heterogeneity in executive impairment in patients with very mild Alzheimer's disease. *Dement Geriatr Cogn Disord.* 2006;22:54-59.

16. Jost BC, Grossberg GT. The evolution of psychiatric symptoms in Alzheimer's disease: a natural history study. *J Am Geriatr Soc.*1996;44:1078-1081.

17. Volicer L, Harper DG, Manning BC, Goldstein R, Satlin A. Sundowning and circadian rhythms in Alzheimer's disease. *Am J Psychiatry.* 2001;158:704-711.

18. Scarmeas N, Brandt J, Blacker D, et al. Disruptive behavior as a predictor in Alzheimer disease. *Arch Neurol.* 2007;64:1755-1761.

19. Aalten J, Verhey FR, Bullock R, et al. Neuropsychiatric syndromes in dementia. Results from the European Alzheimer Disease Consortium: part I. *Dement Geriatr Cogn Disord.* 2007;24:457-463.

20. Starkstein SE, Jorge R, Mizrahi R, Robinson RG. A diagnostic formulation for anosognosia in Alzheimer's disease. *J Neurol Neurosurg Psychiatry.* 2006;77:719-725.

21. Schulte OS, Stephens J, Ann J. Brain function, aging, and dementia. In: Umphred DA, ed. *Neurological Rehabilitation.* 5th ed. St. Louis, MO: Mosby Elsevier; 2007:902-930.

22. Tang-Wai DF, Knopman DS, Geda YE, et al. Comparison of the short test of mental status and the mini-mental state examination in mild cognitive impairment. *Arch Neurol.* 2003;60:1777-1781.

23. Nasreddine ZS, Phillips NA, Bedirian V, et al. The Montreal Cognitive Assessment, MoCA: a brief screening tool for mild cognitive impairment. *J Am Geriatr Soc.* 2005;53:695-699.

24. Kokmen E, Naessens JM, Offord KP. A short test of mental status: description and preliminary results. *Mayo Clin Proc.* 1987;62:281-288.

25. Kokmen E, Smith GE, Petersen RC, Tangalos E, Ivnik RC. The short test of mental status. Correlations with standardized psychometric testing. *Arch Neurol.* 1991;48:725-728.

26. Jette AM, Davies AR, Cleary PD, et al. The Functional Status Questionnaire: reliability and validity when used in primary care. *J Gen Intern Med.* 1986;1:143-149.

27. Pfeffer RI, Kurosaki TT, Harrah CH, Jr, Chance JM, Filos S. Measurement of functional activities in older adults in the community. *J Gerontol.* 1982;37:323-329.

28. Quinn L, Bello-Hass VD. Progressive central nervous system disorders. In: Cameron MH, ed. *Physical Rehabilitation.* St. Louis, MO: Mosby Elsevier; 2007:436-472.

29. Shaw FE, Kenny RA. Can falls in patients with dementia be prevented? *Age Ageing.* 1998;27:7-9.

30. Hauer K, Pfisterer M, Weber C, Wezler N, Kliegel M, Oster P. Cognitive impairment decreases postural control during dual tasks in geriatric patients with a history of severe falls. *J Am Geriatr Soc.* 2003;51:1638-1644.

31. Williams CS, Zimmerman S, Sloane PD, Reed PS. Characteristics associated with pain in long-term care residents with dementia. *Gerontologist.* 2005;45(spec no. 1):68-73.

32. Lewis CB, Bottomley JM. *Geriatric Rehabilitation. A Clinical Approach.* 3rd ed. Upper Saddle River, NJ: Pearson Prentice Hall; 2008.

33. Fuller KS, Wilnkler PA, Corboy JR. Degenerative diseases of the central nervous system. In: Goodman CC, Fuller KS, eds. *Pathology—Implications for the Physical Therapist.* 3rd ed. St. Louis, MO: Saunders Elsevier; 2009:1418-1419.

34. Loewenstein DA, Acevedo A, Czaja SJ, Duara R. Cognitive rehabilitation of mildly impaired Alzheimer disease patients on cholinesterase inhibitors. *Am J Geriatr Psychiatry.* 2004;12:395-402.

35. Simmons-Stern NR, Budson AE, Ally BA. Music as a memory enhancer in patients with Alzheimer's disease. *Neuropsychologia.* 2010;48:3164-3167.

36. Kim EJ, Buschmann MT. The effect of expressive physical touch on patients with dementia. *Int J Nurs Stud.* 1999;36:235-243.

37. Gitlin LN, Hauck WW, Dennis MP, Winter L. Maintenance of effects of the home environmental skill-building program for family caregivers and individuals with Alzheimer's disease and related disorders. *J Gerontol A Biol Med Sci.* 2005;60:368-374.

38. Guerriero Austrom M, Damush TM, Hartwell CW, et al. Development and implementation of non-pharmacologic protocols for the management of patients with Alzheimer's disease and their families in a multiracial primary care setting. *Gerontologist.* 2004;44:548-553.

39. Mittelman MS, Roth DL, Haley WE, Zarit SH. Effects of a caregiver intervention on negative caregiver appraisals of behavior problems in patients with Alzheimer's disease: results of a randomized trial. *J Gerontol B Psychol Soc Sci.* 2004;59:P27-P34.

Cerebrovascular Accident

Sharon L. Gorman
Elizabeth A. Holt

CASE 2

A 41-year-old right-handed male with a history of left basal ganglia ischemic cerebrovascular accident (CVA) 12 weeks ago presented to an outpatient physical therapy clinic. Initially after his stroke, he was hospitalized for 1 week and discharged to his home. He received home health physical therapy for 12 visits and then went to an outpatient physical therapy clinic for 12 more visits. The patient has been improving since his stroke, stating that he feels stronger every week. However, he continues to fatigue easily, suffers from decreased balance, and right-sided upper extremity (UE) and lower extremity (LE) weakness. The proposed mechanism of his stroke was related to his use of warfarin (Coumadin) to treat atrial fibrillation and initiation of a diet high in vitamin K. He was unaware that a diet rich in vitamin K would decrease the effectiveness of warfarin, thus increasing his risk for an ischemic stroke. His health history also indicated he had high cholesterol and sleep apnea. It has been 3 weeks since his last outpatient physical therapy visit. He is returning to outpatient physical therapy because he is unable to walk long distances without fatigue, has difficulty with running or shuffling to play softball, and is unable to throw or hit a softball accurately and consistently. His stated participation restrictions include an inability to walk his dog, coach his daughter's softball team (including demonstrating how to slide into and steal bases), or play sports with his two children.

► What risk factors contributed to this patient's health condition?
► Based on his health condition, what do you anticipate will be the contributors to activity limitations and impairments?
► What are the examination priorities?
► What are the most appropriate physical therapy interventions?
► What outcome measures are best suited to this patient and his presentation?

KEY DEFINITIONS

BASAL GANGLIA: A group of interconnected deep subcortical nuclei comprised of two principal input nuclei (striatum and subthalamic nucleus) and two principal output nuclei (substantia nigra pars reticulata and internal globus pallidus) that help start and control movement

ISCHEMIC STROKE: Disruption of cerebral circulation caused by a blocked artery due to either an embolus or thrombus

VITAMIN K: A fat-soluble vitamin required for blood coagulation

Objectives

1. Describe how a drug–food interaction such as warfarin and a diet rich in vitamin K increases the risk for a cerebrovascular accident.
2. Design a physical examination schema for a higher functioning person poststroke.
3. Compare and contrast selected outcome measures for use with high-functioning individuals poststroke.
4. Incorporate principles of sports rehabilitation into the care of a person poststroke.
5. Describe neuroplasticity principles that should be considered when designing a plan of care for a person poststroke.

Physical Therapy Considerations

PT considerations during management of the high-functioning individual with a stroke in the basal ganglia:

▶ **General physical therapy plan of care/goals:** Increase activity and participation; increase strength and/or normalize muscle tone on involved side; prevent or minimize loss of range of motion (ROM), strength, and aerobic functional capacity; improve quality of life

▶ **Physical therapy interventions:** Neuromuscular re-education; task-specific therapeutic exercise to address participation restrictions; patient safety

▶ **Precautions during physical therapy:** Monitor cardiovascular status; protection of joints on hemiplegic side; protection of skin in insensate areas

▶ **Complications interfering with physical therapy:** Risk for another stroke due to increased physical demands; loss of balance with high-level sporting activities

Understanding the Health Condition

Cerebrovascular accidents (CVA), also known as strokes, are the third leading cause of death in the United States, and represent more serious long-term disability than any other disease.[1] A stroke is an acute brain disorder of vascular origin accompanied by neurologic dysfunction persisting more than 24 hours.[1] In the United States, there are more than 750,000 people who have a stroke each year.[1] Hemorrhagic strokes account for 20% of cases, and are caused by hypertension (HTN), ruptured saccular aneurysm, or arteriovenous malformation. Ischemic strokes, primarily caused by thrombotic changes, account for the remaining 80% of strokes. Potential causes of ischemic stroke include atherosclerotic plaques and HTN or emboli that lodge in an artery and disrupt oxygen supply to the brain. Unmodifiable risk factors for stroke include being African American, Hispanic, or Asian/Pacific Islander, being over the age of 55 years, being male, and having a family history of CVA or transient ischemic attack (TIA).[2] Risk factors that are controllable—either through medical management or through lifestyle changes— include: HTN, atrial fibrillation, high cholesterol, diabetes, atherosclerosis, tobacco use and smoking, sedentary lifestyle, obesity, and excessive alcohol intake.[2]

In the United States, there has been an increase in the incidence of CVA in younger individuals.[3,4] In the 10-year span from 1994-1995 to 2006-2007, hospitals reported a 47% increase in strokes in males between the ages 35 and 44 years (compared to a 36% increase in the same timeframe in females of the same age group).[3] Meanwhile, statistics showed that strokes in the geriatric population dropped due to improved treatment and prevention in this age group.

One factor that can lead to an ischemic CVA is an interaction between warfarin (Coumadin) and vitamin K, which can produce a potentially dangerous hypercoagulability state.[5] Warfarin is an oral anticoagulant (blood thinner) that reduces the blood's ability to clot. Warfarin is one of most commonly prescribed drugs. In persons who are at high risk of forming clots, it is used for chronic anticoagulation in order to prevent pulmonary emboli and venous thromboses.[5] Common uses include: treatment of deep vein thrombosis, pulmonary embolism, acute myocardial infarction; in persons with atrial fibrillation (to decrease the likelihood of thrombus formation in the atria and subsequent emboli); and, in patients with artificial heart valves. Blood clotting (coagulation) is a complicated process, requiring the interaction of more than a dozen factors. Warfarin acts to thin the blood by inhibiting several vitamin-K-dependent factors in the clotting cascade. Vitamin K, on the other hand, promotes clotting by activating several clotting factors in the blood.[5] Therefore, a diet high in vitamin K may counteract the effects of warfarin, potentially resulting in an embolus or thrombus that can cause a CVA, myocardial infarction, pulmonary embolus, and/or deep vein thrombosis. The drug label for warfarin includes a dietary warning to avoid large amounts of leafy green vegetables and other sources of vitamin K (Table 2-1).[5]

Table 2-1 COMMON DIETARY SOURCES OF VITAMIN K	
Dark, leafy green vegetables	Kale
	Spinach
	Lettuce
	Swiss chard
	Brussels sprouts
	Broccoli
	Cabbage

The drug information package insert also advises to "talk to your doctor if you plan to diet and lose weight." While small amounts of vitamin K-rich foods should not change warfarin's effectiveness, patients are advised to monitor their daily intake of vitamin K and not to exceed 120 µg/d for men and 90 µg/d for women. It is also advised that persons taking warfarin maintain a *consistent* intake of vitamin K from day to day.[5] Many individuals taking warfarin may attempt to lead a healthier lifestyle—which may include eating a diet high in green leafy vegetables. However, they often forget the dietary warnings given when they started the drug and neglect to consult their physician or pharmacist. Taking warfarin certainly does not mean individuals should avoid eating leafy greens; however, if the dietary increase in vitamin K is consistent over time, the individual's dosage of warfarin would need to be increased by the physician in order for the drug to effectively prevent clots from forming.

The location of an individual's CVA is important in understanding the resulting impairments. The primary role of the basal ganglia (BG) is in controlling movement. These nuclei are involved in changes in muscle tone, coordination, motor control, postural stability, and possible abnormal/extraneous movement patterns.[1,6] An insult to the BG (such as occurs in Parkinson's disease, Huntington's disease, or occlusion to the region's blood supply) results in different types of movement dysfunction. Patients may find initiation of movement or changing motor programs extremely challenging.[1,6] The BG are activated before the prime movers fire, indicating their role in the initiation and proper smooth sequencing of movements that produce a defined response.[1] This response set is thought to be involved more with internal cueing and complex movement pattern generation. The important role of the BG in postural stability is evident with damage to these nuclei. Individuals can present with a decreased ability to adjust or modify posture, increased difficulty balancing with eyes closed, and loss of postural reflexes. Patients with strokes in the BG may also demonstrate abnormal "motor chunking."[6] In other words, these individuals are less able to organize movements into sequences and they show increased response times during learned motor functions compared to neurologically intact individuals. Thus, while individuals with strokes affecting the BG may have milder motor deficits than those with strokes affecting larger cerebral vessels, they often present with motor initiation difficulties, slower responses, and difficulty with complex movements like running, jumping, and throwing.

Physical Therapy Patient/Client Management

Age at time of stroke matters: younger age at time of stroke indicates increased neuroplasticity.[7] Salience and specificity need to be considered when selecting interventions. Younger individuals may have a higher prior level of function that they want to return to and it is the physical therapists' responsibility to provide interventions that will improve their function. Intensity and repetition matter; performing interventions at the highest possible intensity and with enough repetition to induce change is paramount. A younger brain coupled with more aggressive treatment may increase the likelihood of increased functional gains.

The current patient is now 3 months poststroke to the BG with resultant right-sided weakness, balance deficits, and motor control/movement dysfunction specifically related to complex movement patterns and movement initiation. He is considered a high-functioning person poststroke. At the time of this outpatient examination, he was living at home with his family and had complaints primarily related to his participation restrictions. He was independent with all of his activities of daily living, and presented primarily with fatigue-related gait deficits during community-level ambulation. Because of his higher level of functioning, the therapist was not able to rely on more traditional **standardized outcome measures** such as the Berg Balance Scale, the Stroke Rehabilitation Assessment of Movement (STREAM), or the Performance Oriented Mobility Assessment (POMA, or Tinetti Balance Assessment Tool). Therefore, the therapist evaluated and treated this individual as a middle-aged athlete with motor control and movement dysfunction and chose more appropriate measures not validated in the poststroke population.

Examination, Evaluation, and Diagnosis

The patient's past history consisted of intermittent low back pain with right-sided sciatica and left plantar fasciitis. His specific risk factors for CVA included high cholesterol, obesity, and atrial fibrillation. When he was fatigued, the patient noticed an increase in his neurological symptoms including headache, right foot drop, and right-sided numbness and tingling. An aggravating factor was lack of sleep. Easing factors included sleep and rest between activities. When he begins to feel fatigued or notices deterioration in his gait pattern, he sits for 15 to 20 minutes to decrease symptoms. He states that he is exhausted by 9:00 PM and begins to notice increased neurological signs, including right-sided weakness. Prior to his stroke, he was a client service manager in the billing department of a government organization. His full-time work consisted of sitting at a desk and working on the computer. Currently, he is not working and will continue receiving disability benefits for another 9 months. The patient's goals were to return to: coaching his daughter's softball team, walking the dog, running and exercising with his family, and being "normal."

The patient's prior medical history included atrial fibrillation, hypercholesterolemia, prehypertension, and obesity (body mass index $40.3 \ kg/m^2$). The patient did not report dizziness, vision disturbances, dysphagia, dysarthria, nausea/vomiting, or syncopal episodes. The patient has been taking warfarin (Coumadin; 9 mg daily for 9 years), pantoprazole (Protonix; 40 mg for erosive esophagitis), baby aspirin, folic acid (2 mg), and simvastatin (40 mg for hypercholesterolemia). Major surgeries included right meniscus repair 22 years ago and right anterior cruciate ligament repair 4 years ago. He has lost approximately 30 lb since his stroke and reported no radicular symptoms or bilateral numbness/tingling, and no bowel or bladder problems.

The physical therapist's systems review indicated further cardiovascular and pulmonary examination was required due to his history of CVA. His vital signs at the time of the initial examination were: blood pressure 130/90 mm Hg (prehypertension), heart rate 70 beats per minute (normal), and respiratory rate 15 breaths per minute (normal). Neuromuscular and musculoskeletal systems warranted further examination due to the patient's right hemiparesis, history of low back pain with right-sided sciatica and left plantar fasciitis, reported difficulties with balance and gait, numbness and tingling on his right side, and upper and lower extremity weakness. No further examination was indicated for the integumentary system because the patient's skin was intact. Further examination of the patient's cognition was deferred because the patient was alert and oriented to person, place, time, and purpose and he displayed no signs or symptoms consistent with cognitive deficits during the patient interview.

The therapist's physical examination began with observation. The patient's seated posture demonstrated anterior trunk lean, anterior pelvic tilt, and large abdominal girth. When he walked into the examination room, the therapist observed his gait pattern. He showed decreased right ankle dorsiflexion during swing phase leading to decreased toe clearance with a slight right Trendelenburg sign during stance phase. Next, the therapist conducted a functional movement analysis. A double-leg squat was chosen because it was a skill needed for coaching softball. The patient was able to perform a standing squat without obvious deviations or need for upper extremity support for balance. The therapist then selected a more challenging task. Throwing accuracy was selected as a functional movement analysis of the right upper extremity. The therapist assessed how accurate the patient was with trampoline throws (Fig. 2-1). The patient stood 10 ft from an angled trampoline placed on the floor. He threw a 1-lb PlyoBall at a 9 × 9 inch square marked in the middle of the trampoline. Accuracy was measured by his ability to hit the target during 20 attempts. This functional movement analysis is similar to the Functional Throwing Performance Index (FTPI). The FTPI

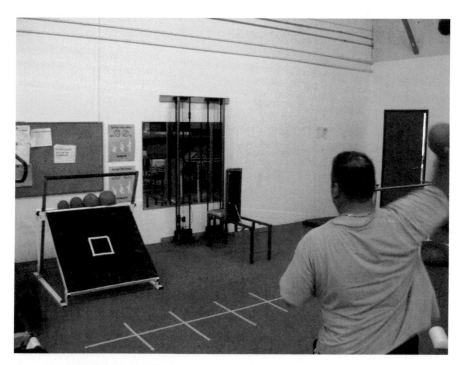

Figure 2-1. Set-up for throwing accuracy.

assesses throwing accuracy of a rubber ball at a target 15 ft away from a target sized 1 ft × 1 ft at a height of 3.94 ft where the number of successful throws in 30 seconds is counted.[8] The therapist used the accuracy with the trampoline throws to create an assessment tool that was achievable in the limited clinic space. This task could also form the basis of a therapeutic exercise to improve the patient's throwing ability. At initial examination, the patient's throwing accuracy was 4 out of 20 attempts.

The therapist administered the Patient Specific Functional Scale (PSFS).[9] The PSFS is a standardized self-report outcome measure in which the patient chooses five to seven items that he feels he cannot perform as well after his injury as he did before the injury. Each of the self-selected activities is scored on a scale 1 to 10 in which a score of 1 indicates the patient is currently unable to perform task and a score of 10 indicates the patient is able to perform task as well as before the injury. A systematic review found that the PSFS was reliable, valid, and responsive in many populations with musculoskeletal conditions, including acute low back pain and neck dysfunction.[9] Because of the similarity between musculoskeletal and neurological rehabilitation programs, individuals with neurological dysfunction would likely benefit from the use of PSFS as a patient-centered outcome measure.[9] The use of the PSFS can assist in determining specific activities to improve the saliency of the task for the patient. If the patient weighs an activity as important on the PSFS and therapeutic exercises/interventions address those items, the patient should demonstrate increased performance during rehabilitation, helping to maximize neuroplasticity during retraining of the specific task.

Table 2-2 describes this patient's PSFS items and scores. The activities the patient selected as currently being more difficult than prior to his stroke were walking, balance, shuffling, running, throwing a ball, and swinging a baseball bat to hit a ball.

Table 2-2 PATIENT-SPECIFIC FUNCTIONAL SCALE (PSFS) RESULTS FOR CASE PATIENT						
	Running	Throwing	Balance	Shuffle	Walking	Hitting
Initial examination	4	4	5	5	7	4
Visit 2	4	5	5	5	7	4
Visit 3	5	6	6	6	7	5
Visit 4	5	6	6	6	6	6
Visit 5	6	7	7	7	7	7
Visit 6	7	7	6	6	6	7
Visit 7	7	8	8	8	8	8
Visit 8	7	8	7	8	8	8
Visit 9	7	8	8	8	8	8
Visit 10	7	9	8	9	9	8
Visit 11	8	9	8	9	9	8
Change (initial to discharge from physical therapy)	4	5	3	4	2	3

The second outcome measure selected by the therapist was the **High-level Mobility Assessment Tool (HiMAT)**.[10,11] The HiMAT is reliable and valid in individuals with traumatic brain injury[11] and demonstrates good internal validity in persons with neurological conditions.[10] The HiMAT is scored using time or distance measures for each item, which are converted and recorded as ordinal levels. The highest score of 5 represents a "normal" time or distance to complete the task item whereas the lowest score of 1 indicates increased time or decreased distance thereby indicating poorer performance. A patient receives a score of 0 if he cannot complete the item successfully. In this clinic, the "Up Stairs" and "Down Stairs" items were adapted because a flight of 14 stairs was not available. Instead, the patient was instructed to perform two trials of 14 step-ups onto an 8-inch step under two conditions: (1) unaffected leg stepping up first and (2) affected leg stepping up first. Time to complete the 14 step-ups was averaged and recorded. Table 2-3 shows the patient's performance on the HiMAT. Overall, the patient performed well on less demanding activities such as walking, but did poorly on higher-level activities like running and skipping.

At this point in the examination, the therapist developed several hypotheses about potential impairments contributing to abnormal activity-level performance found during the initial examination. Impairment level testing was then conducted to rule in/rule out these impairments and their contribution to the patient's movement deficits and activity-level deficits.

Table 2-3   HIGH-LEVEL MOBILITY ASSESSMENT TOOL (HIMAT) RESULTS FOR CASE PATIENT

ITEM	Initial Examination	Visit 4	Visit 8	Visit 11	Change (initial to discharge from physical therapy)
Walk	3	1	2	3	0.46 s
Walk backward	3	2	3	3	0.57 s
Walk on toes	3	3	3	3	0.59 s
Walk over obstacle	2	2	2	3	0.88 s
Run	1	1	1	1	0.23 s
Skip	1	1	1	1	1.96 s
Hop forward (affected)	1	1	1	1	12.39 s
Bound (affected)	2	2	3	3	13 cm
Bound (less-affected)	2	2	3	3	11 cm
Step-up (affected)	23.96 s	20.14 s	15.83 s	16.58 s	6.47 s
Step-up (less-affected)	21.61 s	19.02 s	16.50 s	16.09 s	4.08 s

The Romberg and Sharpened Romberg tests were used to examine static standing balance.[1,12-14] The Romberg test is performed with the patient standing with feet together and arms crossed over the chest for 60 seconds, first with eyes open, and then repeated with eyes closed. If excessive trunk sway or a stepping strategy is used, the therapist stops the stopwatch.[13] Times below 20 seconds correlate with a three-fold increase in falling.[12,13] This patient was able to perform the Romberg test with both eyes open and eyes closed for 60 seconds. The Sharpened Romberg test is a slight modification of the Romberg test in which the patient stands in a tandem heel-to-toe stance with arms crossed over the chest for up to 60 seconds. The patient repeats the test with eyes closed for 60 seconds. Excessive trunk sway or initiating a stepping strategy stops the time.[11] The Sharpened Romberg test has normative values for women between the ages 60 and 64 years (the youngest age range for which normative values are available) for eyes open (56.4 seconds) and eyes closed (24.6 seconds).[15] This patient performed the Sharpened Romberg test with eyes open for 60 seconds (normal). With his eyes closed, he maintained the position for only 4 seconds when his left foot stepped forward to maintain his balance. Because he struggled with the Sharpened Romberg test in the eyes closed condition, the physical therapist reassessed the patient with this test throughout his physical therapy episode of care.

The patient had full and pain-free active ROM in the upper and lower extremities. However, muscle length testing revealed several shortened muscles bilaterally: piriformis, hamstrings (70° straight leg raise), quadriceps, and iliotibial band.[16] These shortened muscles may contribute to his movement or activity limitations. Manual muscle testing (MMT) was performed. The patient's left upper and lower extremity strength was normal (graded 5/5). On the right side, weakness was noted in the upper extremity in the lower and middle trapezius (4/5) and shoulder abductors (4/5). The patient also had proximal and distal right lower extremity weakness. Right hip abduction and extension were graded 4/5, plantarflexion and dorsiflexion were graded 4/5, and great toe extension was graded 3/5. Trunk core strength was tested with a pelvic tilt and graded as 4/5. Grip strength (tested with a grip dynamometer) was normal bilaterally compared to age-matched values.[17] The patient's right-sided weakness may contribute to the functional and movement problems he demonstrated on other tests during the initial examination. It should be noted that recent studies have found that strength testing via manual muscle tests with grades higher than 3 are not as reliable as handheld dynamometer strength testing.[18] Given that this patient needed an assessment of how strong he was (rather than how weak), it may have been more appropriate to use handheld dynamometer testing to get more accurate results.

Because the patient complained of abnormal sensation, the therapist performed additional examination. Proprioception testing and light touch was intact in bilateral lower extremities.[16] The patient also had normal heel-to-shin and fingertip-to-nose movements.[1] These sensory tests ruled out proprioception, light touch, and nonequilibrium coordination deficits as contributing factors to the patient's activity and movement limitations.

The physical therapy diagnosis was a 41-year-old male presenting with deficiencies in: balance, right-sided upper and lower extremity strength, bilateral lower extremity muscle length, and throwing accuracy after having a left CVA in the basal ganglia 3 months ago. The patient is limited in his ability to walk his dog and play softball with his children. He states he is unable to throw, swing a bat, run, or shuffle smoothly to allow for his return to coaching softball. Contributing factors that may hinder progress include his history of low back pain, right-sided sciatica, and left plantar fascia pain.

Plan of Care and Interventions

Neuroplasticity is the inherent ability of the central nervous system to change and adapt to the forces placed upon it.[7,19,20] According to the **principles of neuroplasticity**, interventions must be targeted to the patient's specific deficits and be important to the patient and his return to specific activities in order to enact plasticity and change. Intensity and repetition improve plasticity and should be incorporated into the treatment plan. Neuroplasticity principles pertaining to this case include saliency, specificity, repetition, and intensity. Saliency refers to the fact that a motor skill should be important and/or relevant to the patient to ensure consistency and maintain motivation to improve function. Specificity means that the intervention needs to be specific to the patient's impairments in order to improve that activity. Repetition is incorporated to maximize repetitions of the motor task as much as possible to enforce learning. Intensity refers to the fact that consistent re-examination should be employed to increase the intensity both within each session and between sessions to ensure that it is maximized based on the patient's performance.

Anticipated goals, to be achieved in 3 weeks, were developed in collaboration with the patient. These included: (1) ability to tolerate > 1 hour of walking and standing activity without fatigue to facilitate return to coaching softball; (2) independence with home exercise program (HEP) to promote continued progress and return to prior level of function (PLOF). Expected outcomes, to be met in 6 weeks included: (1) increased strength to 5/5 MMT scores for right upper and lower extremity muscles to improve ability to perform functional and recreational activities; (2) scores on PSFS to improve to > 8 on each of the chosen activities to improve patient's quality of life; (3) minimum of 1 point increase per item on the HiMAT to improve patient's balance and mobility to allow for improved ability to play and coach softball.

The duration of treatment was set at once or twice per week for 6 weeks. The physical therapist felt that the patient's prognosis for achieving the anticipated goals and expected outcomes was good secondary to the patient's younger age, motivation, high prior level of function, and his continued progress since onset of his stroke 3 months ago.

The therapist used results from the HiMAT, PSFS, throwing accuracy, and Sharpened Romberg test to determine appropriate interventions. The PSFS helped determine the activities that would be most relevant for the patient and assist with motivation and neuroplasticity. The HiMAT and Sharpened Romberg were used to determine interventions that were specific to his impairments.

Each session began with a cardiovascular warm-up to increase hamstring flexibility and improve performance.[21] Due to the patient's cardiovascular risk factors, the warm-up also provided a good example of how to begin an aerobic exercise session that the patient could continue after his formal physical therapy concluded and he transitioned to an independent HEP. The therapist took the patient's blood pressure and heart rate before and after the aerobic activity to ensure appropriate physiological responses to exercise. He performed 5 to 10 minutes on an elliptical machine at moderate intensity and no resistance.

Therapeutic exercise consisted of selected lower extremity stretching to muscles identified as shortened. While stretching does not decrease the risk of muscle soreness, prevent injury, or improve sport performance,[22] it was implemented to provide more normal muscle length to allow for improved functional and movement performance. Hamstring stretches were performed using straight leg raise in supine; gastrocnemius/soleus stretches were performed with the patient standing on a slant board to approximately 20° of ankle dorsiflexion with the knee fully extended; piriformis stretches were performed in the supine position (Fig. 2-2). Initially, the therapist incorporated the stretches into his treatment session. After two to three visits, the patient understood positioning, duration, and quantity/quality of each stretch. Therefore, these stretches were transitioned into the patient's HEP with periodic checks during subsequent sessions.

Lower extremity therapeutic exercises were the crux of this patient's interventions and plan of care. Specific therapeutic exercises were chosen to improve his balance, endurance, strength, core stability, and ability to change motor programs (Table 2-4). Upper extremity plyometric training was included. Plyometric training

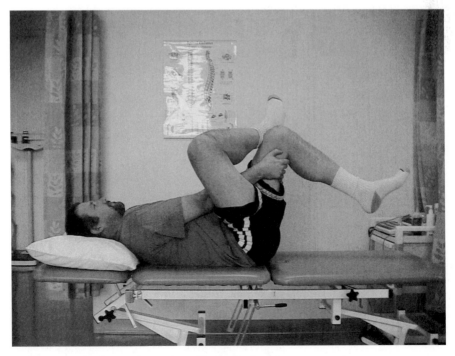

Figure 2-2. Position for stretching right piriformis muscle.

Table 2-4 THERAPEUTIC EXERCISE INTERVENTIONS FOR CASE PATIENT										
	Visit 1	Visit 2	Visit 3	Visit 4	Visit 5	Visit 6	Visit 7	Visit 8	Visit 9	Visit 10
Tandem stance on ½ foam roller	2 sets of 30 s	X	X	X	X	X	X	X	–	–
Stepping over 8-in step	2 sets of 30 s	X	X	X	X	X	X	X	X	X
Plyometric box jumps	30 repetitions	X	X	X	X	X	X	X	X	–
Overhead external rotation with pulley	1 kg × 60 s	–	–	X	X	–	2 kg × 30 repetitions	X	X	X
Karaoke or grapevine (walking sideways while alternating each foot front to back)	5 laps	–	–	X	X	X	X	X	X	X
Jogging with sports cord resistance	–	–	–	3 laps	X	–	X	X	–	–
Bridge curls and jack knives over inflatable ball	20 each	–	X	–	X	X	X	X	X	–
Lunge walks	–	–	–	–	X	X	X	–	X	–

Baseball swings	–	4 kg × 10 swings	X	X	X	X	X	X
Seated inflatable ball chops (bilateral arms move in spiral and diagonal pattern)	–	4 kg × 10 repetitions	–	X	X	–	X	X
Box drills (run, shuffle, back pedal, karaoke)	–	–	–	–	–	3 laps	X	–
Obstacle course requiring rapid changing of motor programs	–	–	–	–	–	X	X	–
Abdominal exercise with fixed upper extremity/upper trunk and flexion of hips/knees to 90°	–	–	–	–	X	X	X	–

One lap = 20 m.

"–" indicates that this item was not performed on this date.

"X" indicates that this item was performed on this date.

utilizes quick, powerful movements of rapid stretching and contraction of muscles to improve the speed and force of muscle contraction and to improve performance in sport-specific activities.[23,24] Plyometric training improves upper extremity proprioception and kinesthesia.[25] Plyometric training of overhead throwing has also been shown to improve performance.[22] Due to the inherent structure of the shoulder, dynamic stability must be trained in the overhead athlete to improve performance and decrease risk of injury.[26] Because throwing was impaired and this patient had a goal to be able to throw in order to coach his daughter's softball team, upper extremity plyometric training was appropriate.

The patient was discharged after 11 visits over 7 weeks. He met five of six anticipated goals and expected outcomes. He became independent with his HEP and tolerated > 60 minutes of continuous activity to facilitate coaching softball. The patient was not able to improve his score by 1 point on each item of the HiMAT. He reported that his ability to coach softball had greatly improved, evident in his ability to throw a softball and swing a bat accurately. He stated that he will continue coaching softball and he is starting a gym routine for continued improvement and maintenance of fitness and function. The patient's throwing accuracy also improved during this episode of care. He advanced from 4/20 to 11/20 accurate throws—a three-fold increase in throwing accuracy over 11 visits.

The patient's scores on the PSFS showed improvement throughout the treatment period (Table 2-2), with minor setbacks in scores due to low back pain (visit 4), right-sided piriformis pain, and left plantar fascia pain (visit 6). For individuals with orthopaedic impairments, the minimal detectable change on the PSFS is 3 on each item or an average change of 2 across items. This patient exceeded the minimal detectable change on five of the six items on the PSFS and exceeded the minimal detectable change across items.[27]

Reassessment of the HiMAT was performed on visits 4, 8, and 11. The patient demonstrated consistent improvement across all items on the HiMAT from initial examination through discharge (Table 2-3). Even though the patient improved his *actual* times/distances on the individual HiMAT items, he did not improve his *overall* HiMAT score over the course of 11 treatment sessions. When the raw timed scores and distances were converted to the ordinal scale, they were not significant enough to change the ordinal scores, hence his overall HiMAT score remained the same. With this patient, the HiMAT may not have been able to capture his changes (due to a floor effect), but it was extremely useful for the therapist in developing, advancing, and revising his interventions, exercise, and HEP. Because the HiMAT was developed to include very high-level, sports-like activities, it also challenged the patient more than other outcome measures may have, leading to improved saliency and intensity, and potentially maximizing the role of neuroplasticity in his recovery.[28]

Strength was re-examined via MMT on the final visit, showing that the patient had no remaining strength deficits. Periodically, the therapist re-examined the patient's performance on the Sharpened Romberg test with eyes closed (Table 2-5). The patient improved with both the left foot forward and right foot forward condition by 26 and 36 seconds, respectively. This improvement indicates a normal result for both the left foot forward and right foot forward using the lowest available

Table 2-5 RESULTS OF SHARPENED ROMBERG WITH EYES CLOSED (IN SECONDS) FOR CASE PATIENT	Left Foot Forward	Right Foot Forward
Initial examination	4	0
Visit 2	50	0
Visit 3	15	13
Visit 4	NT	NT
Visit 5	NT	NT
Visit 6	7	5
Visit 7	2	6
Visit 8	6	7
Visit 9	12	23
Visit 10	20	25
Visit 11	30	36
Change (initial to d/c)	26	36

NT, not tested.

age-matched norm (24.58 seconds in 60-64 year olds). With the increasing number of younger persons having strokes, future investigations should develop age-matched norms for common tests in younger age groups for males and females.

Evidence-Based Clinical Recommendations

SORT: **Strength of Recommendation Taxonomy**

A: Consistent, good-quality patient-oriented evidence

B: Inconsistent or limited-quality patient-oriented evidence

C: Consensus, disease-oriented evidence, usual practice, expert opinion, or case series

1. Use of standardized outcome measures from other areas of physical therapy practice can be useful to document the progress of higher level patients poststroke. **Grade C**

2. The High-level Mobility Assessment Tool (HiMAT) is an 11-task outcome measure that can be used to quantify the ability of individuals with neurological conditions to perform high-level mobility. **Grade B**

3. Incorporation of neuroplasticity principles into the plan of care maximizes recovery in persons with neurologic insults such as strokes. **Grade B**

COMPREHENSION QUESTIONS

2.1 Which of the following is *not* a dietary restriction for patients taking warfarin (Coumadin)?

A. Brussels sprouts

B. Kale

C. Green bell pepper

D. Butter lettuce

2.2 Your patient is a 62-year-old female, status/post stroke to the BG. She wants to return to ballroom dancing with her husband. Which of the following examples does *not* incorporate the principles of neuroplasticity into her plan of care?

A. Using music during step practice

B. Emphasizing increased step length during bouts of gait training

C. Asking the patient to perform sit-to-stand repetitions with increasing speed each session

D. Performing 10 repetitions of toe raises each session

ANSWERS

2.1 **C.** Although green bell peppers are green, they are not considered a dark green, leafy vegetable that contains high concentrations of vitamin K, which are the types to be avoided for individuals taking warfarin (options A, B, and D).

2.2 **D.** Keeping the *intensity* of an exercise consistent across sessions is not consistent with the principles of neuroplasticity. Using a consistent exercise while having the patient attempt to increase the speed of performance demonstrates neuroplasticity adaptation based on *intensity* (option C). *Saliency* is seen by using music during activities on her feet, since this relates to her ballroom dancing goals (option A). *Specificity* is demonstrated with the emphasis on increased step length (option B).

REFERENCES

1. Umphred DA. *Neurological Rehabilitation*. 5th ed. St Louis, MO: Mosby; 2006.

2. National Stroke Association. Stroke risk factors. http://www.stroke.org/site/PageServer?pagename=risk. Accessed August 25, 2012.

3. Jones B. CDC: more strokes hitting young, middle-aged folks. *USA Today*. February 9, 2011. http://yourlife.usatoday.com/health/medical/story/2011/02/CDC-More-strokes-hitting-young-middle-aged-folks-/43513652/1. Accessed February 6, 2012.

4. Neergaard L. Stroke on rise amongst young, middle-aged. *The Chronicle Herald*. February 4, 2012. http://thechronicleherald.ca/science/58946-stroke-rise-amongst-young-middle-aged#.TzAypbGqKH0.email. Accessed February 6, 2012.

5. National Institutes of Health Drug–Nutrient Interaction Task Force. Warren Grant Magnuson Center. Important information you should know when you are taking: Coumadin and Vitamin K. ods.od.nih.gov/pubs/factsheets/coumadin1.pdf. Accessed August 25, 2012.

6. Boyd LA, Edwards JD, Siengsukon CS, Vidoni ED, Wessel BD, Linsdell MA. Motor sequence chunking is impaired by basal ganglia stroke. *Neurobiol Learn Mem.* 2009;92:35-44.

7. Kleim JA, Jones TA. Principles of experience-dependent neural plasticity: implications for rehabilitation after brain damage. *J Speech Lang Hear Res.* 2008;51:S225-S239.

8. Wassinger CA, Myers JB, Gatti JM, Conley KM, Lephart SM. Proprioception and throwing accuracy in the dominant shoulder after cryotherapy. *J Athl Train.* 2007;42:84-89.

9. Horn KK, Jennings S, Richardson G, Vliet DV, Hefford C, Abbott JH. The patient-specific functional scale: psychometrics, clinimetrics, and application as a clinical outcome measure. *J Orthop Sports Phys Ther.* 2012;42:30-42.

10. Williams G, Hill B, Pallant JF, Greenwood K. Internal validity of the revised HiMAT for people with neurological conditions. *Clin Rehabil.* 2012;26:741-747.

11. Williams GP, Greenwood KM, Robertson VJ, Goldie PA, Morris ME. High-Level Mobility Assessment Tool (HiMAT): interrater reliability, retest reliability, and internal consistency. *Phys Ther.* 2006;86:395-400.

12. Agrawal Y, Carey JP, Hoffman HJ, Sklare DA, Schubert MC. The modified Romberg balance test: normative data in U.S. adults. *Otol Neurotol.* 2011;32:1309-1311.

13. Black FO, Wall C, 3rd, Rockette HE, Jr, Kitch R. Normal subject postural sway during the Romberg test. *Am J Otolaryngol.* 1982;3:309-318.

14. Newton R. Review of tests of standing balance abilities. *Br Injury.* 1989;3:335-343.

15. Briggs RC, Gossman MR, Birch R, Drews JE, Shaddeau SA. Balance performance among noninstitutionalized elderly women. *Phys Ther.* 1989;69:748-756.

16. Reese NB. *Muscle and Sensory Testing.* 3rd ed. St. Louis, MO: Elsevier; 2012.

17. Peters MJ, van Nes SI, Vanhoutte EK, et al. Revised normative values for grip strength with the Jamar dynamometer. *J Peripher Nerv System.* 2011;16:47-50.

18. Bohannon RW. Manual muscle testing: does it meet the standards of an adequate screening test? *Clin Rehabil.* 2005;19:662-667.

19. Forrester LW, Wheaton LA, Luft AR. Exercise-mediated locomotor recovery and lower-limb neuroplasticity after stroke. *J Rehabil Res Dev.* 2008;45:205-220.

20. Wolpaw JR, Carp JS. Plasticity from muscle to brain. *Prog Neurobiol.* 2006;78:233-263.

21. O'Sullivan K, Murray E, Sainsbury D. The effect of warm-up, static stretching and dynamic stretching on hamstring flexibility in previously injured subjects. *BMC Musculoskelet Disord.* 2009;10:37.

22. Herbert RD, Gabriel M. Effects of stretching before and after exercising on muscle soreness and risk of injury: systematic review. *BMJ.* 2002;325:468.

23. Bernier J. *Quick Reference Dictionary for Athletic Training.* 2nd ed. Thorofare, NJ: SLACK Inc.; 2005.

24. Kisner C, Colby LA. *Therapeutic Exercise: Foundations and Techniques.* 5th ed. Philadelphia, PA: F.A. Davis; 2007.

25. Swanik KA, Lephart SM, Swanik CB, Lephart SP, Stone DA, Fu FH. The effects of shoulder plyometric training on proprioception and selected muscle performance characteristics. *J Shoulder Elbow Surg.* 2002;11:579-586.

26. Carter AB, Kaminski TW, Douex AT, Jr, Knight CA, Richards JG. Effects of high volume upper extremity plyometric training on throwing velocity and functional strength ratios of the shoulder rotators in collegiate baseball players. *J Strength Cond Res.* 2007;21:208-215.

27. Berghuis-Kelly D, Scherer S. Outcome measures in cardiopulmonary physical therapy: use of the Patient Specific Functional Scale. *Cardiopul Phys Ther J.* 2007;18:21-23.

28. Williams GP, Morris ME. High-level mobility outcomes following acquired brain injury: a preliminary evaluation. *Brain Inj.* 2009;23:307-312.

Parkinson's Disease: Diagnosis

Heather Scott David

A 70-year-old male was diagnosed with Parkinson's disease (PD) 8 years ago with a clinical presentation of a unilateral tremor in the right upper extremity. He now presents to outpatient physical therapy with reports of rigidity, postural instability, falls, and difficulty rising from a chair without falling backward. He requires minimal assistance for all transfers and bed mobility and ambulates within the home (50 ft) with a front-wheeled walker and contact guard assistance. He occasionally requires minimal assistance to limit forward momentum due to a festinating gait. He lives at home with his 65-year-old wife who is in good health and is the patient's primary caregiver. Over the last 3 months, the patient has begun falling regularly and has been unable to participate in weekly bridge games at his community clubhouse because of his decline in mobility. He is unable to get off the ground by himself and his wife has had to call 911 or neighbors to help him up; however, he has not suffered any serious injuries as a result of his falls. The patient presents with a masked face and hypophonia, making it difficult to communicate. He has also begun to experience dysphagia. This patient has been taking carbidopa/levodopa (Sinemet) for 8 years and has begun to experience decreased effectiveness with definitive on and off phases. The patient has just arrived for his first outpatient physical therapy evaluation.

▶ What examination signs may be associated with this diagnosis?
▶ What are the most appropriate physical therapy outcome measures for functional mobility, balance, and gait?
▶ What are possible complications interfering with physical therapy?

KEY DEFINITIONS

DYSPHAGIA: Impaired swallowing; common in patients with PD due to rigidity and decreased mobility

FESTINATING GAIT: Gait pattern common in patients with PD that is characterized by progressively shortened stride lengths and increasing speed

HYPOPHONIA: Decreased voice production resulting in soft speech

MASKED FACE: Decreased facial expressions due to rigidity in patients with PD; also known as hypomimia

ON/OFF PHENOMENON: Transient improvement in symptoms after medication administration with a rapid decline in medication effectiveness; occurs frequently with long-term use of levodopa[1]

RIGIDITY: Increased muscle tone with resistance to passive elongation that is consistent throughout the range of motion, is present in both directions, and is not velocity dependent;[1] there are two types of rigidity: "leadpipe" and "cogwheel"

TREMOR: Slow-frequency involuntary oscillation of a body part; in patients with PD, tremor occurs at rest, begins unilaterally, and often affects the hand

Objectives

1. Describe the cardinal signs of PD.
2. List direct and indirect impairments of PD.
3. Describe how the progression of PD affects the patient's International Classification of Functioning, Disability and Health (ICF) related to body structure and functions, impairments, activity limitations and participation restrictions.
4. Identify reliable and valid outcome measures for the assessment of activity limitations, and participation restrictions in individuals with PD.
5. Identify potential adverse drug reactions (ADRs) that may affect physical therapy examination and interventions and describe possible therapy solutions.

Physical Therapy Considerations

PT considerations during management of the individual with gait instability, balance difficulties, fall history, and decreased functional mobility due to PD:

▶ **General physical therapy plan of care/goals:** Improve transfer safety and independence; improve ability to rise from sitting without loss of balance posteriorly; improve household ambulation independence

▶ **Physical therapy tests and measures:** Assessment of range of motion (ROM) and strength; reliable and valid tools for functional mobility, balance, gait, and participation restrictions

▶ **Precautions during physical therapy**: Close guarding due to patient's high risk of falling; recognize potential ADRs

▶ **Complications interfering with physical therapy:** Orthostatic hypotension; timing of medication dosing

Understanding the Health Condition

PD is the most common form of parkinsonism, which is a group of disorders caused by abnormalities of the basal ganglia. PD is a chronic progressive neurodegenerative disease of the basal ganglia. The etiology is idiopathic in approximately 80% of cases with the remaining 20% referred to as secondary parkinsonism. Secondary parkinsonism can be caused by damage to the basal ganglia as a result of toxicity, encephalitis, vascular disease, tumor, metabolic causes, and other neurodegenerative disorders.[2] The motor deficits present in patients with PD result from a loss of pigmented neurons in the substantia nigra pars compacta. The loss of neurons in the substantia nigra decreases neural projections to the caudate and putamen (collectively referred to as the striatum) and results in a loss of dopamine production from the striatum. The mean age of onset for PD is 57 years.[3] PD affects an estimated 800,000 individuals in the United States with a prevalence of 350 per 100,000.[4] The rate of progression for individuals with PD is variable but is often more rapid in cases of late onset and in individuals with postural instability.[5]

There is no definitive diagnostic test for PD. Instead, the diagnosis is made based on a patient's clinical presentation. **There are four cardinal signs of PD**: resting tremor, bradykinesia (and the extreme form, akinesia), rigidity, and postural instability.[2,5] The pathophysiology of PD is related to decreased dopamine in the substantia nigra of the basal ganglia. This dopamine insufficiency leads to deficits in the direct and indirect pathways of the basal ganglia.[1] The direct pathway of the basal ganglia facilitates output to the thalamus and motor regions of the cortex; disruption of this pathway may be responsible for bradykinesia. The indirect pathway works to suppress movements; disruption in this pathway may be responsible for tremor in individuals with PD.[2]

Tremor is often the first sign that an individual presents with and is often unilateral in early stages of the disease. Tremor associated with PD is typically present at rest. It is often initially localized to one hand as "pill-rolling," a back and forth movement of the thumb over the second finger. Tremor decreases with relaxation and is not present when the individual is sleeping.[2,5] Bradykinesia, hypokinesia, and akinesia are common in patients with PD.[1,6] Bradykinesia is a decrease in movement *speed* and hypokinesia is a decrease in movement *amplitude*. Akinesia is a lack of movement often described as "freezing." Individuals with PD have difficulty initiating and executing all movements, especially complex multistep motor plans.[1,6] Rigidity is increased resistance to passive movement and is present in the agonist and antagonist muscle groups. Rigidity can affect the extremities and trunk and is often asymmetrical in the early stages of PD, progressing from proximal musculature of the shoulders, neck, and hips to distal extremities and the face. Unlike spasticity, rigidity is consistent and *not* velocity dependent. Rigidity can be described as "cogwheel" or "leadpipe." Cogwheel rigidity is characterized by jerky catching and releasing movements throughout the available ROM and leadpipe rigidity is uniform resistance throughout the available ROM.[1,6] Over time, rigidity can contribute to a loss of ROM and development of contractures and postural deformities.[5] Postural instability is one of the most disabling features of PD. Standing postural balance reactions in patients with PD can be assessed with a **retropulsion or "pull test."** In this test, the examiner quickly pulls the individual backward or forward by the shoulders and assesses the individual's balance reaction. Taking more than two steps to recover or the absence of any postural reaction indicates abnormal postural control.[5,7] Inter-rater reliability of the retropulsion test has been reported at 93%; with reported sensitivity of 63% and specificity of 88%.[7]

The four cardinal signs of PD are all direct impairments that are primary manifestations of the disease process. Additional direct impairments can include autonomic, cognitive, and cardiovascular dysfunction.[2] An indirect impairment is a secondary deficit resulting from the impact of one or more direct impairments of the disease. Indirect impairments of PD include postural deformities, ROM limitations, contractures, gait abnormalities, dysphagia, dysarthria, and respiratory impairments. The characteristic stooped posture that is seen with PD is an indirect impairment resulting from rigidity that appears to affect the flexors more than the extensor muscle groups of the trunk.[2,8] This stooped posture contributes to balance impairments by displacing the individual's center of mass forward, placing him at his anterior limit of stability. Individuals with PD may demonstrate a festinating gait pattern, which is a progressive increase in gait speed combined with a shortened step length as the individual attempts to "catch up" with his anteriorly displaced center of mass. Additional gait deviations associated with PD include freezing episodes related to akinesia, short shuffling steps, decreased hip and knee extension, and shortened stride lengths bilaterally.[2]

There is no cure for PD. Interventions are directed at slowing the progression of the disease, preventing indirect impairments, and symptom management.[5] Pharmacological interventions to promote the production of dopamine in the striatum have been successful in managing symptoms of PD.[3] Because dopamine does not cross the blood–brain barrier, levodopa (a precursor of dopamine) is the primary drug used in the treatment of PD.[1,3] The combination of levodopa with carbidopa (Sinemet) increases the amount of dopamine crossing the blood–brain barrier and can increase the effectiveness of the medication.[3,9] Administration of levodopa can also be used to confirm the diagnosis of PD. Within 15 to 30 minutes of administration, an improvement in motor symptoms such as bradykinesia and rigidity can help confirm a diagnosis of PD.[3] Levodopa is more effective in reducing bradykinesia and rigidity than tremor and postural instability.[1,3] Levodopa's effectiveness can begin to decrease as early as 2 years after beginning treatment, resulting in shorter "on" periods in which the individual experiences a reduction in symptom severity and longer "off" periods when symptoms are not improved with medication.[3,9,10] In addition, long-term use of levodopa can lead to ADRs such as increased frequency of involuntary abnormal movements of the limbs and orofacial muscles called dyskinesias.[3,4,9] Levodopa has very few food and drug interactions. However, iron and protein can potentially interfere with its absorption. Iron supplements should be taken 2 hours before or after levodopa.[3] Although levodopa can be taken with meals to decrease nausea, meals high in protein should be avoided to promote maximal levodopa uptake into the central nervous system (CNS). Some patients benefit from taking medication between meals to promote maximal levodopa uptake into the CNS.[3] In addition to nausea and dyskinesias, ADRs can include postural hypotension, sedation, nightmares, and hallucinations.[3]

Surgical management of PD may include deep brain stimulation (DBS) with implanted electrodes. DBS is usually done bilaterally and targets either the globus pallidus interna or the subthalamic nuclei.[11] There is evidence supporting the use of DBS to treat tremor in patients with advanced PD that has been unresponsive to medication. This surgical intervention can help decrease motor symptoms of PD without the motor fluctuations and dyskinesias that are common in response to levodopa.[11-13]

Physical Therapy Patient/Client Management

Physical therapy management for a patient with PD includes teaching the individual how to move more effectively, develop strategies to maintain or improve postural stability, and prevent falls. The physical therapist should promote increased physical activity to manage secondary impairments affecting the musculoskeletal and cardiovascular systems.[14] The physical therapist often works as part of a medical team including primary care physicians, neurologists, occupational therapists, speech therapists, and other allied health professionals. During each therapy session, the physical therapist should ask the patient about potential ADRs including postural hypotension and dyskinesias and communicate these to the prescribing physician. It may also be necessary to refer the individual to other members of the healthcare team, including speech pathologists for communication and swallowing problems and psychologists or psychiatrists for depression.

Examination, Evaluation, and Diagnosis

A physical therapy examination is comprised of specific screening and testing procedures leading to a physical therapy diagnosis and referral to other members of the healthcare team, when appropriate. The physical therapist has multiple tools to evaluate impairments and loss of functional mobility in patients with PD. Physical therapy evaluation of a patient should focus on the individual's current functional limitations and the extent to which impairments such as rigidity, bradykinesia, postural instability, and tremor interfere with the performance of activities of daily living (ADLs) and instrumental ADLs (IADLs).

There are a number of rating scales and outcome measures currently used to evaluate motor impairments and disability in patients with PD, including measures of participation, activity, and body structure and function consistent with the ICF model. The **Unified Parkinson's Disease Rating Scale (UPDRS) and Hoehn and Yahr Scale** are measures of the body structure and function domain of the ICF model. The Hoehn and Yahr Scale and Modified Hoehn and Yahr Scale are both used to document the progression of the disease and have an inter-rater reliability of 0.44 to 0.71.[15] In the Hoehn and Yahr Scale, patients are classified on a scale from 1 to 5. Stage 1 indicates unilateral involvement with minimal to no functional loss and Stage 5 describes an individual who is severely disabled and confined to a bed or wheelchair.[5,15,16] The UPDRS is the most commonly used assessment tool to measure the level of disability and impairments in a person with PD. This assessment tool measures cognitive and emotional status, ADL function, motor abilities, and ADRs. It has a test-rest reliability of 0.89 to 0.95 and is commonly used to measure disease severity and response to drug therapy.[10,17-19] The Hoehn and Yahr Scale and UPDRS can be helpful tools to identify the progression of PD related to levels of disability and impairments. However, they may not be the most appropriate scales for physical therapists to use for treatment planning and to document physical therapy gains.[2,15,17]

Physical therapists can choose from several reliable assessments for functional mobility, gait, balance, and postural stability that have been validated in individuals with PD. Table 3-1 presents the time each test requires to perform, test-retest reliability, and any minimal detectable change (MDC) that has been reported in individuals with PD.[18]

Balance assessment tools include the **Berg Balance Scale (BBS)**[18,20,21] and Functional Reach Test (FRT).[21-23] Gait and functional mobility measures include the **Six-Minute Walk Test (6MWT)**,[18] **10-Meter Walk Test (10MWT)**,[18] **Timed Up and Go (TUG)**,[18,21] and the Dynamic Gait Index (DGI).[19] The BBS is a measure of static balance and fall risk in adult populations using a 14-item test (0 to 4 scale for each item) with higher scores indicating better balance performance. The FRT is an assessment of standing dynamic balance in which the physical therapist measures the distance an individual is able to reach forward and maintain his balance. The 6MWT estimates walking endurance by measuring the distance an individual is able to walk at a self-paced rate in 6 minutes. The 10MWT is a measure of gait

Table 3-1   COMMONLY USED ASSESSMENT TOOLS FOR FUNCTIONAL MOBILITY, GAIT, AND BALANCE IN INDIVIDUALS WITH PARKINSON'S DISEASE

Assessment	Time Required	Test-Retest Reliability	Minimal Detectable Change (MDC)
Berg Balance Scale (BBS)	15-20 min	0.94	5 points
Functional Reach Test (FRT)	< 5 min	0.73	Not reported
Six-Minute Walk Test (6MWT)	6 min	0.96	Not reported
10-Meter Walk Test (10MWT)	< 5 min	0.96-0.97	0.18-0.25 m/s
Timed Up and Go (TUG)	< 5 min	0.85	11 s
Dynamic Gait Index (DGI)	10 min	Not reported	Not reported

speed. The TUG test measures the amount of time it takes an individual to stand up from a chair, walk 10 ft, turn around, walk 10 ft, and sit down again. The DGI assesses an individual's ability to maintain walking balance with a variety of internal and external challenges. There are eight items included in the DGI (*e.g.*, changes in gait speed, gait with head turns, stepping over obstacles). Each item is rated on a 0 to 4 scale with 4 representing the highest balance grade. The DGI demonstrates adequate discriminative validity between fallers and non-fallers with sensitivity of 68% and specificity of 71% with a cut-off score of 18.5.[19]

To gather data about the patient's participation in society—and not simply his physical function—many self-report participation measures can be used. These include the **39-question Parkinson's Disease Questionnaire (39-PDQ), the Medical Outcomes Study 36-Item Short-Form Health Survey (SF-36),**[18,24] **and the Activities Balance Confidence Scale (ABC).**[18,25] The 39-PDQ is a widely used disease-specific self-report questionnaire with 39 questions divided into 8 subscales including: (1) Mobility, (2) ADL, (3) Emotional Well-being, (4) Stigma, (5) Social Support, (6) Cognitions, (7) Communication, and (8) Bodily Discomfort. In a review of health-related quality of life measures by The Movement Disorder Society Task Force, the 39-PDQ was recommended for use in patients with PD.[24] The 39-PDQ was found to have satisfactory content and convergent validity.[24] The SF-36 survey is a questionnaire that can be used to measure quality of life from the patient's point of view and has a test-retest reliability of 0.80 to 0.95 for individuals with PD.[18] The SF-36 is divided into eight domains of physical and mental health including: (1) Physical Functioning, (2) Social Functioning, (3) Role-Physical, (4) Bodily Pain, (5) Mental Health, (6) Role-Emotional, (7) Vitality, and (8) General Health. This survey requires licensing purchase, takes about 10 minutes to complete, and can be self-administered or given in person or by telephone by a trained interviewer.[18] Last, the ABC scale assesses an individual's self-reported confidence with performing 16 functional mobility tasks. Each task is scored from 0% (no confidence) to 100% (full confidence) and the average for all 16 items are taken for an overall score. This test takes approximately 10 minutes to complete and has excellent test-retest reliability of 0.94 and an MDC of 13 for individuals with PD.[18]

Plan of Care and Interventions

A physical therapy plan of care for a patient with PD is described in Case 4.

Evidence-Based Clinical Recommendations

SORT: Strength of Recommendation Taxonomy

A: Consistent, good-quality patient-oriented evidence

B: Inconsistent or limited-quality patient-oriented evidence

C: Consensus, disease-oriented evidence, usual practice, expert opinion, or case series

1. Resting tremor, bradykinesia, postural instability, and rigidity are considered the cardinal signs of Parkinson's disease (PD). **Grade A**

2. An effective test of postural stability for individuals with PD is the retropulsion or "pull test." **Grade B**

3. The Hoehn and Yahr Scale and the UPDRS are helpful tools to identify the progression of Parkinson's disease related to levels of disability and impairments. **Grade A**

4. For individuals with PD, the Berg Balance Scale, 10-Meter Walk Test, and the Timed Up and Go test are reliable and valid assessments of balance, gait speed, and functional mobility that are sensitive to change (*i.e.*, have reported minimal detectable changes). **Grade B**

5. The 39-question Parkinson's Disease Questionnaire (39-PDQ), Medical Outcomes Study 36-Item Short-Form Health Survey (SF-36), and the Activities Balance Confidence Scale (ABC) are reliable and valid measures of participation in patients with PD. **Grade B**

COMPREHENSION QUESTIONS

3.1 Tremor in early Parkinson's disease is:
  A. Typically bilateral
  B. Increased with activity
  C. Present at rest
  D. Usually improved with levodopa

3.2 Which of the following assessment tools would be the *most* appropriate to measure the participation restrictions in an individual with Parkinson's disease?
  A. Berg Balance Scale (BBS)
  B. Six-Minute Walk Test (6MWT)
  C. Medical Outcomes Study 36-Item Short-Form Health Survey (SF-36)
  D. Functional Reach Test (FRT)

ANSWERS

3.1 **C.** Tremor associated with PD is usually present at rest and is diminished with activity. *Unilateral* tremor is often an early sign of PD. Levodopa is more effective at improving bradykinesia and rigidity and less effective in reducing tremor and postural instability.

3.2 **C.** The tool that measures participation restrictions is the SF-36, which assesses quality of life (including physical and mental domains) from the patient's point of view. The BBS, 6MWT, and FRT measure the direct impairments common in patients with PD: functional mobility, gait, balance, and postural stability.

REFERENCES

1. Umphred DA. *Neurological Rehabilitation*. 5th ed. St. Louis, MO: Mosby Elsevier; 2007.

2. O'Sullivan SB, Schmitz TJ. *Physical Rehabilitation*. Philadelphia, PA: FA Davis; 2007.

3. LeWitt PA. Levodopa for the treatment of Parkinson's disease. *N Engl J Med.* 2008;359: 2468-2476.

4. Goodman CC, Fuller KS. Pathology: *Implications for the Physical Therapist.* 3rd ed. Philadelphia, PA: Saunders; 2008.

5. Jankovic J. Parkinson's disease: clinical features and diagnosis. *J Neurol Neurosurg Psychiatry.* 2008;79: 368-376.

6. Ropper AH, Brown RH. *Adams and Victor's Principles of Neurology.* 9th ed. New York: McGraw-Hill Professional; 2009.

7. Munhoz RP, Li JY, Kurtinecz M, et al. Evaluation of the pull test technique in assessing postural instability in Parkinson's disease. *Neurology.* 2004;62:125-127.

8. Schenkman M, Butler RB. A model for multisystem evaluation treatment of individuals with Parkinson's disease. *Phys Ther.* 1989;69:932-943.

9. Stowe RL, Ives NJ, Clarke C, et al. Dopamine agonist therapy in early Parkinson's disease. *Cochrane Database Syst Rev.* 2008;Apr 16(2):CD006564.

10. Antonini A, Martinez-Martin P, Chaudhuri RK, et al. Wearing-off scales in Parkinson's disease: critique and recommendations. *Mov Disord.* 2011;26:2169-2175.

11. Follett KA, Weaver FM, Stern M, et al. Pallidal versus subthalamic deep-brain stimulation for Parkinson's disease. *N Engl J Med.* 2010;362:2077-2091.

12. Deuschl G, Schade-Brittinger C, Krack P, et al. A randomized trial of deep-brain stimulation for Parkinson's disease. *N Engl J Med.* 2006;355:896-908.

13. Nutt JG, Wooten GF. Diagnosis and initial management of Parkinson's disease. *N Engl J Med.* 2005;353:1021-1027.

14. Morris ME, Martin CL, Schenkman ML. Striding out with Parkinson disease: evidence-based physical therapy for gait disorders. *Phys Ther.* 2010;90:280-288.

15. Goetz CG, Poewe W, Rascol O, et al. Movement Disorder Society Task Force report on the Hoehn and Yahr staging scale: status and recommendations. *Mov Disord.* 2004;19:1020-1028.

16. Hoehn MM, Yahr MD. Parkinsonism: onset, progression and mortality. *Neurology.* 1967;17: 427-442.

17. Movement Disorder Society Task Force on Rating Scales of Parkinson's Disease. The Unified Parkinson's Disease Rating Scale (UPDRS): status and recommendations. *Mov Disord.* 2003;18: 738-750.

18. Steffen T, Seney M. Test-retest reliability and minimal detectable change on balance and ambulation tests, the 36-item short-form health survey, and the Unified Parkinson Disease Rating Scale in people with parkinsonism. *Phys Ther.* 2008;88:733-746.

19. Landers M, Backlund A, Davenport J, et al. Postural instability in idiopathic Parkinson's disease: discriminating fallers from nonfallers based on standardized clinical measures. *J Neurol Phys Ther.* 2008;32:56-61.

20. Ebersbach G, Ebersbach A, Edler D, et al. Comparing exercise in Parkinson's disease—the Berlin LSVT BIG study. *Mov Disord.* 2010;25:1902-1908.

21. Tanji H, Gruber-Baldini AL, Anderson KE, et al. A comparative study of physical performance measures in Parkinson's disease. *Mov Disord.* 2008;23:1897-1905.

22. Dibble L, Lange M. Predicting falls in individuals with Parkinson disease: a reconsideration of clinical balance measures. *J Neurol Phys Ther.* 2006;30:60-67.

23. Lim LI, van Wegen EE, de Goede CJ, et al. Measuring gait and gait-related activities in Parkinson's patients own home environment: a reliability, responsiveness and feasibility study. *Parkinsonism Relat Disord*. 2005;11:19-24.

24. Martinez-Martin P, Jeukens-Visser M, Lyons KE, et al. Health-related quality-of-life scales in Parkinson's disease: critique and recommendations. *Mov Disord*. 2011;26:2371-2380.

25. Lohnes CA, Earhart GM. External validation of abbreviated versions of the activities-specific balance confidence scale in Parkinson's disease. *Mov Disord*. 2010;25:485-489.

Parkinson's Disease: Treatment

Heather Scott David

A 70-year-old male was diagnosed with Parkinson's disease (PD) 8 years ago with a clinical presentation of a unilateral tremor in the right upper extremity. He now presents to outpatient physical therapy with reports of rigidity, postural instability, falls, and difficulty rising from a chair without falling backward. He requires minimal assistance for all transfers and bed mobility and ambulates within the home (50 ft) with a front-wheeled walker and contact guard assistance. He occasionally requires minimal assistance to limit forward momentum due to a festinating gait. He lives at home with his 65-year-old wife who is in good health and is the patient's primary caregiver. Over the last 3 months, the patient has begun falling regularly and has been unable to participate in weekly bridge games at his community clubhouse because of his decline in mobility. He is unable to get off the ground by himself and his wife has had to call 911 or neighbors to help him up; however, he has not suffered any serious injuries as a result of his falls. The patient presents with a masked face and hypophonia making it difficult to communicate. He has also begun to experience dysphagia. This patient has been taking carbidopa/levodopa (Sinemet) for 8 years and has begun to experience decreased effectiveness with definitive on and off phases. The physical therapist has completed the initial evaluation of this patient (Case 3) and is initiating the physical therapy plan of care.

▶ Describe a physical therapy plan of care based on this stage of the patient's disease.
▶ Based on the patient's diagnosis, what are appropriate physical therapy interventions?
▶ What precautions should be taken during physical therapy interventions?

Objectives

1. Identify physical therapy interventions to address impairments, activity limitations, and participation restrictions in individuals with PD.
2. Prescribe appropriate assistive devices for individuals with PD.
3. Describe interventions to address postural instability and gait abnormalities that are common in individuals with PD.

Physical Therapy Considerations

PT considerations during management of the individual with gait instability, balance difficulties, positive fall history, and decreased functional mobility due to PD:

▶ **General physical therapy plan of care/goals:** Improve transfer safety and independence; improve ability to rise from sitting without loss of balance posteriorly; improve household ambulation independence

▶ **Physical therapy interventions:** Patient and family education regarding fall prevention; increase range of motion (ROM); gait training, balance exercises, transfer training; Lee Silverman Voice Treatment (LSVT) BIG training

▶ **Precautions during physical therapy interventions:** Close guarding due to patient's high risk of falling; recognize potential ADRs and describe potential therapy solutions

▶ **Complications interfering with physical therapy:** Orthostatic hypotension; timing of medication dosing

Plan of Care and Interventions

The physical therapy plan of care for a patient with PD describes the planned interventions, frequency, and duration of treatment sessions. The plan of care should include measurable and time-specific therapy goals, expected outcomes, and the patient's discharge plan. Physical therapy interventions often include a variety of interventions to promote motor learning, strength, flexibility and ROM, functional mobility, balance, gait, use of assistive devices, and cardiorespiratory function.[1-5] Interventions always include patient and family education. Exercise interventions can be performed in individual and/or group sessions. Additional physical therapy interventions include the use of rhythmic auditory stimulation, Lee Silverman Voice Treatment (LSVT) BIG,[6,7] and body-weight-support treadmill training.

Patients with PD benefit from stretching and ROM activities to minimize the indirect impairments of decreased ROM, stooped posture, and the development of contractures. Stretching and ROM exercises can be targeted for muscle groups frequently affected by rigidity such as hip flexors, knee flexors, ankle plantarflexors, pectoralis muscles, and cervical flexors.[2] Patients with PD benefit from strengthening exercises targeting weak extensor muscle groups to try to counteract the active ROM losses in hip extension, knee extension, ankle dorsiflexion, scapular retraction, and cervical extension.[2] Due to the lack of upper and lower trunk disassociation that occurs as a result of PD-associated rigidity, the therapist should incorporate exercises that promote axial rotation. A systematic review of seven studies of patients with PD supports the use of a **wide variety of exercises for physical improvements** in axial rotation, functional reach, flexibility, balance, muscle strength, gait, and mobility.[8] This systematic review included a variety of exercise interventions including: stretching, progressive exercise training, trunk strengthening and aerobic exercise, relaxation, strength and balance training, gait training, Qigong, and a home exercise program. Frequency and duration varied from 1 to 3 hours per week for 4 to 12 weeks. Cardiovascular decline in patients with PD can contribute to decreased functional mobility and participation restrictions. During bicycling and walking, individuals with PD demonstrate increased oxygen consumption compared to those without PD.[9,10] However, aerobic training can improve maximal oxygen consumption in individuals with PD.[10,11]

To address limitations in functional mobility, task-specific training should be incorporated. This includes repeated sit-to-stand transfers from a variety of surfaces, stair climbing, upper extremity overhead reaching activities, and rolling in bed to emphasis trunk disassociation. The patient in this case requires minimal assistance for all transfers. In fact, patients with PD often have difficulty with the task of rising from a chair. Education and specific training of this activity should occur. The therapist should have the individual scoot to the edge of his chair to promote an adequate anterior trunk lean to unweight his hips and load his feet underneath him. Raising the surface height will decrease the difficulty of this task in the early stages of motor learning. Progressive lowering of the surface height and task practice on a variety of surfaces like toilets, cars, beds, and chairs will increase the patient's ability to carryover the skill to a variety of environments and situations. In addition to functional strength training, patients benefit from education related to restorative and compensatory approaches to functional mobility including bed mobility, transfers, sit-to-stand, gait training, and fall recovery. One therapeutic approach designed to improve movement perception and increase movement scaling in patients with PD is called Lee Silverman Voice Treatment (LSVT) BIG program. This exercise approach is based on the LSVT LOUD program—a treatment approach that has been used to increase voice production in patients with PD experiencing hypophonia.[6] The LSVT BIG approach focuses on high-amplitude movements, multiple repetitions, high intensity, and increasing difficulty. This intervention is typically performed for 1 hour, 4 times per week for 4 weeks.[6] In a randomized controlled trial of 60 individuals with PD, the LSVT BIG group (using the frequency and duration described above) demonstrated greater improvements in Unified Parkinson's Disease Rating Scale (UPDRS) motor scores and improved times on the Timed Up and Go and 10-Meter Walk tests compared to both a walking program group and a home exercise program group.[6]

Gait training and assistive device prescription is an important component of physical therapy management for patients with PD. Common gait deviations include decreased stride length, reduced velocity, cadence abnormalities, increased double limb support time, insufficient dorsiflexion, insufficient hip and knee extension, difficulty turning, festinating gait, freezing of gait, and difficulty with motor and cognitive dual tasking.[2] Gait training should be specific to the needs of the patient and his lifestyle and may include walking in crowds, through obstacles, through doorways, over curbs, and across different surfaces. An individual experiencing difficulty walking may benefit from the use of an assistive device to increase mobility, improve stability, and decrease risk of falling. There are many devices available. The physical therapist should carefully consider each option based on the evidence in the literature and careful assessment of the patient's gait pattern with the use of each. Three types of assistive devices available for patients with PD include canes and walking sticks, walkers, and wheelchairs. A single point cane may prevent falls in patients with mild imbalance, but will not likely help with falls due to retropulsion.[12] A tall walking stick may be appropriate for use in patients with PD to prevent the stooped posture that can occur with use of an assistive device. In patients with moderate to severe postural instability, a single point cane is unlikely to prevent falls; these patients may need to use a walker to assist with safe ambulation. A standard four-point walker may provide stability for patients with PD; however, this type of walker is also not likely to prevent falls due to retropulsion and may contribute to a worsening of freezing episodes.[12,13] A study comparing the use of standard walkers with front-wheeled walkers found the use of both mobility aids increased stability and confidence.[13] However, the use of the devices decreased walking speed compared to walking without an assistive device. The authors found that the front-wheeled walker did not worsen freezing episodes, while the use of a standard walker did.[13] A four-wheeled walker provides hand brakes and may provide improved mobility with increased ease of turning; however, these walkers are less stable than traditional aluminum front-wheeled walkers. Front-wheeled walkers and four-wheeled walkers may provide stability without worsening freezing episodes but may not be appropriate for patients with festinating gait. A patient with festinating gait may be unable to stop the forward momentum that can occur with the use of a wheeled walker. This may decrease stability and *increase* a patient's risk of falling. For the current patient who has a history of falling backward and festinating gait, choosing the best assistive device can be very challenging. A single point cane would likely not prevent retropulsion and a front-wheeled walker may be unsafe due to a potential increase in forward momentum. Another option for this patient is a walker that requires the user to squeeze the brake handles to disengage the brakes, causing the walker to stop forward motion when the user lets go of the brakes. This may help prevent uncontrolled forward momentum and provide more stability than a single point cane. The use of a manual or power wheelchair may increase functional mobility for patients with PD that are not safe ambulating without physical assistance. Power wheelchairs and scooters require individuals to have the cognitive ability to safely use the device in their living environments. Joystick sensitivity and speed limitations can be modified to accommodate patients with tremor or bradykinesia.[12]

Gait training in patients with PD can be enhanced with the use of rhythmic auditory stimulation (RAS), visual cues, and body-weight-supported treadmill training. Rhythmic auditory stimulation (RAS) can be used as a tool during gait training. This is performed with the use of music or a metronome set at a specific tempo for the patient to match his gait to. Studies using RAS for gait training in patients with PD have demonstrated increased stride length, gait velocity, and cadence compared to control groups.[14-18] **Auditory cues to assist with gait training** for patients with PD can also include verbal cueing. Verbally cueing patients to increase step length and arm swing can result in short-term improvement in these gait parameters.[19] The use of visual cues may improve gait in patients with PD, including the use of floor markings, specialized canes, and specialized walkers.[2] Patients with freezing of gait may benefit from the use of a cane or walker with a laser light beam or an inverted cane with a curved end that the patient can step over. Devices like these can provide a visual cue that may help overcome freezing episodes.[12] A systematic review of the use of visual cues found that floor markers improved stride length; however, this review did not find sufficient evidence to support the use of other visual cues including light beams, flashing lights on spectacles, and walking aids.[20] A recent Cochrane review of eight randomized controlled trials testing the effectiveness of treadmill training with and without body-weight-support for patients with PD found that treadmill training improved gait speed, stride length, and walking distance, but not cadence.[21]

Postural instability is one of the cardinal features of PD. Postural instability includes impaired standing postural control strategies, impaired reactive balance strategies to an unexpected destabilizing force, and postural instability during voluntary mobility activities. Individuals with PD demonstrate a loss of feedforward and feedback postural strategies.[5] Balance training may be effective in improving postural stability in patients with PD. **Balance training for individuals with PD** should include activities that promote a variety of movement strategies in a range of environmental conditions. Anticipatory balance activities including reaching outside the individual's base of support to improve limits of stability can be combined with reactive balance training with perturbations. In a randomized controlled trial, individuals with PD who participated in balance training aimed at improving feedforward and feedback balance abilities demonstrated significant improvements on the Berg Balance Scale, Activities Specific Balance Confidence Scale, functional transfer ability, and a test of center of foot pressure displacement. The control group that performed stretching and active ROM activities performed in supine, sitting, and standing did not demonstrate significant improvements on these primary outcome measures.[5]

Falls are a significant problem in the PD population. In a prospective study of falls and fall risk, individuals with PD had a fall rate of almost 70% with recurrent falls in approximately 50% of individuals within 1 year.[22] Studies with shorter follow-up times demonstrated proportionally lower fall rates. Patients and caregivers should be taught how to get up after a fall. The therapist should teach the patient to have a way to call for help if he will be home alone; if an injury occurs as a result of a fall, the individual should not try to get up without assistance. Instead, he should call for help. If the individual is not injured, he can crawl on hands and knees to a stable piece of furniture and transition from quadruped to half-kneeling then standing or sitting on a stable sofa or chair. Such fall recovery training should be incorporated into the plan of care. Caregivers should also be taught how to assist a patient up from the floor as appropriate.[2]

Patient and family education is an integral part of the physical therapist's role in the care of a patient with PD. Physical therapists provide education to patients, families, and caregivers related to disease progression, symptom management, movement strategies, energy conservation, strategies to perform ADLs and recreational activities, fall prevention strategies, fall recovery strategies, and additional PD resource identification.[2] Individuals with PD often experience psychosocial problems such as depression, anxiety, social isolation, loss of control, and difficulty coping with disability. Caregivers are often family members and partners who also experience psychosocial stresses.[23] A European consortium (EduPark) developed a program for standardized patient and caregiver education to address psychosocial issues experienced by patients and caregivers. The Patient Education Program Parkinson (PEPP) provides patients and caregivers with knowledge and skills designed to improve quality of life.[24] The physical therapist may be able to provide information about locally available support groups and exercise groups. National PD associations can provide educational materials, newsletters, and information about support group locations.

Evidence-Based Clinical Recommendations

SORT: Strength of Recommendation Taxonomy

A: Consistent, good-quality patient-oriented evidence

B: Inconsistent or limited-quality patient-oriented evidence

C: Consensus, disease-oriented evidence, usual practice, expert opinion, or case series

1. Exercise improves overall physical performance in individuals with Parkinson's disease. **Grade B**

2. Auditory cueing with gait training leads to short-term improvements in gait velocity in individuals with Parkinson's disease. **Grade B**

3. Balance training improves postural stability in individuals with Parkinson's disease. **Grade B**

COMPREHENSION QUESTIONS

4.1 A physical therapist is evaluating a patient with Parkinson's disease. The patient and his caregivers report the patient has begun falling and they would like to know what would be the best assistive device. During your evaluation, you note that the patient requires moderate assistance for loss of balance and demonstrates freezing of gait. He does not demonstrate festinating gait. Which assistive device would be the *most* appropriate for this patient?

    A.   Front-wheeled walker

    B.   Single point cane

    C.   Standard four-point walker

    D.   Inverted cane

4.2 During a physical therapy evaluation, a patient with Parkinson's disease tells the therapist he is having difficulty rising from a chair and getting off the toilet. What would be the *most* appropriate intervention to address this problem?

A. Lower extremity strength training in seated position

B. Balance training

C. Sit-to-stand training from various height surfaces

D. Rhythmic auditory stimulation

4.3 A physical therapist is working with a patient with advanced Parkinson's disease. The patient has lost weight and his family is concerned about his ability to speak clearly and swallow effectively. Which of the following would be the appropriate referral for additional services?

A. Speech-language pathologist

B. Psychologist

C. Occupational therapist

D. Social worker

ANSWERS

4.1 **A.** A front-wheeled walker can be used in patients with freezing of gait to decrease the risk of falls, but this device may be unsafe for patients with festinating gait. This patient does not demonstrate festinating gait, therefore a front-wheeled walker is the best choice for him. A single point cane (option B) will likely be insufficient to prevent falls in a patient with balance impairments requiring moderate assistance for recovery of balance. An inverted cane (option D) is used to provide a visual cue for a patient with freezing gait, but will likely be insufficient to decrease the risk of a fall for this patient. A standard walker (option C) can worsen freezing episodes and will not help with retropulsion-related falls.

4.2 **C.** Task-specific functional mobility training to improve sit-to-stand performance can effectively be done with sit-to-stand training. Having the patient practice from a variety of surface heights will help with transfer of training.

4.3 **A.** A referral to a speech-language pathologist (SLP) to evaluate this patient's swallowing abilities is appropriate. A speech-language pathologist can address the possibility of dysphagia, which could be potentially life-threatening as it can lead to aspiration pneumonia. The SLP can also evaluate his ability to speak clearly. Patients with Parkinson's disease frequently have difficulty related to speech production.

REFERENCES

1. Umphred DA. *Neurological Rehabilitation*. 5th ed. St. Louis, MO: Mosby Elsevier; 2007.

2. O'Sullivan SB, Schmitz TJ. *Physical Rehabilitation*. Philadelphia, PA: FA Davis; 2007.

3. Morris ME, Martin CL, Schenkman ML. Striding out with Parkinson disease: evidence-based physical therapy for gait disorders. *Phys Ther*. 2010;90:280-288.

4. American Physical Therapy Association. *Guide to Physical Therapist Practice*. 2nd ed. *Phys Ther*. 2001;81:9-746.

5. Smania N, Corato E, Tinazzi M, et al. Effect of balance training on postural instability in patients with idiopathic Parkinson's disease. *Neurorehabil Neural Repair*. 2010;24:826-834.

6. Ebersbach G, Ebersbach A, Edler D, et al. Comparing exercise in Parkinson's disease—the Berlin LSVT BIG study. *Mov Disord*. 2010;25:1902-1908.

7. Farley BG, Koshland GF. Training BIG to move faster: the application of the speed–amplitude relation as a rehabilitation strategy for people with Parkinson's disease. *Exp Brain Res*. 2005;167:462-467.

8. Crizzle AM, Newhouse IJ. Is physical exercise beneficial for persons with Parkinson's disease? *Clin J Sport Med*. 2006;16:422-425.

9. Protas EJ, Stanley RK, Jankovic J, MacNeill B. Cardiovascular and metabolic responses to upper- and lower-extremity exercise in men with idiopathic Parkinson's disease. *Phys Ther*. 1996;76:34-40.

10. Christiansen CL, Schenkman ML, McFann K, Wolfe P, Kohrt WM. Walking economy in people with Parkinson's disease. *Mov Disord*. 2009;24:1481-1487.

11. Bergen JL, Toole T, Elliott RG, Wallace B, Robinson K, Maitland CG. Aerobic exercise intervention improves aerobic capacity and movement initiation in Parkinson's disease patients. *NeuroRehabilitation*. 2002;17:161-168.

12. Constantinescu R, Leonard C, Deeley C, Kurlan R. Assistive devices for gait in Parkinson's disease. *Parkinsonism Relat Disord*. 2007;13:133-138.

13. Cubo E, Moore CG, Leurgans S, Goetz CG. Wheeled and standard walkers in Parkinson's disease patients with gait freezing. *Parkinsonism Relat Disord*. 2003;10:9-14.

14. Thaut MH, McIntosh GC, Rice RR, Miller RA, Rathbun J, Brault JM. Rhythmic auditory stimulation in gait training for Parkinson's disease patients. *Mov Disord*. 1996;11:193-200.

15. Willems AM, Nieuwboer A, Chavret F, et al. The use of rhythmic auditory cues to influence gait in patients with Parkinson's disease, the differential effect for freezers and non-freezers, an explorative study. *Disabil Rehabil*. 2006;28:721-728.

16. del Olmo MF, Cudeiro J. Temporal variability of gait in Parkinson disease: effects of a rehabilitation programme based on rhythmic sound cues. *Parkinsonism Relat Disord*. 2005;11:25-33.

17. McIntosh GC, Brown SH, Rice RR, Thaut MH. Rhythmic auditory-motor facilitation of gait patterns in patients with Parkinson's disease. *J Neurol Neurosurg Psychiatry*. 1997;62:22-26.

18. Howe TE, Lövgreen B, Cody FW, Ashton VJ, Oldham JA. Auditory cues can modify the gait of persons with early-stage Parkinson's disease: a method for enhancing parkinsonian walking performance? *Clin Rehabil*. 2003;17:363-367.

19. Behrman AL, Teitelbaum P, Cauraugh JH. Verbal instructional sets to normalise the temporal and spatial gait variables in Parkinson's disease. *J Neurol Neurosurg Psychiatry*. 1998;65:580-582.

20. Lim I, van Wegen E, de Goede C, et al. Effects of external rhythmical cueing on gait in patients with Parkinson's disease: a systematic review. *Clin Rehabil*. 2005;19:695-713.

21. Mehrholz J, Friis R, Kugler J, Twork S, Storch A, Pohl M. Treadmill training for patients with Parkinson's disease. *Cochrane Database Syst Rev*. 2010;Jan 20:CD007830.

22. Wood BH, Bilclough JA, Bowron A, Walker RW. Incidence and prediction of falls in Parkinson's disease: a prospective multidisciplinary study. *J Neurol Neurosurg Psychiatry*. 2002;72:721-725.

23. A'Campo LE, Wekking EM, Spliethoff-Kamminga NG, Le Cessie S, Roos RA. The benefits of a standardized patient education program for patients with Parkinson's disease and their caregivers. *Parkinsonism Relat Disord*. 2010;16:89-95.

24. Macht M, Gerlich C, Ellgring H, et al. Patient education in Parkinson's disease: formative evaluation of a standardized programme in seven European countries. *Patient Educ Couns*. 2007;65:245-252.

Normal Pressure Hydrocephalus

Annie Burke-Doe

A 78-year-old male was referred to a neurologist due to complaints of difficulty with gait, feeling unsteady, and urinary urgency. His wife reported that over the last year he has had progressive difficulty with memory and has been unable to manage financial matters for the household. Prior medical history was unremarkable. Neurologic examination revealed impaired memory and visuospatial skills and difficulty with calculations. The rest of the neurologic examination was notable for diminished postural reflexes and magnetic gait with *en block* turning. Laboratory tests did not reveal any treatable cause of dementia (*e.g.*, vitamin B_{12} deficiency or thyroid toxicity). Magnetic resonance imaging (MRI) demonstrated large ventricles and hypodensity of white matter. A spinal tap was performed with normal opening pressure and 35 cc of cerebrospinal fluid (CSF) was collected. The CSF analysis was normal. The patient's gait transiently improved after the spinal tap. A diagnosis of normal pressure hydrocephalus was made based on the MRI results and on the presence of the characteristic clinical triad: gait impairment, cognitive decline, and urinary urgency. The patient was admitted to the hospital and underwent ventriculoperitoneal (VP) shunting. The physical therapist is asked to evaluate and treat the patient to assist in determining the effect of the VP shunt on the patient's functional abilities.

- Based on his health condition, what do you anticipate will be the contributors to activity limitations?
- What are the examination priorities?
- What is his rehabilitation prognosis?
- What are the most appropriate physical therapy outcome measures for gait and balance?
- What are possible complications interfering with physical therapy?

KEY DEFINITIONS

EN BLOCK TURNING: Lack of trunk rotation when walking and turning around, resulting in movements that are "in mass" or as a whole

MAGNETIC GAIT: Walking as if feet are attached to floor by a magnet; each step is initiated in a "wrestling" motion that carries the foot upward and forward

NORMAL PRESSURE HYDROCEPHALUS (NPH): Accumulation of cerebrospinal fluid that causes the ventricles in the brain to become enlarged, sometimes with little or no increase in intracranial pressure

Objectives

1. Describe normal pressure hydrocephalus.
2. Identify key questions to determine the history of the present illness, prior level of function, and presence of factors at home/work such as stairs, ramps, thresholds that may interfere with gaining access to these environments.
3. Identify reliable and valid outcome tools to measure gait and functional mobility.
4. Discuss appropriate components of the examination for the individual with NPH.

Physical Therapy Considerations

PT considerations during management of the individual with gait instability, history of falls, general motor and balance difficulties, and decreased endurance due to normal pressure hydrocephalus:

▶ **General physical therapy plan of care/goals:** Assess gait and possible benefits of VP shunt placement; maximize functional independence and safety while minimizing secondary impairments

▶ **Physical therapy interventions:** Patient education on level of assistance required for safe execution of tasks, anticipated progression of condition, relevant precautions, and home exercise program; therapeutic exercise, functional mobility training, endurance conditioning, gait training

▶ **Precautions during physical therapy:** Clamping of spinal tap drains prior to mobility; close physical supervision to decrease risk of falls; monitor vital signs

▶ **Complications interfering with physical therapy:** Subdural hematoma, falls, intracranial infections, stroke, shunt failure

Understanding the Health Condition

Normal pressure hydrocephalus (NPH) is an accumulation of CSF that causes the ventricles in the brain to become enlarged, sometimes with little or no increase in intracranial pressure (ICP).[1] In the majority of cases, ventricular enlargement results from an obstruction of CSF flow around the brain convexities and insufficient absorption through the arachnoid granulations and arachnoid villi of the superior sagittal sinus.[2] Usually, it is not clear what causes the CSF absorptive pathways to become blocked. The resultant initial elevation in ICP causes enlargement of the ventricles, creating a new balance with normal pressure.[3] Ventricular enlargement reduces compliance of the brain, which compresses and stretches the periventricular white matter.[2] NPH is sometimes called communicating or nonobstructive hydrocephalus because the lateral, third, and fourth ventricle are not obstructed.[4] Most commonly diagnosed in older adults, NPH is accompanied by some or all of the following clinical triad: gait disturbance, mild dementia, and impaired bladder control.

NPH is most prevalent during the sixth and seventh decades and is rare in people younger than 60 years of age.[5] However, young patients ranging from neonates to young adults with secondary NPH have been reported.[6] The true prevalence in the population is unknown because some patients may present with only gait impairment and without cognitive deficits.[2] Gait is also influenced by the progression of NPH. In early stages, the gait may be wide-based[5] and ataxic. However, in later stages, the gait may be characterized by short, shuffling steps and the patient may appear frozen.[7] Postural instability is also common, which increases the risk for falls. Turning is awkward and *en block* with multiple steps. Patients often complain about leg weakness, fatigue, and sensory changes. The neurologic evaluation may reveal a mild degree of spasticity with increased stretch reflexes in the lower extremities and Babinski's signs may also be present.[2] Motor impairment may also involve the upper limbs (*e.g.*, dysdiadochokinesia).

Cognitive decline varies widely, but is characterized by prominent attention deficit, memory impairment, and executive (frontal lobe) dysfunction. Early urinary involvement is due to a loss of voluntary supraspinal control resulting in bladder hyperactivity and detrusor instability, which is manifested by urgency. Late frank incontinence also has a frontal component manifested by a lack of concern. Many of the symptoms of cognitive decline (deficits in attention, initiation, and executive functions) can be accounted for by compression of the frontal white matter.[2]

Diagnosis is typically determined through signs and symptoms, neuroimaging studies, and evaluation of CSF composition, pressure, and drainage (prolonged or continuous). A routine spinal tap may be performed to rule out other conditions. Normal CSF concentrations of protein and glucose with a white blood cell count of ≤ 5 cells/μL and opening pressure of < 200 mm H_2O suggest that NPH may be the cause of the neurologic symptoms.[8] An intermittent high volume tap that removes 30 to 60 mL of CSF can be used to compare neurological symptoms before and after the tap. Improvement of symptoms with removal of CSF may indicate the eventual positive response to VP shunting.[8]

The most common treatment for NPH is ventriculoperitoneal (VP) shunting.[8] In VP shunting, a catheter is placed into one of the lateral ventricles and attached to a cap and valve positioned under the scalp. Tubing is tunneled subcutaneously from the valve to the abdomen, where CSF is deposited into the sterile peritoneal cavity for continuous drainage.[8]

It is difficult to determine the prognosis for patients who have had VP shunt placement. The proportion of patients with long-term improvement after a VP shunt varies from 25% to 80%. Improvement depends on the indications for the VP shunt placement, experience of the neurosurgeon, and preoperative conditions.[9,10] In 2000, Vanneste[7] described the factors that predicted a good surgical outcome. These included: gait disturbance preceding mental impairment, short history of slight or moderate mental impairment, known cause of NPH, and substantial clinical improvement after one or several spinal taps. Factors related to poor surgical outcomes included: a predominance of severe dementia, dementia as the first neurological sign, and MRI revealing marked cerebral atrophy with widespread white matter involvement.

Since walking difficulties and postural imbalance are usually the first signs of NPH and are also the signs most likely to improve after placement of a VP shunt,[5,11-13] physical therapists are poised to assist in: (1) the diagnosis of probable NPH; (2) determining the effectiveness of CSF drainage; (3) determining the likelihood of benefit from shunt surgery; and, (4) assessing the course of improvement following shunt surgery.

Physical Therapy Patient/Client Management

A patient with NPH typically presents with dementia, gait abnormality, and incontinence. The only established treatment is the surgical implantation of a VP shunt.[8] Physical therapists may be asked to assess changes in functional status over the course of NPH and its treatment. The primary physical therapy goal is to maximize functional independence and minimize secondary impairments.

Examination, Evaluation, and Diagnosis

Prior to seeing this patient, the physical therapist needs to acquire information from the chart, including history, diagnostic testing, medications, prior level of function, and current complaints. When gathering information about the history of the present illness, examples of questions a therapist may ask the patient and/or caregiver or spouse may include: "When did you start to notice a change in function and/or walking ability?" "Specifically, *how* has function and/or walking ability changed?" "Have you had any falls in the last year?" "Do you have any stairs, ramps, thresholds at work or home that may interfere with access to these environments?"

During the examination, the physical therapist assesses mental status, posture, gait, strength, balance, and performs functional tests. When assessing gait in patients with NPH, it is important to note that improvement in gait often precedes improvement in incontinence or cognition after VP shunt surgery.[14,15] The therapist can determine the most appropriate assistive device using both qualitative (observational) and quantitative (spatial and temporal) measures. In 2008, Feick et al.[16] found that the **Timed Up and Go** (TUG) and the **Tinetti Assessment Tool of Gait and Balance**[17] were sensitive to differential gait changes in this population. The TUG is a reliable and valid performance-based measure of functional mobility initially developed to identify mobility and balance impairments in older adults.[18] The TUG requires the subject to rise from a chair, stand up, walk 3 m, turn around, walk back to the chair, and sit down. The test score is the time it takes the subject to compete the task. The TUG score is strongly correlated to level of functional mobility (*i.e.*, the more time taken, the more dependent the person would be in activities of daily living), fall risk, gait speed, balance, and the ability to go out in the community. Scores on the TUG can also mirror changes in patients' functional status over time. To interpret the results: < 10 seconds is considered normal; < 20 seconds is indicative of good mobility without an assistive device; < 30 seconds indicates problems with gait, and the individual cannot safely ambulate in the community and requires an assistive device.[17,18] A score of ≥ 14 seconds has been shown to indicate high risk for falls.[17,18] The Tinetti Assessment Tool of Gait and Balance is a reliable and valid measure of observed performance of mobility and fall risk.[19] The scale has two components: balance and gait. For balance, the Tinetti includes subtests of sitting balance, sit-to-stand, immediate standing balance, balance with eyes closed, turning 360°, and sitting down. For gait, the Tinetti includes subtests of gait initiation, step length, step symmetry and continuity, path deviation, trunk stability, and walking stance. The maximum score for the balance and gait components are 16 points and 12 points, respectively. The maximum total score is 28 points. Higher scores are correlated with better mobility.[19,20] In general, patients who score < 19 points are at a high risk for falls.

Postural imbalance is also considered one of the first signs of NPH.[7] Balance should be assessed in sitting, standing, and during ambulation. Balance can be expected to degrade under conditions of narrowing base of support, or in response to perturbations.[21] The Romberg test, tandem walking, and single leg stance are three assessments that require patients to vary their base of support. Perturbation tasks that can be used to challenge balance include self-initiated movements (*e.g.*, arm raise, bending-reach, Functional Reach Tests,[22] or the Multidirectional Reach Test[23]).

Plan of Care and Interventions

Specific physical therapy goals are set after the evaluation. Goals should be based on the individual's current status and history of functional abilities. Identification of impairments, dysfunction, and functional limitations such as presence of headache, impairments of strength, range of motion, endurance, posture, and gait as well as decreased independence will assist the therapist in determining goals and interventions. Interventions most commonly used for treating patients with NPH include therapeutic exercise, functional mobility training, balance training, gait training with **visual and auditory cueing (*e.g.*, marching to a metronome[24])**, and prescription of assistive devices that relate to the identified impairments.

Evidence-Based Clinical Recommendations

SORT: Strength of Recommendation Taxonomy

A: Consistent, good-quality patient-oriented evidence

B: Inconsistent or limited-quality patient-oriented evidence

C: Consensus, disease-oriented evidence, usual practice, expert opinion, or case series

1. Physical therapists can use the Timed Up and Go (TUG) assessment to identify functional mobility, fall risk, gait speed, balance impairments, and the ability for safe community ambulation in older adults. **Grade A**

2. Physical therapists can use the Tinetti Assessment Tool of Gait and Balance to determine functional mobility, gait deviations, balance impairments, and fall risk. **Grade A**

3. Visual and auditory cueing improves gait in individuals with NPH. **Grade C**

COMPREHENSION QUESTIONS

5.1 A physical therapist is working with a patient who is 3 days status/post VP shunt placement for treatment of NPH. The patient has a past medical history of hypertension, atrial fibrillation, hypercholesterolemia, and diffuse atherosclerosis. The patient is confused, has weakness and sensory loss on the left side of the body, and difficulty with speech. Which of the following potential complications of a VP shunt placement is most likely related to the clinical signs and symptoms present?

   A. Shunt failure

   B. Increased intracranial pressure

   C. Meningitis

   D. Stroke

5.2 A physical therapist is treating a patient with NPH status/post VP shunt placement. The patient presents with cognitive and perceptual impairments, upper extremity tone, and difficulty with activities of daily living. Which of the following would be the appropriate referral for additional services?

   A. Speech-language pathologist

   B. Psychologist

   C. Occupational therapist

   D. Care coordinator

ANSWERS

5.1 **D.** Key signs and symptoms of stroke are one-sided weakness and decreased sensation and dysarthria. Certain patients are at risk for vascular disease including ischemic stroke. When the history is taken, patients should be asked if they have any of the following common vascular risk factors: hypertension, diabetes, hypercholesterolemia, cigarette smoking, and family or personal history of stroke or other vascular disease. In addition, certain cardiac disorders are important risk factors for stroke, especially atrial fibrillation.

5.2 **C.** A patient may benefit from occupational therapy when clinical presentation includes cognitive or perceptual impairments, upper extremity weakness and tone, or any impairment that affects the patient's ability to perform activities of daily living independently. Occupational therapists also assist patients who have upper extremity splinting or adaptive equipment needs.

REFERENCES

1. National Institutes of Neurologic Disease and Stroke. Normal pressure hydrocephalus. http://www.ninds.nih.gov/disorders/normal_pressure_hydrocephalus/normal_pressure_hydrocephalus.htm. Accessed October 31, 2010.

2. Hedera P, Friedland RP, Farlow M. Normal pressure hydrocephalus. In: Gilman S, ed. *MedLink Neurology*. San Diego: MedLink Corporation. www.medlink.com. Accessed October 1, 2010.

3. Simon RP, Greenberg DA, Aminoff MJ. Chapter 1: Disorders of cognitive function. *Clinical Neurology*. 7th ed. http://www.accessmedicine.com/content.aspx?aID=5143601. Accessed October 31, 2010.

4. Ropper AH, Samuels MA. Disturbances of cerebrospinal fluid and its circulation, including hydrocephalus, pseudotumor cerebri, and low-pressure syndromes. In: *Adams and Victor's Principles of Neurology*. 9th ed. http://www.accessmedicine.com/content.aspx?aID=3635067. Accessed October 31, 2010.

5. Fisher CM. Hydrocephalus as a cause of disturbances of gait in the elderly. *Neurology*. 1982;32: 1358-1363.

6. Barnett GH, Hahn JF, Palmer J. Normal pressure hydrocephalus in children and young adults. *Neurosurgery*. 1987;20:904-907.

7. Vanneste JA. Diagnosis and management of normal-pressure hydrocephalus. *J Neurol*. 2000;247:5-14.

8. Verrees M, Selman WR. Management of normal pressure hydrocephalus. *Am Fam Physician*. 2004;70:1071-1078.

9. Vanneste J, Augustijn P, Dirven C, Tan WF, Goedhart ZD. Shunting normal-pressure hydrocephalus: do the benefits outweigh the risk? A multicenter study and literature review. *Neurology*. 1992;42: 54-59.

10. Poca MA, Mataro M, Del Mar Matarin M, Arikan F, Junque C, Sahuquillo J. Is the placement of shunts in patients with idiopathic normal-pressure hydrocephalus worth the risk? Results of study based on continuous monitoring of intracranial pressure. *J Neurosurg*. 2004;100:855-866.

11. Soelberg-Sorensen PS, Jansen EC, Gjerris F. Motor disturbances in normal pressure hydrocephalus. Special reference to stance and gait. *Arch Neurol*. 1986;43:34-38.

12. Sudarsky L, Simon S. Gait disorder in late-life hydrocephalus. *Arch Neurol*. 1987;44:263-267.

13. Graff-Radford NR, Godersky JC. Normal-pressure hydrocephalus. Onset of gait abnormality before dementia predicts good surgical outcome. *Arch Neurol*. 1986;43:940-942.

14. McGirt MJ, Woodworth G, Coon AL, Thomas G, Williams MA, Rigamonti D. Diagnosis, treatment, and analysis of long-term outcomes in idiopathic normal-pressure hydrocephalus. *Neurosurgery*. 2005;57:699-705.

15. Marmarou A, Young HF, Aygok GA, et al. Diagnosis and management of idiopathic normal-pressure hydrocephalus: a prospective study in 151 patients. *J Neurosurg*. 2005;102:987-997.

16. Feick D, Sickmond J, Liu L, et al. Sensitivity and predictive value of occupational and physical therapy assessment in the functional evaluation of patients with suspected normal pressure hydrocephalus. *J Rehabil Med*. 2008;40:715-720.

17. Podsiadlo D, Richardson S. The timed "Up & Go": a test of basic functional mobility for frail elderly persons. *J Am Geriatr Soc*. 1991;39:142-148.

18. Shumway-Cook A, Brauer S, Woollacott M. Predicting the probability for falls in community-dwelling older adults using the Timed Up & Go Test. *Phys Ther*. 2000;80:896-903.

19. Tinetti ME, Williams TF, Mayewski R. Fall risk index for elderly patients based on number of chronic disabilities. *Am J Med.* 1986;80:429-434.

20. Lin MR, Hwang HF, Hu MH, Wu HD, Wang YW, Huang FC. Psychometric comparisons of the timed up and go, one-leg stand, functional reach, and Tinetti balance measures in community-dwelling older people. *J Am Geriatr Soc.* 2004;52:1343-1348.

21. O'Sullivan S. Parkinson disease. In: O'Sullivan S, Schmitz TJ, eds. *Physical Rehabilitation.* 5th ed. Philadelphia, PA: FA Davis Company; 2007.

22. Duncan PW, Weiner DK, Chandler J, Studenski S. Functional reach: a new clinical measurement of balance. *J Gerontol.* 1990;45:M192-M197.

23. Newton RA. Validity of the multi-directional reach test: a practical measure for limits of stability in older adults. *J Gerontol A Bio Sci Med Sci.* 2001;56:M248-M252.

24. Ropper AH, Samuels MA. Chapter 7. Disorders of stance and gait. *Adams and Victor's Principles of Neurology.* 9th ed. http://www.accessmedicine.com/content.aspx?aID=3630849. Accessed October 31, 2010.

Coccidioidomycosis Meningitis

Delisa Rideout
Terrence M. Nordstrom
Rolando Lazaro

CASE 6

The patient is a 60-year-old Hispanic male employed as a farm worker in an orchard in Kern County, California. His work primarily involves pruning trees, which entails maneuvering through tight spaces, climbing ladders, and handling farm machinery and gardening equipment. The patient was brought to the hospital emergency department with complaints of severe headache, dizziness, nausea and vomiting, and an inability to walk. For the last 2 months, he has had a chronic cough, occasional shortness of breath, generalized weakness, and joint pain. On physical examination, the patient was noted to have skin lesions on his nose and arms. Further medical work-up including blood tests and magnetic resonance imaging (MRI) of the brain and spinal cord indicated that the patient had coccidioidomycosis with resulting pneumonia, meningitis, and hydrocephalus. The MRI scan showed a dilated lower half of the fourth ventricle. Cystic lesions that were likely cocci granulomas were identified in the C1-C2, C6-C7, and T6-T7 spinal cord segments. Medical interventions included antifungal medications and ventriculo-peritoneal (VP) shunt placement. On the third day of hospitalization, the patient was referred to physical therapy to address limitations in functional mobility, transfers, and gait. Prior to the hospitalization, the patient lived at home with his wife. He was active in the community and had no history of drug or alcohol abuse. At the time of examination, there were no bowel/bladder changes, no headache, and no nausea or vomiting. Although the patient's primary language is Spanish, he speaks some English. When asked about his goals, the patient stated "I want to be able to walk again." His current medications include acetaminophen, bisacodyl suppository (Dulcolax), chlorhexidine, clotrimazole topical (Lotrimin), famotidine (Pepcid), heparin, voriconazole, fluconazole, and prednisone.

- ▶ Based on his health condition, what do you anticipate will be the contributors to activity limitations?
- ▶ What are the examination priorities?
- ▶ What are the most appropriate physical therapy outcome measures for gait and balance?
- ▶ What are possible complications interfering with physical therapy?

KEY DEFINITIONS

CEILING EFFECT: Psychometric property of an outcome measure in which the instrument is unable to detect a further increase in score for the highest-scoring individuals

PART-TO-WHOLE TASK PRACTICE: Method of structuring therapeutic interventions based on motor control and motor learning theories whereby a task is broken down into smaller components that the individual practices with gradual progression toward performing the whole task

VENTRICULOPERITONEAL (VP) SHUNT: Surgically placed drain that runs subcutaneously between the fourth ventricle and the abdominal cavity; used to treat hydrocephalus and increased intracranial pressure caused by excessive cerebrospinal fluid

Objectives

1. Describe the typical signs and symptoms of coccidioidomycosis affecting the central nervous system.
2. List pertinent tests and measures used in a physical therapy examination for a hospitalized patient with meningitis and hydrocephalus secondary to coccidioidomycosis.
3. Discuss appropriate physical therapy interventions for a person with movement dysfunctions secondary to coccidioidomycosis.

Physical Therapy Considerations

PT considerations during management of the individual with balance dysfunction, gait instability, and weakness due to coccidioidomycosis meningitis:

▶ **General physical therapy plan of care/goals:** Close monitoring of vital signs and upper motor neuron signs especially in the early stages of disease resolution; prevent deleterious effects of inactivity (skin breakdown, decreased joint mobility and strength); improve sitting and standing balance, functional mobility, transfers, and gait

▶ **Physical therapy interventions:** Sitting balance training, functional mobility training, gait training using appropriate assistive devices, therapeutic exercise to improve function

▶ **Precautions during physical therapy:** Increased intracranial pressure, changes in level of consciousness, increased fall risk

▶ **Complications interfering with physical therapy:** Worsening of vital signs; signs/symptoms of increased intracranial pressure; development of pressure sores; falls

Understanding the Health Condition

Coccidioidomycosis is also known as valley fever and is caused by inhalation of spores from *Coccidioides immitis*, a fungus that is present in the soil.[1,2] This condition is endemic to the western United States, with cases reported mainly in Arizona, California, Nevada, New Mexico, and Texas. The highest incidence of coccidioidomycosis in California has been reported in Kern county (155 new cases/100,000 individuals).[3,4] It has been reported that the majority of cases of coccidioidomycosis resolve spontaneously with no medical intervention needed. However, Filipinos and African Americans have an increased risk of severe disease and dissemination of the infection.[1,5] Coccidioidomycosis may affect the skin, lungs, central nervous system (*e.g.*, meninges), bones, and joints.[1] Meningitis can lead to hydrocephalus and may require VP shunt placement.[6] The signs and symptoms of coccidioidomycosis usually present within 1 to 3 weeks after exposure and persist for weeks to months. Signs and symptoms include fatigue, lower extremity swelling, fever, cough, night sweats, joint pain or stiffness, loss of appetite, weight loss, neck stiffness, altered mental state, headache, nausea, vomiting, and painful skin rash or lesion.[1,2] Diagnostic tests include sputum culture or smear, serological testing, imaging studies, bronchoscopy, biopsy (bone marrow and muscle), lumbar puncture, and skin testing.[2] Medical treatment includes **antifungal medications** (topical, oral, and/or intravenous) and/ or surgical debridement (for serious skin lesions).[1,5] There is no vaccination available against *Coccidioides immitis*.[7] Medical prognosis is variable and depends on many factors including severity of disease, degree of progression, timely and appropriate medical treatment, and anatomical region(s) or body system(s) affected. Often, initial acute coccidioidomycosis is mild, but individuals may take months or longer to completely recover. In a retrospective examination of the morbidity and mortality of disseminated coccidioidomycosis (the most serious form of the condition in which the infection spreads beyond the lungs to other parts of the body), researchers found that 15 of 91 patients hospitalized because of the infection died during that hospitalization.[8] In addition, the authors concluded that resolution of symptoms did not guarantee resolution of complications secondary to the original infection. Acute infection can become chronic and persistence of residual plaques (nodular skin lesions) from disseminated infection can persist for years following initial diagnosis and treatment.

Physical Therapy Patient/Client Management

There is no literature describing the physical rehabilitation of individuals with coccidioidomycosis. Patient presentation is variable, but when the infection affects the nervous system, individuals can present like those with other diagnoses involving neurological damage such as cerebrovascular accidents (CVA) or traumatic brain injury (TBI). Due to the presence of cocci spores in the spinal cord, the patient may also present with signs and symptoms consistent with spinal cord injury (SCI). Physical rehabilitation may be guided by medical/surgical procedures common in these patients, including neurosurgical procedures such as VP shunt insertion and craniotomies. Therefore, it is important to conduct a comprehensive neurologic examination to determine the extent of neurological involvement secondary to meningeal inflammation and to monitor the patient for complications after VP shunt placement. Due to the VP shunt placement, the patient's level of consciousness must be consistently reassessed during each patient encounter.

Examination, Evaluation, and Diagnosis

The examination should focus on the patient's functional abilities. This aids the physical therapist in the selection of appropriate interventions to optimize function and support the patient's goal of regaining his ability to ambulate. Once the therapist has identified what the patient is and is not able to do, the next step is to postulate the potential impairments causing his activity limitations. In the case of a patient with a possible upper motor neuron dysfunction, potential impairments causing activity limitations include muscle tone abnormalities, motor control deficits, decreased strength, and limitations in joint range of motion (ROM). The presence of brain swelling necessitates close monitoring of vital signs and symptoms indicative of increased intracranial pressure (increased headache, nausea, vomiting, decreased cognition, changes in pupillary responses). The therapist must periodically assess the patient's level of consciousness and cognitive status and report any signs of deterioration to the medical team immediately.

The patient required only minimum assistance to roll in bed; he was able to assist by using the bedrails. He required moderate assistance transferring from supine to sitting, with assistance provided at the trunk and pelvis and verbal cues provided for using his right arm to push into the mattress from the sidelying position. Once upright in sitting, he complained of a headache that subsided after several minutes. His vital signs were stable. The patient required maximum assistance for scooting to the edge of the bed, where he demonstrated poor static and dynamic sitting balance and required moderate assistance to support his head and trunk in sitting. In sitting, the patient demonstrated thoracic kyphosis, forward head, lateral head tilt to the left, cervical flexion, left trunk lean and bilateral scapular winging. During the examination, the patient was able to maintain 30 seconds of continuous upright and midline cervical posture with manual facilitation of cervical extensors. The patient required verbal cues such as "lean forward" or "sit up tall." Returning from sitting to supine, the patient required moderate assistance with his lower extremities and trunk. The patient assisted with crossing his right leg under his left leg. The therapist decided to defer examination of standing balance and gait due to the patient's poor endurance, low level of function, and safety issues.

It is important for the therapist to identify and implement an appropriate standardized functional measure to track patient progress and to document the effectiveness of physical therapy interventions. The goal, therefore, was to find an outcome measure that was appropriate for the patient's current physical condition and whose results would offer guidance for future physical therapy sessions. Sitting was the focus for choosing a standardized outcome measure because it is a functional task integral to the performance of activities of daily living and a variety of interventions can be performed in this position. Outcome measures that were considered included the Performance Oriented Mobility Assessment[9] (POMA; also referred to as Tinetti Balance Assessment Tool), Berg Balance Scale (BBS),[10] the Stroke Rehabilitation Assessment of Movement (STREAM),[11] the Trunk Impairment Scale (TIS),[12] and the **Function in Sitting Test (FIST)**.[13] The physical therapist decided that several of these outcome measures would not be appropriate at this time for this patient. The POMA has only one sitting balance item and would not have been appropriate for demonstrating functional progress in sitting because it is not sensitive enough to measure improvements in sitting.[14] Because many of the test items on the BBS are more advanced than what the patient could currently achieve (e.g., dynamic standing balance tasks), this outcome measure would not be a good indicator of the patient's progress, especially during his acute hospitalization.[15] The sitting items on the STREAM would have been reasonable for the patient to perform, but the patient's significant hypotonicity and muscle weakness in the left upper extremity would have limited his ability to complete some of the test items. Moreover, this outcome measure would only highlight impairments that were already determined through examination. The TIS would also not have been appropriate because it measures the quality of completing activities at a higher level than the patient was able to achieve at the time of initial examination. The starting position (sitting at the edge of the test surface without back or arm support) would not have been possible because the patient required upper extremity support and assistance in static sitting. Given these considerations regarding potential outcome measures, the therapist chose the FIST as the most appropriate tool for this patient. The FIST was developed by Gorman and colleagues in 2010.[13] It is a bedside test that takes approximately 8 to 10 minutes to complete and consists of 14 functional tasks in sitting. (Detailed instructions on implementation and scoring of the FIST can be found at http://www.samuelmerritt.edu/fist.) **Better sitting balance** is positively correlated with improved functional mobility outcomes and initial balance and disability can be a predictor of recovery after a CVA.[16] Specific functional sitting balance activities (e.g., supported sitting balance, static sitting balance, dynamic sitting balance)[17] are well correlated with reliable and valid balance outcome measures such as the Berg Balance Scale, Motor Assessment Scale,[18] and the Rivermead Mobility Index.[19] The current patient presented similarly to an individual after an acute stroke, which is the population in which the FIST has been validated. The FIST seemed to best match the patient's current activity tolerance and low level of functional mobility, would likely *not* present a ceiling effect, and focused on quantifying sitting ability—a critically important functional task and one with which the patient was not independent. On initial examination, the patient scored 13/56 on the FIST with major limitations identified in multiple test items (Table 6-1).

Following the examination of activities, the therapist performed several tests to determine if impairments were contributing to the patient's decreased functional performance. Passive ROM of the upper and lower extremities was within functional limits. Since the patient appeared to have selective motor control of the upper and lower extremities, manual muscle testing was performed to determine strength deficits. The right upper extremity and lower extremity were graded 4/5 (good), the left

	Item	Initial Exam	Week 2	Week 4 (discharge)
	Table 6-1 PATIENT'S FUNCTION IN SITTING TEST (FIST) RESULTS DURING INPATIENT EPISODE OF CARE			
1	Anterior nudge	1 (max)	4	4
2	Posterior nudge	1 (max)	4	4
3	Lateral nudge	1 (max)	4	4
4	Static sitting	1 (max)	4	4
5	Sitting, shake no	1 (max)	4	4
6	Sitting, eyes closed	1 (max)	4	4
7	Sitting, lift foot	1 (max)	4	4
8	Pick up object from behind	1 (max)	3	4
9	Forward reach	1 (max)	1 (mod)	2
10	Lateral reach	1 (max)	1 (min)	4
11	Pick up object from floor	1 (max)	3	4
12	Posterior scooting	0	4	4
13	Anterior scooting	1 (max)	4	4
14	Lateral scooting	1 (max)	4	4
	Total	13/56	48/56	54/56

0, dependent; 1, needs physical assistance; 2, requires use of upper extremities; 3, increased time/needs verbal cues; 4, normal; max, maximum physical assistance ($\geq$ 75%); mod, moderate physical assistance (26%–74%); min, minimal physical assistance ($\leq$ 25%).
Reproduced with permission from Gorman SL. Function in Sitting Test. Available at http://www.samuelmerritt.edu/fist/documentation. Retrieved April 10, 2013.

upper extremity was graded 2+/5 (poor +), and the left lower extremity was graded 2/5 (poor).

The therapist also assessed functional balance grades in sitting according to the protocol described by O'Sullivan and Schmidt.[20] The patient presented with poor (1/4) static sitting balance (*i.e.*, he required moderate to maximal assistance to maintain upright sitting position) and poor dynamic sitting balance (*i.e.*, he was unable to move without losing his balance). When the patient lost his balance in sitting, he tended to lean backward. Additional tests were performed specific to the patient's neuromuscular signs and symptoms. The patient had diminished sharp/dull discrimination sensation on the left upper and lower extremities with deficits more pronounced distally than proximally. He also had decreased proprioception in the left thumb, knee, ankle, and big toe; no deficits were noted in the right upper and lower extremities. Cranial nerve testing (CN II-XII) was performed, and noted to be intact.

Plan of Care and Interventions

The therapist identified important deficits that could be improved with physical therapy interventions: poor sitting posture, impaired sitting balance/postural control, weakness of the left upper and lower extremities, and decreased functional mobility.

The physical therapy diagnosis was limited bed mobility, decreased ability to transfer, and inability to ambulate due to global weakness (left side greater than right side), and poor balance consistent with coccidioidomycosis meningitis that prevented the patient from returning to independent living and participating in farm work.

The anticipated goals for the patient to achieve in 2 weeks included: (1) minimal assistance to transfer from sitting back and forth to supine; (2) good static and dynamic sitting balance; (3) strength of left upper extremity muscles 3+/5 and strength of lower extremity muscles 3/5; and (4) moderate assistance with safe transfers to/from bed to wheelchair or chair. At 4 weeks, the expected outcomes for the patient were: (1) independent with all bed mobility to minimize risk of skin breakdown; (2) independent with safe transfers to/from a level surface to wheelchair/chair to improve mobility; (3) independent with wheelchair set-up and positioning for transfers to better access hospital community; and (4) independent self-propulsion of wheelchair 200 ft for household locomotion. Because the patient was highly motivated to participate in physical therapy sessions, and he demonstrated no signs and symptoms of activity intolerance or complications during current physical therapy visits, the physical therapist determined that his prognosis to achieve the stated goals was good. On initial examination, he was able to complete 13 of the 14 items on the FIST. Thus, he had good potential for improved function in sitting in these areas, which may indicate good potential for improvements in other functional mobility tasks. The patient participated in physical therapy sessions twice per day, 5 d/wk for 4 weeks (40 sessions total).

Therapeutic exercises were prescribed to improve the patient's mobility and strength. Progressive resistance exercises were performed using manual resistance, Thera-Band, and weights. The patient was also given an exercise program to perform by himself to augment the exercises performed during the therapy sessions. Specific exercises included isometric quadriceps sets and short arc quads to improve quadriceps strength and single-leg bridging to improve gluteal and lower extremity strength. He was instructed to perform active assisted range of motion (AAROM) exercises using a cane to improve upper extremity mobility and strength in shoulder external rotation, abduction, and flexion.

Based on the patient's ability to accomplish some sitting tasks during the FIST, sitting balance activities were the initial focus of interventions. The therapist initially concentrated on static postural exercises in sitting to improve posture, balance, and upright tolerance. Exercises included chin tucks to activate cervical flexors and scapular pinches and neck and trunk extension exercises to improve upright endurance. Proprioceptive neuromuscular facilitation exercises were performed as appropriate to provide proprioceptive input to activate postural muscles and improve sitting posture and balance. While the patient was sitting with optimal postural alignment, the therapist provided approximation throughout the shoulders to increase proprioceptive input and encourage co-contraction of postural muscles. As the patient was able to perform these exercises with less tactile and verbal cueing from the therapist, dynamic sitting balance activities were introduced. Activities included sitting up straight, aligning to midline, weight shifting, and finally reaching outside his base of support. Improving his endurance to increase sitting tolerance was an interprofessional focus. The physical therapist worked with the occupational therapist and nursing staff to ensure that the patient was out of bed for short periods of time with supervision and assistance, including during meals, morning activities of daily living and hygiene, and when family visited. Initially, he required a high-back wheelchair to provide support in sitting, but as his sitting balance improved, the physical therapist progressed him to a standard wheelchair.

Bed mobility training included bridging/scooting up in bed and rolling to decrease the assistance he would require upon returning home. Practice was initially sequenced as part-task to whole-task because of the patient's decreased strength and endurance. The therapist assisted his performance as needed, and gradually decreased the assistance as the patient developed the strength and motor control to perform the activity. Transfer training was incorporated into the plan of care to allow the patient to get out of bed and improve mobility. The patient was taught how to scoot laterally, forward, and backward. Scooting was included because it was an area of weakness identified by the FIST and because it was necessary for self-repositioning. As the patient's performance improved, he was progressed to partial stands, and then finally to squat pivot transfers from bed to wheelchair or bed to regular chair. Eventually, the therapist increased the difficulty by having the patient transfer from different surfaces and seat heights.

Wheelchair training activities were performed to allow the patient a way to improve locomotion using a wheelchair. Initially, the patient was given a high-back wheelchair with elevating leg rests because he had poor trunk control and needed leg rests to assist with positioning his weak left lower extremity. He was instructed to use his right hand and leg to propel the chair. He was also taught wheelchair safety, such as locking and unlocking the wheelchair brakes. As his trunk mobility, balance, and strength improved, he was transitioned to a standard wheelchair.

The patient demonstrated improvement in all areas of function and was progressed to activities that involve standing and gait. The patient did not have goals pertaining to standing and gait during the initial examination, but his considerable improvement allowed him to progress to ambulation, and this goal was added to his plan of care. To start, standing balance and pre-gait activities were performed to increase weightbearing on the weaker left lower extremity. Next, a pre-gait sequence of lateral weight shifting was implemented, followed by single-leg stepping with the left side. Activities were also performed to facilitate weight acceptance on the left side as the patient took a full step with the right leg. All activities were progressed based on principles of motor learning to provide the appropriate amount of challenge.[21] During the patient's last week in the hospital, gait training was initiated. The patient was able to ambulate using a front-wheeled walker for 100 ft with minimum assistance of one person by the time he was discharged from the hospital.

At the time of hospital discharge, the patient demonstrated improvement in all areas of functional mobility, transfers, and wheelchair mobility. Table 6-1 shows the FIST results on initial examination, at week 2, and at week 4 (hospital discharge). Table 6-2 shows the patient's progress related to areas of functional mobility. Upon discharge from the hospital, the patient met all of his anticipated goals and expected outcomes. He was discharged to his home and continued his rehabilitation with home health physical therapy for 2 weeks, followed by outpatient physical therapy for another 4 weeks, where he demonstrated continued progress. At 4 months after initial admission to the hospital, the patient was able to return to work and had achieved full functional ability.

Table 6-2   PATIENT'S FUNCTIONAL MOBILITY TESTING DURING INPATIENT EPISODE OF CARE

Activity	Initial Exam	Week 2	Week 4 (discharge)
Rolling side-to-side	Min A	Min A	I
Sit to supine	Mod A	Min A	SBA
Supine to sit	Mod A	Min A	SBA
Scooting to the edge of bed	Max A	CGA	SBA
Squat pivot transfer to wheelchair	Mod A × 2	Min A	CGA
Sit to stand	Unable to attempt	Min A	CGA

Abbreviations: Min A, minimal physical assistance (≤ 25%) provided; Mod A, moderate physical assistance (50%) provided; Max, maximal assistance (≥ 75%) provided; × 2, two person assistance needed; CGA, contact guard assistance (hands on) provided for balance; SBA, stand-by assistance provided for safety; I, independent, no assistance needed[22]

Evidence-Based Clinical Recommendations

SORT: Strength of Recommendation Taxonomy

A: Consistent, good-quality patient-oriented evidence

B: Inconsistent or limited-quality patient-oriented evidence

C: Consensus, disease-oriented evidence, usual practice, expert opinion, or case series

1. Antifungal medications are the treatment of choice in patients with coccidioidomycosis. **Grade A**

2. The Function in Sitting Test (FIST) is an appropriate tool to assess sitting balance in individuals with coccidioidomycosis meningitis. **Grade C**

3. Improvements in sitting balance are positively correlated with improved functional mobility outcomes. **Grade B**

COMPREHENSION QUESTIONS

6.1 Which of the following patients may be *most* appropriate for examination using the Function in Sitting Test (FIST)?

   A. Patient is able to ambulate with assistive device and minimal physical assistance.

   B. Patient is able to stand on right lower extremity for 10 seconds and left lower extremity for 29 seconds.

   C. Patient can sit with upper extremity support at the edge of the bed for 20 seconds before requiring contact guard assistance.

   D. Patient is comatose.

6.2 The physical therapist is working with a patient who has difficulty with sit-to-stand transfers. The therapist decides to teach the patient the skill by breaking it down into smaller components, having the patient practice these components, then asking the patient to put the components together in one complete movement. This type of practice is called

A. Distributed practice

B. Part-to-whole task practice

C. Random practice

D. Massed practice

ANSWERS

6.1 **C.** The FIST is indicated for persons with sitting balance deficits who are not able to stand or ambulate (options A and B). Patients who are dependent with static sitting may be too low level for the FIST (option D).

6.2 **B.** Part-to-whole task practice was used in this example, as the patient practiced the component tasks first and then practiced the entire task.

REFERENCES

1. DiCuado DJ. Coccidioidomycosis: a review and update. *J Am Acad Dermatol.* 2006;55:929-942.

2. National Center for Emerging and Zoonotic Infectious Diseases. Coccidioidomycosis. http://www.cdc.gov/nczved/divisions/dfbmd/diseases/coccidioidomycosis/. Accessed February 15, 2012.

3. Centers for Infectious Diseases. Epidemiologic summary of coccidioidomycosis in California, 2001-2008. http://www.vfce.arizona.edu/resources/pdf/Epidemiologic_summary_of_Coccidipoidomycosis_in_California, 2001-2008.pdf. Updated November 5, 2011. Accessed January 30, 2012.

4. Centers for Disease Control and Prevention. Increase in coccidioidomycosis—California, 2000-2007. *MMWR Morb Mortal Wkly Rep.* Feb 13, 2009. http://www.cdc.gov/mmwr/preview/mmwrhtml/mm5805a1.htm#content_area. Accessed January 30, 2012.

5. Galgiani JN, Ampel NM, Blair JE, et al. Coccidioidomycosis. *Clin Infect Dis.* 2005;41:1217-1223.

6. Barnes NP, Jones SJ, Hayward RD, Harkness JW, Thompson D. Ventriculoperitoneal shunt block: what are the best predictive clinical indicators? *Arch Dis Child.* 2002;87:198-201.

7. Magee D, Cox R, eds. Vaccine development for coccidioidomycosis. In: Esser K, Bennett J. *The Mycota: A Comprehensive Treatise on Fungi as Experimental Systems for Basic Applied Research.* 12th ed. Berlin, Germany: Springer, 2004:243-257.

8. Adam RD, Elliot SP, Taljanovic MS. The spectrum and presentation of disseminated coccidioidomycosis. *Am J Med.* 2009;122:770-777.

9. Tinetti ME. Performance-oriented assessment of mobility problems in elderly patients. *J Am Geriatr Soc.* 1986;34:119-126.

10. Berg KO, Wood-Dauphinee SL, Williams JI, Maki B. Measuring balance in the elderly: validation of an instrument. *Can J Pub Health.* 1992;83:S7-S11.

11. Ashburn A. A physical assessment for stroke patients. *Physiotherapy.* 1982;68:109-113.

12. Verheyden G, Nieuwboer A, Mertin J, Preger R, Kiekens C, De Weerdt W. The Trunk Impairment Scale: a new tool to measure motor impairment of the trunk after stroke. *Clin Rehabil.* 2004;18:326-334.

13. Gorman SL, Radtka S, Melnick ME, Abrams GM, Byl NN. Development and validation of the Function in Sitting Test in adults with acute stroke. *J Neurol Phys Ther.* 2010;34:150-160.

14. Faber MJ, Bosscher RJ, van Wieringen PC. Clinimetric properties of the performance-oriented mobility assessment. *Phys Ther.* 2006;86:944-954.

15. Blum L, Korner-Bitensky N. Usefulness of the Berg Balance Scale in stroke rehabilitation: a systematic review. *Phys Ther.* 2008;88:559-566.

16. Tyson S, Hanley M, Chillala J, Selley AB, Tallis RC. The relationship between balance, disability, and recovery after stroke: predictive validity of the Brunel Balance Assessment. *Neurorehabil Neural Repair.* 2007;21:341-346.

17. Gorman SL. Function in Sitting Test. Samuel Merritt University. http://www.samuelmerritt.edu/fist. Accessed August 11, 2012.

18. Carr JH, Shepherd RB, Nordholm L, Lynne D. Investigation of a new motor assessment scale for stroke patients. *Phys Ther.* 1985;65:175-180.

19. Collen FM, Wade DT, Robb GF, Bradshaw CM. The Rivermead Mobility Index: a further development of the Rivermead Motor Assessment. *Int Disabil Stud.* 1991;13:50-54.

20. O'Sullivan S. Stroke. In: O'Sullivan S, Schmitz TJ, eds. *Physical Rehabilitation.* 5th ed. Philadelphia, PA: FA Davis; 2007:705-769.

21. VanSwearingen JM, Parera S, Brach JS, Wert D, Studentski SA. Impact of exercise to improve gait efficiency on activity and participation in older adults with mobility limitations: a randomized controlled trial. *Phys Ther.* 2011;91:1740-1751.

22. O'Sullivan S. Examination of functional status and activity level. In: O'Sullivan S, Schmitz TJ, eds. *Physical Rehabilitation.* 5th ed. Philadelphia, PA: FA Davis; 2007:373-400.

Concussion

Christopher Ivey

CASE 7

A 22-year-old male Division I football wide receiver was diagnosed with a concussion following a helmet-to-helmet hit during a game 2 days ago. Initially following the injury, the athlete exhibited disequilibrium as he slowly walked to the sidelines. The sideline examination was performed by the team physical therapist. The therapist's assessment of concussion-related symptoms, postural control, and neurocognitive function was consistent with a concussion injury. The athlete was not allowed to return to play in the game. During the postgame injury clinic, the team physician confirmed the diagnosis of a concussion.

▶ What are the most appropriate physical therapy goals?
▶ What precautions should be taken during the physical therapy examination and interventions?
▶ What are possible complications interfering with physical therapy?

KEY DEFINITIONS

CONCUSSION: Complex pathophysiological process affecting the brain, induced by traumatic biomechanical forces. Several common features include: (1) may be caused either by a direct blow to the head, face, neck, or elsewhere on the body with an "impulsive" force transmitted to the head; (2) typically results in rapid onset of short-lived impairment of neurologic function that resolves spontaneously; however, in some cases, symptoms and signs may evolve over a number of minutes to hours; (3) may result in neuropathological changes, but acute clinical symptoms largely reflect functional disturbance rather than structural injury and, as such, no abnormality is seen on standard structural neuroimaging studies; (4) results in graded set of clinical symptoms that may or may not involve loss of consciousness; resolution of the clinical and cognitive symptoms typically follows sequential course, however, it is important to note that in some cases symptoms may be prolonged.[1]

POST-CONCUSSIVE SYNDROME: Symptoms that occur following concussion; symptoms lasting ≥ 3 months following a concussion are classified as persistent post-concussive syndrome.[2]

SECOND IMPACT SYNDROME: Condition that occurs within minutes of a concussion in someone who is still experiencing symptoms from a prior brain injury, which may have occurred earlier during the same event. Vascular engorgement leads to a massive increase in intracranial pressure and brain herniation, which can result in severe brain damage or death.[2]

Objectives

1. Discuss appropriate components of the examination of the athlete with a potential concussion.
2. Describe potential complications during the early recovery period and over a longer period of time.
3. Identify reliable and valid outcome tools to measure an athlete's appropriateness for return to play.
4. Describe the phases of rehabilitation in concussion management.

Physical Therapy Considerations

PT considerations for management of the individual with a diagnosis of concussion:

▶ **General physical therapy goals:** Monitoring of the athlete for signs and symptoms that indicate any potential decline warranting further medical evaluation; rehabilitation progression based upon the individual athlete's symptom resolution

▶ **Physical therapy interventions:** Patient education regarding signs and symptoms of post-concussive syndrome; implementation of rehabilitation program beginning with physical and cognitive rest and progressing through aerobic exercise, resistance exercise, sport-specific exercise, noncontact training drills, full contact practice, and return to play

▶ **Precautions during physical therapy:** Recovery course is longer for younger athletes; advancement in the rehabilitation stage is not recommended in an individual with post-concussive symptoms

▶ **Complications interfering with physical therapy:** Persistent symptoms associated with post-concussive syndrome alter progression of the rehabilitation stages and may affect the return-to-play timeline

Understanding the Health Condition

It is estimated that 1.6 to 3.8 million people sustain a traumatic brain injury (TBI) during sports activities each year in the United States.[3] The majority of these injuries are categorized as mild traumatic brain injuries (mTBI). Many are classified as concussions. Children have the highest annual incidence, occurring in 692 of 100,000 American children younger than 15 years of age.[4] Epidemiological data are most likely conservative, given the large number of individuals who do not seek medical attention following this type of injury. With increasing numbers of sports participants and improved awareness of mTBI, the number of diagnosed concussions will likely increase.

Much of the research regarding the pathophysiology of concussion has been performed on animal models. After a concussion, a sudden release of the excitatory neurotransmitter glutamate occurs—resulting in a rapid loss of intracellular potassium and influx of calcium.[5,6] In order to restore the normal resting membrane potential of injured neurons, the sodium-potassium pump works overtime, which increases cerebral glucose metabolism.[5,6] Unfortunately, this increase in cerebral glucose metabolism occurs during a time of diminished cerebral blood flow, creating a cellular energy crisis.[5] Furthermore, the influx of calcium disrupts oxidative metabolism within injured neurons thereby inhibiting mitochondrial activity and increasing the mismatch of energy supply and demand.[6] This mismatch may increase vulnerability to a second insult during the recovery process—such as a second impact syndrome.[2] After the initial period of increased glucose metabolism, there is a much longer period of decreased aerobic metabolism of glucose in the injured neurons, which typically lasts 7 to 10 days.[7] In animal models, this neurometabolic cascade following a concussion represents a *functional* change in the nervous system rather than structural damage. Evidence from animal models is consistent with findings that x-rays or magnetic resonance imaging are of little value in diagnosing concussions.

Many signs and symptoms associated with a concussion are vague. Common concussion signs and symptoms are listed in Table 7-1.[8] The four categories include physical, cognitive, emotional, and sleep disturbances. An individual diagnosed with a concussion can experience symptoms in one or more of these categories. While loss of consciousness (LOC) can occur with this type of injury, less than 10% of diagnosed concussions are associated with LOC.[9]

Table 7-1 COMMON CONCUSSION SIGNS AND SYMPTOMS[8]			
Physical	Cognitive	Emotional	Sleep
Headache	Feeling mentally "foggy"	Irritability	Drowsiness
Nausea	Feeling slowed down	Sadness	Sleeping less than usual
Vomiting	Difficulty concentrating	More emotional	Sleeping more than usual
Balance problems	Difficulty remembering	Nervousness	Trouble falling asleep
Dizziness	Forgetful of recent information		
Visual problems	or conversations		
Fatigue	Confused about recent events		
Sensitivity to light	Answers questions slowly		
Sensitivity to noise	Repeats questions		
Numbness/tingling			
Dazed or stunned			

While concussion symptoms generally improve in a predictable pattern within 7 to 10 days, some individuals have persistent symptoms.[10] Symptoms that last 3 months or longer following a concussion are classified as persistent post-concussive syndrome.[2] These symptoms can be vague and nonspecific, which can make the diagnosis difficult. The World Health Organization established a definition of postconcussive syndrome as the presence of three or more of the following symptoms after a head injury: headache; dizziness; fatigue; irritability; difficulty with concentrating and performing mental tasks; impairment of memory; insomnia; and reduced tolerance to stress, alcohol, or emotional excitement.[11]

Returning to play while individuals are still symptomatic is not recommended. Athletes who have a history of concussion have an increased risk of having a second concussion.[9] Neurocognitive effects of repetitive concussions were initially recognized in boxers in a syndrome classified as dementia pugilistica (punch drunk syndrome). In addition, parkinsonism (pugilistic parkinsonism) can also be associated with this type of repetitive injury.[12] As evidence of the adverse neurocognitive effects of repetitive concussions accumulates, it has become apparent that cumulative effects of head injury are not specific to boxing. The term chronic traumatic encephalopathy (CTE) has become more widely used in sports including football and wrestling. The first autopsy report from a professional football player demonstrating the effects of CTE occurred in 2005.[13] CTE is a progressive neurodegenerative disease secondary to cumulative brain trauma. The initial signs and symptoms generally do not manifest until decades after the trauma, which is usually in the fifth or sixth decade of life. The incidence and prevalence of CTE is unknown[1] because the condition is diagnosed on autopsy by distinctive immunoreactive stains of the brain for tau protein. However, CTE is not the same disease as Alzheimer's disease.[2] The typical signs and symptoms of CTE include a decline in recent memory and executive function; mood and behavioral disturbances such as depression, aggressiveness, and suicidal behavior; and progression to dementia.[2] A small subset of individuals with CTE have developed chronic traumatic encephalomyopathy, a progressive motor neuron disease similar to amyotrophic lateral sclerosis characterized by profound weakness, atrophy, spasticity, and fasciculation.[2]

As many as 25 sets of criteria to grade concussions have been developed, and none have been validated.[14] The current recommendations advise abandoning management of concussion based on these grading scales.[10] Rather, return-to-play criteria should rely on symptoms as a guide rather than on a timeline based on grading.[15,16]

Physical Therapy Patient/Client Management

Concussion requires a multidisciplinary approach for effective management. The medical professional involved in the sideline assessment depends on who is present at the sporting event. Initial evaluation of the athlete may be performed by a physical therapist, athletic trainer, physician, or an emergency medical technician (EMT). Early recognition of concussion symptoms is imperative, and **the athlete should not return to play on the same day**.[2] When available, results from baseline neurocognitive and balance tests performed during the preparticipation examination should be compared to the results of those tests following the injury. The athlete should be examined by a physician to confirm the diagnosis, which generally occurs in the postgame injury clinic or during an office visit the following day. The initial treatment recommendations following the diagnosis of a concussion emphasize rest with a gradual, monitored return to activity. As the athlete progressively increases his activity, the physical therapist is often involved in order to monitor and safely progress his return to play. Once the athlete has completed the graduated return-to-play protocol, a physician who is trained in concussion management should be involved in the return-to-play decision.

Examination, Evaluation, and Diagnosis

The examination of the injured athlete may be performed by several healthcare providers including the athletic trainer, physician, or physical therapist and at several time points after the initial injury. The identification of a concussion is perhaps the most difficult component of the assessment because most athletes often do not inform medical personnel of concussion symptoms due to fear that they will be removed from the game or event.[17] While LOC is a readily identifiable sign of a possible concussion injury, less than 10% of athletes have an associated episode of LOC.[9] The immediate assessment of this patient is the primary survey, which can occur on the field of play. If an athlete is found to be unconscious, a cervical spine injury should be suspected with the appropriate precautions maintained. First, the level of consciousness must be determined. The Glasgow Coma Scale (GCS) can be used to assess the level of consciousness. If LOC occurs, the duration should be recorded.

The primary survey continues with an assessment of the athlete's airway, breathing, and circulation. Once the athlete regains consciousness, he can be taken to the sidelines for further evaluation provided that the probability of more severe injuries, such as injuries to the cervical spine, is low.[18] Balance problems or unsteadiness may be noted during transfer from the field of play to the sidelines. If the athlete does not regain consciousness, transportation to the nearest medical facility is necessary.

The initial sideline evaluation includes an assessment of the athlete's symptoms, a neurologic examination, and an evaluation of cognition. Several sideline assessment tools are available including: a graded system checklist, the Maddocks questions, the **Standardized Assessment of Concussion (SAC), the Balance Error Scoring System (BESS)**, and the Sport Concussion Assessment Tool 2 (SCAT2). The SCAT2 is an updated version of the original SCAT and it includes the majority of accepted sideline assessments in one comprehensive evaluation. The SCAT2 was designed to be administered by healthcare professionals. The SCAT2 contains sections for a graded system checklist, GCS, Maddocks Score, SAC, and BESS. Although the SCAT2 has not been validated, it contains a section to calculate the SAC, which has been validated in detecting mental status changes after a concussion injury among athletes.[19] The SCAT2 is available for free download.[20] Table 7-1 demonstrates the variability of signs and symptoms that can occur with a concussion. The graded system checklist allows the examiner to track symptoms over time. The athlete should complete the graded system checklist at the initial evaluation and at each follow-up assessment until all signs and symptoms have cleared at rest and during physical exertion.[21] The symptoms are scored on a scale of 0 to 6, where 0 = not present, 1 = mild, 3 = moderate, and 6 = most severe.

The examiner must be aware that the standard orientation questions such as time, place, and person have been shown to be *unreliable* in assessing for concussion in athletes during sport when compared to a more complete memory assessment.[22] For that reason, brief neuropsychological tests such as the Maddocks questions and the SAC can be utilized as practical and effective evaluation tools.[23] The Maddocks questions are a qualitative measure used to evaluate orientation as well as short- and long-term memory related to the sport and current game.[22] An athlete's inability to answer Maddocks questions correctly should raise suspicion for the presence of a concussive injury. For the current case patient, a particularly relevant Maddocks question is "what venue are we at today?" The SAC is a brief screening tool used to assess neurocognition. The SAC does not require training in psychometric testing to administer or interpret.[24] The SAC requires approximately 5 minutes to perform; orientation, immediate memory, concentration, and delayed recall are measured.[25] Multiple variations of the SAC are used, which results in little to no practice effect.[19] In other words, the use of multiple variations prevents the athlete from memorizing the answers to the SAC in advance or with repeated testing. The results of the sideline assessment can be compared to those from a baseline assessment that was performed earlier in the season or preseason. Any decrease from the baseline score on the SAC was found to be 95% sensitive and 76% specific for a concussion.[26]

Balance disruption is common with concussion. The BESS is an assessment of postural stability that is easy to administer, inexpensive, and requires approximately 5 to 7 minutes to complete.[26] It was developed to provide healthcare professionals with an inexpensive and objective way to assess postural stability outside the laboratory.[27] Much like the SAC, the results of the BESS test can be compared to a baseline assessment. Three stances (narrow double-leg stance, single-leg stance, and tandem stance) and two footing surfaces (firm surface/floor and medium density foam) are used to perform the test. Each stance is held, with hands on hips and eyes closed, for 20 seconds. Point deductions are given for specific errors including opening eyes, lifting hands off hips, stepping, stumbling, falling, moving stance hip into more than 30° of flexion or abduction, lifting forefoot or heel, or remaining out of the testing position for more than 5 seconds.[28] There is a maximum score of 60 points if both floor surfaces are used, or 30 points if only one surface is used. It is important to note that the BESS seems to have a practice effect resulting in improved scores from repeatedly performing the same test.[29] In addition, the BESS can be influenced by fatigue.[27] The BESS has been validated against the Sensory Organization Test in the concussion population.[28] The intra-tester and inter-tester reliability for the BESS ranges from 0.6 to 0.92 and 0.57 to 0.85, respectively. The test-retest reliability is moderate.[30] The specificity of the BESS ranges from 91% to 96% on days 1 to 7 following a concussion injury; however, the sensitivity of the BESS is poor—34% being the highest value at the time of injury.[30] Thus, the BESS would not be a good tool to rule *out* a concussion. Athletes experiencing impaired postural stability following concussion typically return to their baseline BESS scores within 3 to 5 days following injury.[31] The SCAT2 utilizes a modified BESS that is performed on one surface (which should match the surface of the baseline test). At present, no reported reliability, sensitivity, or specificity studies are available for the modified BESS.

Neuropsychological (NP) testing in athletes began in the 1980s as a tool to identify cognitive impairment and assist in documenting recovery from a concussive injury.[28] With the availability of computerized neuropsychological (CNP) testing, the use of NP testing has expanded. Several CNP testing programs are currently utilized, including: ANAM (Automated Neuropsychological Assessment Metrics), CogState, HeadMinder, and ImPACT. The athlete can take a CNP test that is monitored by a medical professional such as a physical therapist, athletic trainer, or physician who is familiar with the software.[32] In addition, the athlete can take a paper and pencil NP test administered by a neuropsychologist. Cognitive impairments may last longer than subjective symptoms, and while NP testing has not been validated as a diagnostic tool for concussion, it has the ability to identify cognitive impairments in the otherwise asymptomatic athlete.[30,33] Interpretation of the tests should be performed by a neuropsychologist or a physician who is experienced with the test and concussion management. Additional research is needed to create evidenced-based guidelines or validated protocols concerning when to administer CNP following a concussion.

Plan of Care and Interventions

The immediate treatment of the post-concussive patient population should emphasize education to the athlete as well as to the coach, parents, spouse, and/or caregivers. Education includes signs and symptoms that should be monitored that indicate any potential decline warranting further medical evaluation. The typical recovery process should also be discussed. When individuals who had sustained a concussion injury were provided education about concussion injury and treatment, they experienced fewer sleep disturbances and less anxiety and psychological stress compared to those that did not receive the education.[34]

Current guidelines recommend physical and cognitive rest for the treatment of concussion.[35] As previously mentioned, an earlier return to sport could have serious adverse effects such as second impact syndrome.[2] Physical rest includes removal from the competitive sport as well as other aerobic activities and resistance training. The athlete should avoid these activities until symptoms are no longer present when he is at rest. This rest period is followed by a gradual increase in physical activity. If symptoms occur during the gradual increase in physical activity, the athlete should return to the previous level at which he was symptom-free. Cognitive rest is achieved by minimizing activities that require concentration and attention, including reading, schoolwork, video games, text messaging, and working online.[35] Academic accommodations should be considered during the recovery process of student athletes. These accommodations facilitate cognitive rest and may preserve the patient's grades, which are likely to be affected during the recovery process.

Guidelines for returning to play should also follow a gradual progression. Table 7-2 presents the gradual progression of activity that is supported by the American Medical Society for Sports Medicine and the National Athletic Trainers Association.[26,36] The rehabilitation protocol takes approximately 1 week and each rehabilitation stage should take approximately 24 hours.[2] The recovery course is longer for younger athletes than for collegiate and professional athletes and warrants a more conservative approach.[37] If symptoms occur with advancement in the rehabilitation stage, the athlete should return to the previous asymptomatic stage. Progression to the next stage is attempted after the next 24-hour rest has occurred.

Table 7-2 GRADUATED RETURN TO PLAY PROTOCOL[26,36]		
Rehabilitation Stage	Functional Exercise at Each Stage of Rehabilitation	Objective of Each Stage
1. No activity	Complete physical and cognitive rest	Recovery
2. Light aerobic exercise	Walking, swimming, or stationary cycling–keeping intensity at 70% of age-predicted maximum heart rate No resistance training	Increase heart rate
3. Sport-specific exercise	Skating drills in ice hockey, running drills in soccer. No head impact activities	Add movement
4. Noncontact training drills	Progression to more complex training drills (e.g., passing drills in football and ice hockey) May start progressive resistance training	Exercise, coordination, and cognitive load
5. Full contact practice	Following medical clearance participate in normal training activities	Restore confidence and assess functional skills by coaching staff
6. Return to play	Normal game play	

Evidence-Based Clinical Recommendations

SORT: Strength of Recommendation Taxonomy

A: Consistent, good-quality patient-oriented evidence

B: Inconsistent or limited-quality patient-oriented evidence

C: Consensus, disease-oriented evidence, usual practice, expert opinion, or case series

1. Athletes diagnosed with a concussion should not return to play on the same day. **Grade C**

2. Athletes' performance on sideline tests such as the Standardized Assessment of Concussion (SAC) and the Balance Error Scoring System (BESS) should be compared to their performance on preinjury baseline tests. **Grade C**

3. To decrease the likelihood of serious adverse effects such as second impact syndrome, an athlete should not engage in physical or cognitive activities that increase symptoms during the early stages of concussion recovery. **Grade B**

4. Returning to play after a concussion should be individualized, gradual, and progressive. **Grade C**

COMPREHENSION QUESTIONS

7.1 The sideline assessment for concussion should include which of the following tests?

    A. Standard orientation questions such as time, place, and person

    B. Computerized neuropsychological testing

    C. Maddocks questions

    D. Sensory Organization Test

7.2 A physical therapist is working with an athlete who sustained a concussion injury 4 days ago. As the athlete progressed to stage 3 of the graduated return-to-play protocol, she reported the onset of a headache. Given this situation, what recommendations should the physical therapist make to this athlete?

    A. Continue the current treatment with a reassessment of symptoms the following day

    B. Have the athlete stop stage 3 and continue with stage 2

    C. Progress the athlete to stage 4

    D. Have the athlete stop stage 3 and continue with stage 1

ANSWERS

7.1 **C.** Maddocks questions are a qualitative measure used to evaluate orientation as well as short- and long-term memory related to the sport and the current game. Standard orientation questions such as time, place, and person are unreliable in assessing concussion in athletes during sport (option A). Computerized neuropsychological testing and the Sensory Organization Test are not practical assessments for the sideline examination (options B and D). The SAC and BESS tests should also be considered as sideline assessments.

7.2 **B.** If symptoms occur with advancement to the next rehabilitation stage, the athlete should return to the previous asymptomatic stage. Progression to the next stage is attempted after the next 24-hour rest has occurred.

REFERENCES

1. McCrory P, Meeuwisse WH, Aubry M, et al. Br J Sports Med 2013;47:250-258.

2. Herring SA, Cantu RC, Guskiewicz KM, et al. Concussion (mild traumatic brain injury) and the team physician: a consensus statement—2011 update. Med Sci Sports Exerc. 2011;43:2412-2422.

3. Langlois JA, Rutland-Brown W, Wald MM. The epidemiology and impact of traumatic brain injury: a brief overview. J Head Trauma Rehabil. 2006;21:375-378.

4. Guerrero JL, Thurman DJ, Sniezek JE. Emergency department visits associated with traumatic brain injury: United States, 1995–1996. Brain Inj. 2000;14:181-186.

5. Giza CC, Hovda DA. The neurometabolic cascade of concussion. J Athl Train. 2001;36:228-235.

6. DeLellis SM, Kane S, Katz K. The neurometabolic cascade and implications of mTBI: mitigating risk to the SOF community. J Spec Oper Med. 2009;9:36-42.

7. Giza CC, DiFiori JP. Pathophysiology of sports-related concussion: an update on basic science and translational research. Sports Health. 2011;3:46-51.

8. US Department of Health and Human Services, Centers for Disease Control and Prevention. Heads Up: Facts for Physicians About Mild Traumatic Brain Injury (MTBI). www.cdc.gov/NCIPC/pub-res/tbi_toolkit/physicians/mtbi/mtbi.pdf. Accessed November 15, 2012.

9. Guskiewicz KM, McCrea M, Marshall SW, et al. Cumulative effects associated with recurrent concussion in collegiate football players: the NCAA concussion study. JAMA. 2003;290:2549-2555.

10. Brooks D, Hunt B. Current concepts in concussion diagnosis and management in sports: a clinical review. BCMJ. Nov 2006;48(9):453-459.

11. The ICD-10 Classification of Mental and Behavioural Disorders Diagnostic criteria for research. www.who.int/classifications/icd/en/GRNBOOK.pdf. Accessed February 5, 2013.

12. DeKosky ST, Ikonomovic MD, Gandy S. Traumatic brain injury—football, warfare, and long-term effects. N Engl J Med. 2010;363:1293-1296.

13. Omalu BI, DeKosky ST, Minster RL, et al. Chronic traumatic encephalopathy in a National Football League player. Neurosurgery. 2005;57:128-134.

14. McCrory P. The eighth wonder of the world: the mythology of concussion management. Br J Sports Med. 1999;33:136-137.

15. Aubry M, Cantu R, Dvorak J, et al. Summary and agreement statement of the 1st International Symposium on Concussion in Sport, Vienna 2001. Clin J Sport Med. 2002;12:6-11.

16. McCrory P, Johnston K, Meeuwisse W, et al. Summary and agreement statement of the 2nd international conference on Concussion in Sport, Prague 2004. Clin J Sport Med. 2005;15:48-55.

17. McCrea M, Hammeke T, Olsen G, Leo P, Guskiewicz K. Unreported concussion in high school football players: implications for prevention. *Clin J SportMed*. 2004;14:13-17.

18. Broglio SP, Guskiewicz KM. Concussion in sports: the sideline assessment. *Sports Health*. 2009:1: 361-369.

19. McCrea M, Kelly JP, Randolph C, Cisler R, Berger L. Immediate neurocognitive effects of concussion. *Neurosurgery*. 2002;50:1032-1042.

20. SCAT2 Sport Concussion Assessment Tool 2. www.cces.ca/files/pdfs/SCAT2[1].pdf. Accessed January 30, 2013.

21. Guskiewicz KM, Bruce SL, Cantu RC, et al. National Athletic Trainers' Association position statement: management of sport-related concussion. *J Athl Train*. 2004;39:280-297.

22. Maddocks DL, Dicker GD, Saling MM. The assessment of orientation following concussion in athletes. *Clin J Sport Med*. 1995;5:32-35.

23. McCrory P, Meeuwisse W, Johnston K, et al. Consensus Statement on Concussion in Sport: the 3rd International Conference on Concussion in Sport held in Zurich, November 2008. *Br J Sports Med*. 2009;43(suppl 1):i76-i90.

24. McCrea M, Kelly JP, Randolph C. *Standardized Assessment of Concussion (SAC): Manual for Administration, Scoring and Interpretation*. 3rd ed. Waukesha, WI: Comprehensive Neuropsychological Services; 2000.

25. McCrea M. Standardized mental status testing on the sideline after sport-related concussion. *J Athl Train*. 2001;36:274-279.

26. Harmon KG, Drenzer JA, Gammons M, et al. American Medical Society for Sports Medicine position statement: concussion in sport. *Br J Sports Med*. 2013;47:15-26.

27. Wilkins JC, Valovich McLeod TC, Perrin DH, Gansneder BM. Performance on the Balance Error Scoring System decreases after fatigue. *J Athl Train*. 2004;39:156-161.

28. Guskiewicz KM, Ross SE, Marshall SW. Postural stability and neuropsychological deficits after concussion in collegiate athletes. *J Athl Train*. 2001;36:263-273.

29. Valovich TC, Perrin DH, Gansneder BM. Repeat administration elicits a practice effect with the Balance Error Scoring System but not with the Standardized Assessment of Concussion in high school athletes. *J Athl Train*. 2003;38:51-56.

30. McCrea M, Barr WB, Guskiewicz K, et al. Standard regression-based methods for measuring recovery after sport-related concussion. *J Int Neuropsychol Soc*. 2005;11:58-69.

31. Bell DR, Guskiewicz KM, Clark MA, Padua DA. Systematic review of the balance error scoring system. *Sports Health*. 2011;3:287-295.

32. Overview and Features of the ImPACT Test. http://www.impacttest.com/about/background. Accessed January 30, 2013.

33. Makdissi M, Darby D, Maruff P, et al. Natural history of concussion in sport: markers of severity and implications for management. *Am J Sports Med*. 2010;38:464-471.

34. Ponsford J, Willmott C, Rothwell A, et al. Impact of early intervention on outcome following mild head injury in adults. *J Neurol Neurosurg Psychiatry*. 2002;73:330-332.

35. Meehan WP 3rd. Medical therapies for concussion. *Clin Sports Med*. 2011;30:115-124.

36. McCrory P, Meeuwisee W, Johnston K, et al. Consensus statement on concussion in sport: the 3rd international Conference on Concussion in Sport held in Zurich, November 2008. *J Athl Train*. 2009;44:434-448.

37. Halstead ME, Walter KD. The Council on Sports Medicine and Fitness. American Academy of Pediatrics. Clinical report—sport-related concussion in children and adolescents. *Pediatrics*. 2010;126:597-615.

Conversion Disorder

Rolando T. Lazaro
Sharon L. Gorman
Anthony R. Novello
Gail L. Widener

CASE 8

The patient is a 25-year-old female who presented to the emergency department with chest pain, back pain, and a headache. She was admitted to the hospital for medical management and continued work-up. She then developed left-sided numbness and tingling and blurry vision in both eyes. Two hours after admission, her symptoms progressed and she reported an inability to move her left lower extremity and complete blindness. Given her admission presentation and presumptive medical diagnosis of "rule out stroke," the neurologist ordered a physical therapy evaluation. In the subsequent 2 days, the patient underwent diagnostic imaging of the brain and spinal cord and had many laboratory panels performed; all were negative for neurologic pathology. Her primary care physician and neurologist concluded that they could not find any organic cause of the patient's current complaints, and a psychiatric consult was requested. The psychiatric evaluation revealed a past history of physical abuse by her father, although the patient stated that her home life had improved. At this time, the medical team considered the possibility that the patient may have conversion disorder. The patient lives in a single-story home with her mother. Prior to hospitalization, she was a student in a nearby community college and also worked as a grocery clerk. She enjoys dancing in her spare time and stated that she would like to get stronger so she could go back to school and work.

► What are the examination priorities?
► What are the most appropriate physical therapy outcome measures for gait and balance?
► What are possible complications interfering with physical therapy?
► What is her rehabilitation prognosis?

KEY DEFINITIONS

ASTASIA-ABASIA: Unstable, abnormal manner of standing and walking in which a person demonstrates dramatic and unusual sways while attempting to walk; the person tends to recover his/her balance at the last moment, or fall when a family member or a soft object is nearby[1]

COLLABORATIVE MODEL: Approach to therapeutic goal setting that allows the patient (and potentially family and/or significant others) to work with the therapist to determine anticipated goals and expected outcomes; agreement of goals by therapist and patient is required, and not assumed; model differs from the team approach in which collaboration is usually limited to members of the interprofessional team (*e.g.*, physiatrist, therapies, nursing, social work)

KNOWLEDGE OF RESULTS: Type of feedback given after a skill is performed; information about the *outcome* of the performance of a skill is given, rather than about the specific movements or quality of movements comprising the skill

TASK-ORIENTED APPROACH: Therapeutic, functional approach to retraining movement in which practice is task-specific and context-specific with an overall goal of functional independence; derived from concepts of motor control, motor learning, dynamical systems theory, and neuroplasticity

Objectives

1. Describe the common clinical features of conversion disorder.
2. List pertinent impairment, activity, and participation level tests and measures for a patient with the diagnosis of conversion disorder.
3. Discuss appropriate physical therapy interventions for a person with the diagnosis of conversion disorder.

Physical Therapy Considerations

PT considerations during management of the individual with gait instability, weakness, blindness, and balance dysfunction due to conversion disorder:

▶ **General physical therapy plan of care/goals:** Improve activity and participation through functional mobility and gait training activities; coordinate care with other members of the interprofessional healthcare team

▶ **Physical therapy interventions:** Functional mobility training; gait training and stair training with appropriate assistive devices; task-oriented approach to intervention addressing issues of decreased motor control

▶ **Precautions during physical therapy:** Appropriate guarding during physical therapy interventions to minimize risk of falls; maintenance of rapport and trust during interactions with patient and family

▶ **Complications interfering with physical therapy:** Adherence to psychiatric plan of care regarding nonconfrontation pertaining to the physical manifestations of conversion disorder

Understanding the Health Condition

The Diagnostic and Statistical Manual for Mental Disorders, 4th edition, Text Revision (DSM-IV-TR) describes conversion disorder as a condition in which an individual experiences decreased motor or sensory function voluntarily, with associated psychological factors.[2] The symptoms are not intentionally produced, are not limited to pain, cannot be caused by a general diagnosable medical condition, and must cause a clinically significant impact in social and occupational functioning. Impairments in persons with conversion disorder are not produced by physiological problems at the cell or tissue level. Rather, observed impairments are considered an extension of the individual's psychological state and are presented without his/her purposeful or conscious control. This is in contrast to individuals who are malingering, as individuals who malinger are consciously presenting with impairments, usually for some type of external gain (*e.g.*, financial, attention).[2] A person with conversion disorder truly believes he/she has impairments. Common clinical symptoms include muscular weakness or paralysis, sensory impairments that do not follow any anatomical patterns, loss of vision or hearing, spastic-like features or dystonic-like posturing, pain, and aphonia. Patients with conversion disorder may also demonstrate astasia-abasia, which is a form of unsteady gait that resembles ataxia and is characterized by bizarre incoordination while walking or standing still.[1] Individuals who demonstrate astasia-abasia may stagger or sway acrobatically while walking, but rarely fall or injure themselves during a fall because this presentation tends to occur when they are near soft objects or persons who can assist them with their balance.

A core feature of conversion disorder is the *absence* of a neurologic or organic basis that may explain the presenting signs and symptoms. It is thought of as an unconscious expression of a psychological conflict or need, reinforced by avoiding underlying emotional stress. The disorder was previously termed hysterical neurosis, conversion type, before the American Psychiatric Association (APA) changed the term to conversion disorder in 1980.[3] In the United States, the annual incidence of conversion disorder is 22 cases per 100,000 people.[2] Prevalence has been reported as 1% to 14% of general medical/surgical inpatients.[4,5] Risk factors include female sex (2:1 compared to males), history of physical and sexual abuse with the patient having difficulty expressing the distress caused by said abuse, economically disadvantaged background, and underlying psychological discord (frequently depression or anxiety).[6,7] In terms of prognosis, current literature reports that 60% of those diagnosed with conversion disorder recover within 2 weeks, while 98% recover within a year.[8,9]

Physical Therapy Patient/Client Management

There are a few case reports that have been published regarding physical therapy management of individuals with conversion disorder.[7,8,10] The following are major recommendations based on these published cases and other resources addressing interventions for persons with conversion disorder.[4-14] First, the physical therapist must immediately establish trust and rapport with the patient and family, primarily to establish a supportive environment that is focused on the achievement of optimum levels of patient activity and participation. From the physical therapist's perspective, it is best to **avoid confrontation with the patient regarding the psychi-atric nature of her presenting signs and symptoms**. It is important to address the physical manifestations of the condition, including any impairments manifested, but not through confrontation about the psychological nature of the impairments. Telling a patient with conversion disorder that her symptoms are "all in her head" or that she does not have anything wrong with her and should move a paralyzed limb is counterproductive to overall recovery. The patient's ability to perform functional movement must be emphasized, including the use of positive feedback for success. While working with the patient, the therapist must withdraw all attention to the ill-ness symptoms. For example, the therapist should not directly address this patient's complaints of weakness but rather focus on the patient's ability to use what strength she does have to perform a task such as rolling in bed. This **emphasis on knowledge of results** also encourages the therapist to provide feedback related to how much of the task the patient was able to perform. For this patient, the therapist consistently validated the patient's attempts at functional movement and provided positive feed-back regarding how much of the task the patient could complete, such as "Great job rolling to the right. You were able to get all the way to the right side, and needed less help than the last attempt." The therapist must also establish clear and collaborative goals. Last, the patient must be **weaned off of assistive and/or supportive devices as soon as safely possible**.[8] Use of an assistive device by the individual with conversion disorder, especially in the longer term, is not appropriate due to the lack of physi-ological need for the device. A person with conversion disorder does not have physiological impairments (*e.g.*, decreased strength, decreased range of motion, impaired balance, impaired coordination, etc.) derived from a medical condition; rather, she has a physiologic or psychiatric manifestation of paralysis or sensory loss resulting in impaired ambulation ability. In this case, the patient's blindness and hemiparesis are the physical manifestation of her psychiatric conflict, most likely related to her history of sexual abuse by a family member. Allowing the patient to develop a psychological need or reliance on an assistive device is counterproductive to the ultimate goal of the patient regaining her prior level of function and asserting more control over her life and circumstances. Long-term use of assistive devices may become a true "crutch" impeding the patient's psychological healing. Psychologi-cal healing is accompanied by improved function and decreased manifestations of aphysiologic impairments.

Examination, Evaluation, and Diagnosis

A thorough chart review is important to obtain information regarding the inter-professional medical management of this patient. In this case, referrals were also made to a neurologist, psychiatrist, and occupational therapist. The discharge plan played a major role in coordinating the patient's care because many disciplines were involved during the patient's hospitalization.

Next, it would be appropriate to examine the patient's functional performance in bed mobility, transfers, and ambulation. The patient required supervision with bed mobility, moderate assistance with sit-to-stand transfers, and maximum assistance of two persons with ambulation on level surfaces. The two-person assistance during gait was thought to be more appropriate and safe and would model interventions to be carried out after the examination. The patient exhibited gait characteristics consistent with astasia-abasia, which when considered with her blindness, also explained her need for two-person assistance.

Impairment testing should follow the functional performance examination. In persons with conversion disorder, it is important to screen multiple systems to guide specific impairment-level testing, since the diagnosis itself does not provide much information about possible impairment-level manifestations or presentations. Range of motion and strength testing provide baseline information, which could serve as a springboard for goals and plan of care. This patient demonstrated full passive range of motion in all major joints bilaterally. On manual muscle testing,[15] the patient had normal (5/5) strength in both upper extremities and the right lower extremity. The left hip flexors and knee flexors were graded as trace (1/5) and left knee extensors and dorsiflexors were graded as zero (0/5). Sensory discrimination was normal to light touch and superficial pain (tested using pinprick) for both upper extremities and the right lower extremity, and absent in the left lower extremity. Because of the impact of balance on safety, balance should be thoroughly assessed to allow the therapist to collaborate with the patient on appropriate goals and to devise a plan of care that will be safe for the patient. This patient demonstrated fair dynamic sitting balance (tolerated minimal challenge; maintained balance while turning her head and her trunk) and poor dynamic standing balance (unable to accept challenge or move without loss of balance).[16] Following the examination, the patient's physical therapy diagnosis indicated she presented with limitations to functional mobility and ambulation. Impairments in strength and static/dynamic balance, as well as sensory impairments may contribute to her functional problems due to a medical diagnosis of conversion disorder.

Plan of Care and Interventions

After the examination and evaluation, goals were established that guided the interventions. The patient and her mother were involved in setting goals using a collaborative model. It was agreed that the physical therapy interventions would be focused on achieving independence in bed mobility and transfers and ambulation with only handheld assistance by hospital discharge. Accomplishment of these goals would allow safe discharge of the patient back home with her mother.

Interventions were focused on function using primarily a task-oriented approach. The patient was encouraged to get up out of bed with as little assistance from the therapist as possible, often with the therapist stating the importance of this function in achieving the patient's goal of being able to get out of bed by herself. The focus of the feedback was on the patient's performance of the task, not on what she did that was "wrong." This knowledge of results feedback was also employed with the sit-to-stand transfer training. The therapist emphasized telling the patient that she completed the motion successfully with less assistance, and not that the motion was "jerky."

Ambulation was started in the parallel bars with the goal of getting the patient to feel secure with taking initial steps, but was quickly progressed from the parallel bars to a front-wheeled walker, then to a single point cane. The therapist consistently reminded the patient to focus on her goal of having only handheld assistance by discharge, especially during the phases of the intervention when an assistive device was being used.

During the entire inpatient episode of care, a consistent collaborative approach was emphasized, often focusing on the mutually agreed upon goals and plan of care. Each session was started with an overview of the interventions planned for that session and how these related to the expected outcomes by discharge. The therapist also made sure to include trusted family members during the entire care process.

The patient was in the hospital for 5 days. At discharge, she required supervision in bed mobility, supervision in transfers, and ambulated 80 ft with a single point cane with minimum assistance of one person. She was discharged home and continued her physical therapy as an outpatient.

Evidence-Based Clinical Recommendations

SORT: Strength of Recommendation Taxonomy

A: Consistent, good-quality patient-oriented evidence

B: Inconsistent or limited-quality patient-oriented evidence

C: Consensus, disease-oriented evidence, usual practice, expert opinion, or case series

1. Confronting an individual regarding the psychiatric link to his/her physical manifestations of conversion disorder is not recommended during physical therapy examination and interventions. **Grade B**

2. Task-oriented approach to intervention planning is feasible and recommended for persons with conversion disorder because it encourages collaborative goal setting and more emphasis on results and function during therapy. **Grade C**

3. When providing interventions for a person with conversion disorder, the use of assistive devices for gait should be discontinued as soon as possible. **Grade C**

COMPREHENSION QUESTIONS

8.1 Which of the following is the *most* appropriate intervention strategy when providing physical therapy to a person with conversion disorder?

    A. Emphasize that there is no medical reason for the patient's signs and symptoms.

    B. When providing feedback, emphasize knowledge of results rather than knowledge of performance.

    C. Encourage use of assistive and supportive devices to facilitate functional recovery.

    D. Emphasize the presence of illness symptoms when talking to the patient as a way to motivate the patient to improve performance.

8.2 The use of the sit-to-stand practice as a method of strengthening the lower extremities is an example of what type of intervention?

A. Knowledge of performance

B. Results-based

C. Task-oriented

D. Impairment-based

8.3 The recommended approach for therapeutic goal setting for persons with conversion disorder involves a focus on clearly defined goals that are constantly reinforced using which of the following methods?

A. Collaboration with patient and family

B. Interprofessional team consensus

C. Therapist's experience and professional judgment

D. Derived from psychiatric assessment

ANSWERS

8.1 **B.** The therapist should provide feedback regarding the *outcome* of the particular skill being practiced, rather than the performance or quality of each component of the skill. It is not productive to emphasize the symptoms of the illness (option D) or the lack of organic reason for these signs and symptoms to the patient (option A). While assistive devices can be used to facilitate safe functional mobility, it is recommended that patients be weaned off of assistive and/or supportive devices as soon as safely possible (option C).

8.2 **C.** Using a functional task that is specific, both in regards to the task and the context is the hallmark of the task-oriented approach. While the intervention may be *aimed* at addressing impairments, functional movements are emphasized in the task-oriented approach (option D). Knowledge of performance is a method of giving patient feedback (option A).

8.3 **A.** The collaborative model of goal setting is recommended as a primary way of giving the patient a voice in her recovery and to begin allowing her to assume some degree of control in the therapeutic plan. While the interprofessional team's input can be valuable, it is not the primary method to approach goal setting for a person with conversion disorder (option B). While the judgment of the therapist and psychiatrist must be considered (options C and D), ensuring the involvement of the patient (and potentially trusted family members) is recommended.

REFERENCES

1. Kim HJ, Lee JY, Beom GS. Episodic astasia-abasia associated with hyperperfusion in the subthalamic region and dorsal brainstem. *Neurology Asia.* 2010;15:279-281.

2. American Psychiatric Association. *Diagnostic and Statistical Manual of Mental Disorders.* 4th ed, text revision (DSM IV-TR).Washington, DC: American Psychiatric Association; 2000.

3. Owens C, Dein S. Conversion disorder: the modern hysteria. *Adv Psychiatric Treatment.* 2006;12:152-157.

4. Letonoff EJ, Williams TR, Sidhu KS. Hysterical paralysis: a report of three cases and a review of the literature. *Spine*. 2002;27:E441-E445.

5. Stefansson JG, Messina JA, Meyerowitz S. Hysterical neurosis, conversion type: clinical and epidemiological considerations. *Acta Psychiatr Scand*. 1976;53:119-138.

6. Teasdell RW, Shapiro A. Rehabilitation of conversion disorders: a programmatic experience. *Phys Med Rehabil*. 2002;16:45-53.

7. Deaton AV. Treating conversion disorders: is a pediatric rehabilitation hospital the place? *Rehabil Psychol*. 1998;43:56-62.

8. Ness D. Physical therapy management for conversion disorder: case series. *J Neurol Phys Ther*. 2007;31:30-39.

9. Binzer M, Kullgren G. Motor conversion disorder: a prospective 2- to 5-year follow-up study. *Psychosomatics*. 1998;39:519-527.

10. Carlson ML, Archibald DJ, Gifford RH, Driscoll CL. Conversion disorder: a missed diagnosis leading to cochlear reimplantation. *Otol Neurotol*. 2011;32:36-38.

11. Heruti RJ, Levy A, Adunski A, Ohry A. Conversion motor paralysis disorder: overview and rehabilitation model. *Spinal Cord*. 2002;40:327-334.

12. Trieschmann RB, Stolov WC, Montgomery ED. An approach to the treatment of abnormal ambulation resulting from conversion reaction. *Arch Phys Med Rehabil*. 1970;51:198-206.

13. Brazier DK, Venning HE. Conversion disorders in adolescents: a practical approach to rehabilitation. *Br J Rheumatol*. 1997;36:594-598.

14. Speed J. Behavioral management of conversion disorder: a retrospective study. *Arch Phys Med Rehabil*. 1996;77:147-154.

15. Reese NB. *Muscle and Sensory Testing*. 3rd ed. St. Louis, MO: Elsevier; 2012.

16. O'Sullivan SB, Schmitz TJ. *Physical Rehabilitation: Assessment and Treatment*. 5th ed. Philadelphia, PA: F.A. Davis Company; 2007: 254.

Benign Paroxysmal Positional Vertigo—Posterior Semicircular Canal

Kristen M. Johnson

A 52-year-old male experienced an acute onset of vertigo immediately following a Valsalva maneuver when he was performing a bench press. His primary physician referred him to outpatient physical therapy because his symptoms have been persistent for more than 3 weeks despite taking meclizine (a common drug for vertigo) for the past 5 days. He has been purposefully limiting his cervical range of motion because he reports that movement of his head up and to the right causes his vertigo. He is still able to work as a mechanical engineer, which involves working at a desk and computer to view drawings. However, he has been taking frequent rest breaks throughout the day. He has also limited his driving because he experiences symptoms when he turns his head to change lanes. Currently, his coworker transports him to and from work. The patient is married and has three school-aged children and lives in a two-story home. His spouse is becoming quite frustrated at his limited assistance with caring for the children and household chores since the onset of his vertigo.

▶ What are the most appropriate examination tests?
▶ What are the examination priorities?
▶ What are the most appropriate physical therapy interventions?
▶ What is his rehabilitation prognosis?

KEY DEFINITIONS

AMPULLA: Widened portion of semicircular canal (SCC) that is near the utricle and contains the sensory hair cells

BONY LABYRINTH: Bony shell filled with perilymphatic fluid, which is similar in composition to cerebrospinal fluid (high sodium, low potassium); includes the three semicircular canals, the cochlea, and the vestibule

CANALITH REPOSITIONING PROCEDURE/EPLEY MANEUVER: Clinical technique used in treating the canalithiasis form of benign paroxysmal positional vertigo

CANALITHIASIS: Type of benign paroxysmal positional vertigo in which otoconia are floating free in the semicircular canals

CRISTA AMPULLARIS: Sensory structure (including hair cells) that senses angular movement within the semicircular canals

CUPULA: Bulbous, gelatinous mass that surrounds hair cells of cristae within semicircular canals

DIX-HALLPIKE MANEUVER: Clinical test for diagnosing benign paroxysmal positional vertigo in the anterior and/or posterior semicircular canals

MEMBRANOUS LABYRINTH: Structure filled with endolymph that is suspended within the bony labyrinth by fluid and connective tissue; contains membranous portion of the three semicircular canals, utricle, and saccule

NYSTAGMUS: Involuntary back-and-forth or cyclical eye movements; movements may be rotary, horizontal, or vertical

OTOCONIA (OTOLITHS): Calcium carbonate crystals in utricle and saccule that cause stimulation of the hair cells when the otoconia are stimulated by linear acceleration

SACCULE: Otolith structure in inner ear that detects vertical translation motion of head

SEMICIRCULAR CANALS: Three fluid-filled loops in the inner ear that measure angular acceleration; includes anterior (superior), posterior (inferior), and horizontal (lateral) canals

UTRICLE: Otolith structure in inner ear that detects horizontal translation and tilt of head

VERTIGO: Illusion of movement; a sense of spinning

Objectives

1. Describe basic vestibular anatomy.
2. Describe benign paroxysmal positional vertigo (BPPV) as a clinical syndrome.
3. Describe the most appropriate assessment and treatment for posterior canal BPPV.
4. Identify the appropriate use of medications for an individual with a diagnosis of BPPV.

Physical Therapy Considerations

PT considerations during management of the individual with complaints of vertigo due to BPPV that are causing activity and participation restrictions:

▶ **General physical therapy plan of care/goals:** Assess and treat BPPV symptoms; monitor secondary impairments of limited cervical range of motion (ROM)

▶ **Physical therapy interventions:** Canalith repositioning procedure

▶ **Precautions during physical therapy:** Close guarding and monitoring, as the patient could have impaired postural control with nausea and vomiting; caution with patients who have hypomobility or hypermobility in the cervical spine

▶ **Complications interfering with physical therapy:** Use of vestibular suppressant medications; multiple semicircular canal involvement

Understanding the Health Condition

To understand benign paroxysmal positional vertigo (BPPV), it is necessary to understand basic anatomy of the peripheral vestibular system (Fig. 9-1).[1,2] The peripheral vestibular system has a threefold purpose: to stabilize images on the fovea of the retina during head movement, to assist in postural control, and to assist with spatial orientation. The peripheral vestibular system contains the membranous labyrinth filled with endolymphatic fluid and the bony labyrinth filled with perilymphatic fluid, as well as hair cells that function to detect head motion. The membranous labyrinth is contained within the bony labyrinth and lies just inside the petrous portion of the temporal bone. The membranous labyrinth is composed of five sensory structures that detect head motion. There are three semicircular canals (SCCs) that sense angular acceleration and two otolithic organs (utricle and saccule) that sense linear acceleration and static head tilt. The SCCs are aligned such that the left and right peripheral vestibular systems function as coplanar pairs and endolymphatic fluid flows in response to head motion. Each SCC has a widened base called the ampulla. The importance of the ampulla is that it contains the cupula—a gelatinous membrane to which hair cells are projected up from the primary sensory structure called the crista ampullaris. Movement of the endolympatic fluid within the SCC causes hair cells to bend. This information is then transmitted into neural firing such that the coplanar pairs of the SCCs work together. For example, if you turn your head to the left, the movement of the hair cells within the SCC on the left causes an increase in neural activity and the movement of the hair cells within the coplanar pair within the opposite SCC causes a decrease in neural activity. The otolithic organs, the utricle and the saccule, are located within the membranous labyrinth. These organs also have hair cells contained within the primary sensory structure called the macula. The hair cells of the macula project up into a gelatinous otolithic membrane. Resting above and within the otolithic membrane are the otoliths or calcium carbonate crystals. The otoliths have a greater mass than

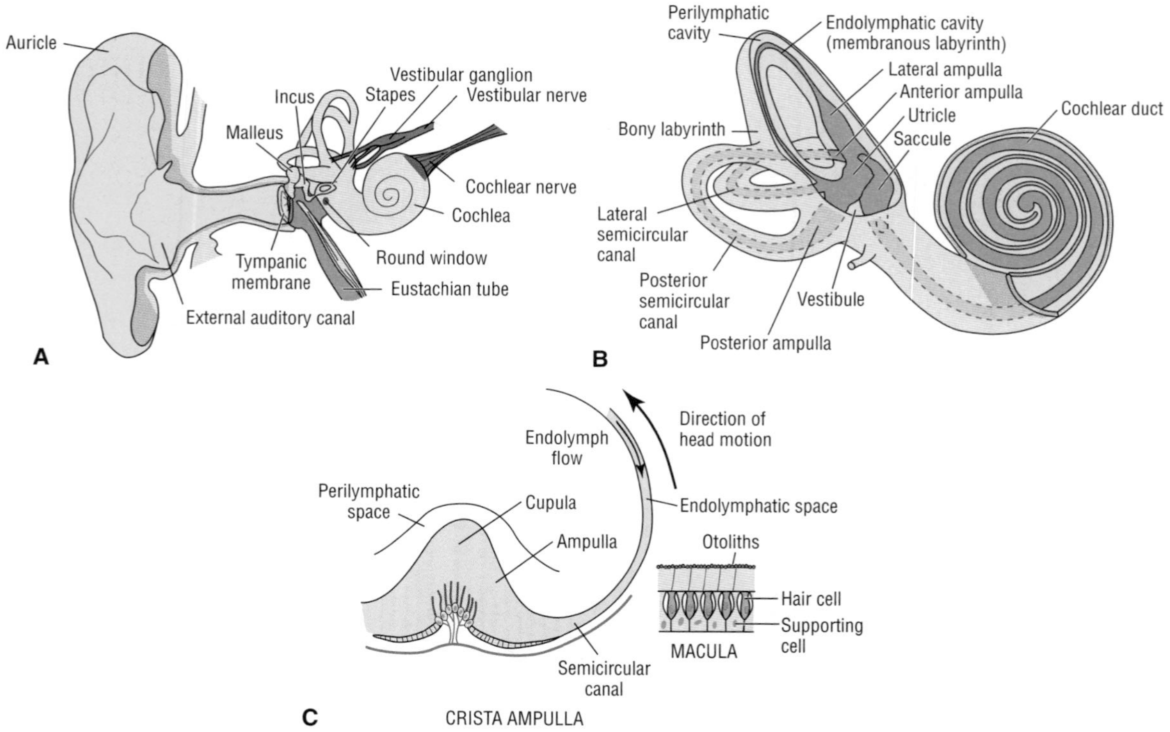
Auricle
Incus
Malleus
Stapes
Vestibular ganglion
Vestibular nerve
Cochlear nerve
Cochlea
Round window
Tympanic
membrane
Eustachian tube
External auditory canal
A
Perilymphatic
cavity
Endolymphatic cavity
(membranous labyrinth)
Lateral ampulla
Anterior ampulla
Utricle
Saccule
Cochlear duct
Bony labyrinth
Lateral
semicircular
canal
Posterior
semicircular
canal
Vestibule
Posterior ampulla
B
Endolymph
flow
Direction of
head motion
Perilymphatic
space
Cupula
Endolymphatic space
Ampulla
Otoliths
Hair cell
Supporting
cell
MACULA
Semicircular
canal
C
CRISTA AMPULLA

Figure 9-1. **A.** The right ear showing the external ear, auditory canal, middle ear, and the inner ear with its semicircular canals. **B.** The main parts of the inner ear. **C.** The crista ampulla, which is the specialized sensory epithelium of a semicircular canal. The crista senses displacement of the endolymph during head rotation. Direction of head rotation is indicated by the large upward arrow and the direction of the endolymph is indicated by the small downward arrow. The macula is within the utricle and saccule. The tips of the hair cells are in contact with the otoliths, which are embedded in the gelatinous cupula. (Reproduced with permission from Ropper AH, Samuels MA, eds. *Adams and Victor's Principles of Neurology*. 9th ed. New York: McGraw-Hill; 2009. Figure 15-1A, B, and D.)

the cupula, which forces the macula to be more sensitive to the pull of gravity and linear movements of the head.

With a lifetime prevalence of 2.4%, BPPV is the most common cause of vertigo.[1-5] Estimates range from 10.7 to 64 cases per 100,000 individuals. BPPV is more common in adults with the highest frequency occurring between the fifth and sixth decades of life.[2,4-7] Due to the high prevalence of this clinical condition, Bhattacharyya et al.[4] calculated the direct and indirect costs of BPPV to the healthcare system. They estimated that BPPV causes activity limitations and participation restrictions in 86% of those that suffer from this health condition with costs approaching $2 billion per year—simply for arriving at a definitive diagnosis.[8,9]

BPPV is best characterized by brief episodes of vertigo related to changes in head position, and may also include nausea with or without vomiting, and decreased postural control.[1] Individuals with BPPV often report vertigo symptoms when changing positions such as rolling over in bed and looking upward and/or downward while performing functional activities. Common examples of activities that precipitate vertigo include putting away groceries on a top shelf, washing hair in the shower, or reaching down to tie a shoe.[1,2] The onset of this condition can be idiopathic, but may also occur following labyrinthitis, ischemia within the vascular distribution of the peripheral vestibular system, or following head trauma.[2]

BPPV is a mechanical, peripheral vestibular disorder in which the otoconia are displaced from the otolithic organs and are then contained within a SCC. The two proposed forms of BPPV are canalithiasis and cupulolithiasis.[1,2] Canalithiasis, the more commonly encountered form, is characterized by otoconia freely flowing within the SCC.[10] With movement of the head into a provoking position, the otoconia move within the endolymphatic fluid of the SCC, thus deflecting the cupula. In an individual with canalithiasis, the onset of symptoms typically declines within 60 seconds of assuming the provocative head position. This temporal decline in symptoms relates to the decreased movement of the endolymph and position of the otoconia.[1,2,4] Cupulolithiasis was first theorized by Schuknecht in 1969.[11] He proposed that pieces of the otoconia were adherent to the cupula and as long as a person remained in the provoking position, symptoms persisted due to continual deflection of the cupula. Patients suffering from cupulolithiasis typically report the onset of symptoms *immediately* following provocative head movements and symptoms remain as long as the provoking head position is maintained.[1,2]

Physical Therapy Patient/Client Management

Physical therapists have a distinct role in the diagnosis and treatment of BPPV. Because BPPV is the most common cause of potentially disabling vertigo and early diagnosis can facilitate rapid and effective interventions and decrease healthcare costs, every practicing physical therapist should be proficient with both assessment and treatment procedures. In addition, a physical therapist can collaborate with other members of the healthcare team to make recommendations against the long-term use of vestibular suppressant medications and to increase the awareness of effective canalith repositioning maneuvers.[4] Common adverse drug reactions of vestibular suppressant medications such as meclizine include drowsiness, dizziness, and incoordination, all of which potentially increase the risk for falls. The role of the physical therapist is to assist in accurate diagnosis of BPPV and to apply appropriate interventions to resolve symptoms that can greatly impact the patient's functional abilities and quality of life.

Examination, Evaluation, and Diagnosis

The examination of a patient who reports vertigo mandates a multifactorial examination. The physical therapist must identify key components within the history including the onset and duration of symptoms. First, it is important to differentiate between vertigo and other complaints such as dizziness.[1,2] Many patients use the general term "dizziness" to describe their symptoms. However, this term is vague and can be interpreted in a variety of ways. While determining the cause of dizziness can be very challenging, the physical therapist must determine specifically what symptoms the patient is experiencing and elucidate whether he is experiencing true vertigo that may be caused by BPPV. The complaint of a spinning sensation in the *absence* of lightheadedness has been shown to be predictive of BPPV (sensitivity 59% and specificity 98%).[12] However, positional testing is still required to make the appropriate diagnosis.

The examination and diagnosis of BPPV involves multiple positional maneuvers to assess involvement of each of the semicircular canals. The current patient presented with symptoms most suggestive of involvement of the posterior semicircular canal as indicated by his symptoms being provoked by head movement up and to the right. Thus, this case only covers the **Dix-Hallpike maneuver**. This test has been considered the gold standard for the diagnosis of posterior canal BPPV because of its high sensitivity (82%) and specificity (71%).[13] Prior to initiating the Dix-Hallpike maneuver, the physical therapist must educate the patient about the possible side effects of nausea, vomiting, and vertigo that can occur during the assessment and that these symptoms, if present, will cease in 60 seconds.[4] This positional test involves the physical therapist passively rotating the head 45° while the patient is seated and then quickly lowering his head and body so the head is extended 20° below the horizontal. The patient is instructed to keep his eyes open and not to fixate or focus on any one particular object within the environment. While supporting the patient's head in this test position, the physical therapist looks for nystagmus and asks the patient to report any vertigo symptoms. The patient and therapist should remain in this position for 60 seconds and then the patient is assisted back to a seated position. The Dix-Hallpike maneuver is then repeated with the head rotated 45° to the opposite side.[1-5] A positive Dix-Hallpike for the right posterior SCC would involve head rotation 45° to the right with upbeating and torsional nystagmus while in this provoking head position.[1-5] In addition, the form of BPPV (canalithiasis or cupulolithiasis) can be determined. In this case example, a diagnosis of right posterior SCC *canalithiasis* involves upbeating, torsional nystagmus with complaints of vertigo that has a latency period of 5 to 20 seconds, and symptoms that fatigue over approximately 60 seconds.[1-5] If the Dix-Hallpike was performed and the direction of nystagmus was the same, except that the symptoms had a latency effect (coming on after 20 seconds) and were sustained, then the diagnosis of right posterior SCC *cupulolithiasis* would be made.[1-5]

The remainder of the examination can include additional tests and measures that are sensitive to additional impairments in ROM and strength (especially of the cervical spine), as well as those that capture both activity limitations and participation restrictions.[1,2]

Plan of Care and Interventions

The treatment plan for posterior SCC canalithiasis should focus on returning otoconia to the otolithic organs, improving postural control, decreasing complaints of vertigo with head movement, and normalizing cervical ROM.[1,2] Posterior SCC canalithiasis is the most common form of BPPV, and there is strong evidence to support the **canalith repositioning procedure (CRP)** for resolution of the condition.[4,5,14-19] Prior to initiation of treatment, the patient should be educated on the possible side effects of nausea, vomiting, and vertigo that often occur during the intervention.[4]

The CRP for right posterior canalithiasis BPPV involves placing the patient's head in four specific and consecutive positions. In the first treatment position, the therapist moves the patient from a seated position into a right Dix-Hallpike position (maintaining 45° of rotation to the right and 20° of cervical extension) and maintains this position until the nystagmus and complaints of vertigo cease (Fig. 9-2A).[2] For the second treatment position, the therapist rotates the patient's head past midline into a left Dix-Hallpike position, and again maintains the same degrees of head movement as the first position. The patient remains in this second position until any symptoms resolve (Fig. 9-2B). The third position involves moving the patient's head into a nose-down position by having the patient roll onto his side (Fig. 9-2C). During the third position, the therapist maintains the 45° of cervical rotation and again holds the patient in this position until the symptoms cease. If no symptoms are present, the position should be held a minimum of 20 to 30 seconds. For the fourth and final position, the therapist maintains the patient's neck in 45° of cervical rotation toward the left (same as third position), but asks the patient to move from a sidelying position to a seated position (Fig. 9-2D). Once seated upright, the patient can slowly look straight ahead. Upon completion of one CRP cycle (approximately 2-4 minutes for all four positions), the patient can now move freely. Post-procedure precautions (*e.g.*, avoiding sleeping or lying flat for the first 24 hours and avoiding extreme neck flexion and extension) are no longer indicated to improve the efficacy of the CRP or prevent reoccurrences of BPPV.[20-23]

Patients are frequently prescribed **vestibular suppressant medications for BPPV.** This patient has been taking a vertigo-inhibiting medication (meclizine) for 5 days as prescribed by his primary physician. Meclizine is a central and peripheral antagonist at histamine H1 receptors. It has several adverse drug reactions including drowsiness, incoordination, and dizziness that can interfere with the assessment and treatment of the individual with BPPV. Meclizine can interfere with central compensation and recovery from vertigo.[4] In addition, it may cause decreased cognition,

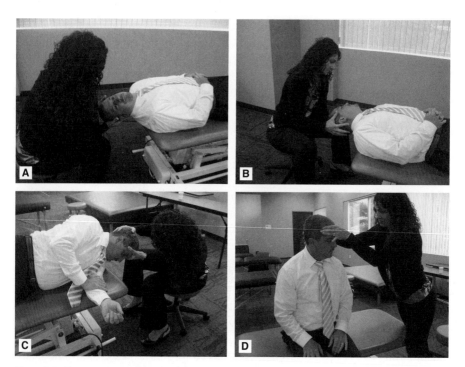

Figure 9-2. Four positions of the canalith repositioning procedure used to treat right posterior canalithiasis BPPV. **A.** With right cervical rotation maintained at 45°, the therapist moves the patient from a seated to supine position and then moves the patient's head into 20° of cervical extension. **B.** Therapist rotates the patient's head past midline into a left Dix-Hallpike position (45° left rotation with 20° extension). **C.** While the patient rolls onto his side, the therapist moves his head into a nose-down position. **D.** As the patient moves from a sidelying to seated position, the therapist maintains the patient's neck in 45° of left cervical rotation.

altered vision, and constipation. According to a recent clinical practice guideline, vestibular suppressant medications are not recommended for long-term management of BPPV.[4] It is within the scope of practice for the physical therapist to communicate with the referring physician regarding how these medications may be contributing to a patient's clinical presentation and make recommendations accordingly.

Successful management of BPPV includes **patient education**. Patients benefit from education about the diagnosis, recurrence rates, and follow-up care, as needed. Although the performance of one CRP has a reported success rate of 67% to 94% in treating BPPV, recurrence after initial assessment and treatment is possible.[24] Nunez and colleagues[25] have estimated the recurrence rate of BPPV to be 15%. Due to potential recurrence, patients should be educated regarding how best to access healthcare providers in order to minimize additional secondary impairments and long-term activity and participation restrictions. In addition, because the BPPV diagnosis can place the patient at a greater risk for falls, patients and families should be educated regarding this consideration and fall risk reduction strategies.

Further education and follow-up should be provided with recommendations to additional healthcare providers, especially if the patient's symptoms persist and/or are combined with atypical symptoms, such as hearing loss or further gait disturbances.[26]

Additional interventions for the individual with BPPV should include treatment for secondary loss of cervical ROM, declines in postural control, and muscle imbalance. Impairments beyond the BPPV diagnosis can greatly impact both the patient's activity limitations and participation restrictions.

Evidence-Based Clinical Recommendations

SORT: Strength of Recommendation Taxonomy

A: Consistent, good-quality patient-oriented evidence
B: Inconsistent or limited-quality patient-oriented evidence
C: Consensus, disease-oriented evidence, usual practice, expert opinion, or case series

1. The gold standard for diagnosis of posterior canal BPPV is the Dix-Hallpike maneuver. **Grade A**

2. The canalith repositioning procedure (CRP) is an effective treatment for posterior SCC canalithiasis. **Grade A**

3. Vestibular suppressant medications are not recommended for long-term management of BPPV. **Grade B**

4. To increase safety and mitigate activity limitations and participation restrictions, physical therapists should educate patients regarding the potential recurrence and impact of BPPV. **Grade C**

COMPREHENSION QUESTIONS

9.1 A physical therapist is evaluating a patient with BPPV involving the posterior semicircular canal. The maneuver with the *best* diagnostic accuracy for this condition is the:

A. Dix-Hallpike maneuver

B. Roll test

C. Epley maneuver

D. Semont Liberatory maneuver

9.2 Education of patients suffering from BPPV should include which of the following?

A. Fall prevention

B. Importance of follow-up

C. Recurrence risk

D. All of the above should be included in patient education.

9.3 If a patient with BPPV is taking a vestibular suppressant medication such as meclizine, the evidence suggests that the physical therapist should:

A. Collaborate with the prescribing physician in support of vestibular suppressant medications

B. Continue with the plan as initially determined by the physician

C. Make a recommendation to the physician against the use of vestibular suppressant medications

D. Tell the patient to immediately discontinue use of vestibular suppressant medications

ANSWERS

9.1 **A.** The Dix-Hallpike maneuver should be used to diagnose posterior canal BPPV when the patient has symptoms of vertigo and nystagmus in the provoking test position.

9.2 **D.** Because of the complaints of vertigo, nystagmus, and altered postural control, patients with BPPV are at a higher risk for falls.[27] It is also important that patients know how and when to contact their physical therapist in the event that symptoms recur.[25]

9.3 **C.** Clinical practice guidelines for BPPV recommend *against* the use of vestibular suppressant medications. The physical therapist should make recommendations to the prescribing physician regarding these guidelines. In addition, there is no evidence in the literature that recommends vestibular suppressant medications as effective treatment for BPPV.[28-32]

REFERENCES

1. O' Sullivan SB, Schmitz TJ. *Physical Rehabilitation*. Philadelphia, PA: FA Davis; 2007.

2. Herdman SJ. *Vestibular Rehabilitation*. 3rd ed. Philadelphia, PA: FA Davis; 2000.

3. Herdman SJ, Clendaniel RA. *Vestibular Rehabilitation*: a competency based course sponsored by Emory School of Medicine and American Physical Therapy Association. Atlanta, GA; 2004.

4. Bhattacharyya N, Baugh RF, Orvidas L, et al. Clinical practice guideline: benign paroxysmal positional vertigo. *Otolaryngol Head Neck Surg*. 2008;139:S47-S81.

5. Fife TD, Iverson DJ, Lempert T, et al. Practice parameter: therapies for benign paroxysmal positional vertigo (an evidence-based review). *Neurology*. 2008;70:2067-2074.

6. Froehling DA, Silverstein MD, Mohr DN, Beatty CW, Offord KP, Ballard DJ. Benign positional vertigo: incidence and prognosis in a population-based study in Olmsted county, Minnesota. *Mayo Clin Proc*. 1991;66:596-601.

7. Baloh RW, Honrubia V, Jacobson K. Benign positional vertigo: clinical and oculographic features in 240 cases. *Neurology*.1987;37:371-378.

8. von Brevern M, Radtke A, Lezius F, et al. Epidemiology of benign paroxysmal positional vertigo: a population based study. *J Neurol Neurosurg Psychiatry*. 2007;78:710-715.

9. Li JC, Li CJ, Epley J, Weinberg L. Cost-effective management of benign positional vertigo using canalith repositioning. *Otolaryngol Head Neck Surg*. 2000;122:334-339.

10. Hall SF, Ruby RR, McClure JA. The mechanics of benign paroxsymal vertigo. *J Otolaryngol.* 1979;8:151-158.

11. Schuknecht HF. Cupulolithiasis. *Arch Otolaryngol.*1969;90:765-778.

12. Oghalai JS, Manolidis S, Barth JL, Stewart MG, Jenkins HA. Unrecognized benign paroxysmal in elderly patients. *Otolaryngol Head Neck Surg.* 2000;122:630-634.

13. Lopez-Escamez JA, Lopez-Nevot A, Gamiz MJ, et al. Diagnosis of common causes of vertigo using a structured clinical history. *Acta Otorrinolaringol Esp.* 2000;51:25-30.

14. Herdman SJ, Tusa RJ, Zee DS, Proctor LR, Mattox DE. Single treatment approaches to benign paroxysmal positional vertigo. *Arch Otolaryngol Head Neck Surg.* 1993;119:450-454.

15. Epley JM. The canalith repositioning procedure: for treatment of benign paroxysmal positional vertigo. *Otolaryngol Head Neck Surg.* 1992;107:399-404.

16. Lynn S, Pool A, Rose D, Brey R, Suman V. Randomized trial of the canalith repositioning procedure. *Otolaryngol Head Neck Surg.* 1995;113:712-720.

17. Hilton M, Pinder D. The Epley (canalith repositioning) manoeuvre for benign paroxysmal positional vertigo. *Cochrane Database Syst Rev.* 2004;2:CD003162.

18. Froehling DA, Bowen JM, Mohr DN, et al. The canalith repositioning procedure for the treatment of benign paroxysmal positional vertigo: a randomized controlled trial. *Mayo Clin Proc.* 2000;75:695-700.

19. Yimtae E, Srirompotong S, Srirompotong S, Saie-Seaw P. A randomized trial of the canalith repositioning procedure. *Laryngoscope.* 2003;113:828-832.

20. Massoud EA, Ireland DJ. Post-treatment instructions in the nonsurgical management of benign paroxysmal positional vertigo. *J Otolaryngol.* 1996;25:121-125.

21. Roberts RA, Gans RE, DeBoodt JL, Lister JJ. Treatment of benign paroxysmal positional vertigo: necessity of postmanuever patient restrictions. *J Am Acad Audiol.* 2005;16:357-366.

22. Tusa RJ, Herdman SJ. BPPV: controlled trials, contraindications, post-maneuver instructions, complications, imbalance. *Audiological Med.* 2005;3:57-62.

23. DiGirolamo S, Paludetti G, Briglia G, Cosenza A, Santarelli R, Di Nardo W. Postural control in benign paroxysmal positional vertigo before and after recovery. *Acta Otolaryngol.* 1998;118:289-293.

24. Blakley BW. A randomized, controlled assessment of the canalith repositioning maneuver. *Otolaryngol Head Neck Surg.* 1994;110:391-396.

25. Nunez RA, Cass SP, Furman JM. Short- and long-term outcomes of canaltih repositioning for benign paroxysmal positional vertigo. *Otolaryngol Head Neck Surg.* 2000;122:647-652.

26. Rupa V. Persistent vertigo following particle repositioning maneuver: an analysis of causes. *Arch Otolaryngol Head Neck Surg.* 2004;130:436-439.

27. Brandt T, Dieterich M. Vestibular falls. *J Vestib Res.* 1993;3:3-14.

28. Frohman EM, Kramer PD, Dewey RB, Kramer L, Frohman TC. Benign paroxysmal positioning vertigo in multiple sclerosis: diagnosis, pathophysiology and therapeutic techniques. *Mult Scler.* 2003;9:250-255.

29. Hain TC, Uddin M. Pharmacological treatment of vertigo. *CNS Drugs* 2003;17:85-100.

30. Carlow TJ. Medical treatment of nystagmus and ocular motor disorders. *Int Ophthalmol Clin.* 1986;26:251-264.

31. Cesarani A, Alpini D, Monti B, Raponi G. The treatment of acute vertigo. *Neurol Sci.* 2004;25:S26-S30.

32. Fujino A, Tokumasu K, Yosio S, Naganuma H, Yoneda S, Nakamura K. Vestibular training for benign paroxysmal positional vertigo. Its efficacy in comparison with antivertigo drugs. *Arch Otoleryngol Head Neck Surg.* 1994;120:497-504.

Benign Paroxysmal Positional Vertigo—Lateral Semicircular Canal

Kristen M. Johnson

CASE 10

A 68-year-old retired elementary school teacher reported dizziness and vertigo when rolling over in bed 2 days ago. Since then, she has fallen while in the shower. Although she did not report any injuries, she became increasingly concerned about her "unsteadiness." On the third day, she called 911 because her symptoms had become severe. She was admitted through the emergency department for further medical work-up. Results from all neuroradiographic imaging were negative. Her symptoms persisted, particularly when she was rolling in the hospital bed. She lives alone and is recently widowed. She is concerned about her ability to be able to return home and care for herself. She enjoys gardening and playing bridge with residents that live in her retirement community. She is a breast cancer survivor (initial diagnosis made 8 years ago) and has mild complaints of osteoarthritis in both knees. She only takes over-the-counter medicine (acetaminophen) as needed for arthritis pain. Her medical history is otherwise unremarkable.

► What are the most appropriate examination tests?
► What are the most appropriate physical therapy interventions?

KEY DEFINITIONS

APOGEOTROPIC NYSTAGMUS: Horizontal nystagmus beating *away* from the ground or uppermost ear that is indicative of lateral canal benign paroxysmal positional vertigo (thought to be caused by otoliths adhering to the cupula)

CENTRAL VESTIBULE: Location where all three semicircular canals join within the membranous labyrinth

FORCED PROLONGED POSITIONING: Clinical technique used in treating lateral semicircular canal benign paroxysmal positional vertigo (BPPV)

GEOTROPIC NYSTAGMUS: Horizontal nystagmus beating *toward* the ground or undermost ear that is indicative of lateral canal BPPV (thought to be caused by free-floating otoliths in the posterior arm of the lateral semicircular canal)

ROLL MANEUVER/LEMPERT MANEUVER/BARBECUE ROLL MANEUVER: Clinical technique used in treating lateral semicircular canal BPPV (canalithiasis form)

SUPINE ROLL TEST: Clinical test for diagnosing BPPV in the lateral semicircular canals

Objectives

1. Describe how to differentiate lateral canal BPPV from posterior or anterior canal BPPV.

2. Describe the most appropriate assessment and treatment for lateral canal BPPV (canalithiasis).

3. Identify appropriate standardized outcome measures for an individual with a diagnosis of BPPV that capture activity limitations and participation restrictions domains of the International Classification of Functioning, Disability and Health (ICF) model.

Physical Therapy Considerations

PT considerations during management of the individual with vertigo due to lateral canal BPPV that is causing activity and participation restrictions:

▶ **General physical therapy plan of care/goals:** Assess and treat BPPV symptoms; monitor secondary impairments of limited gait and postural control

▶ **Physical therapy interventions:** Roll maneuver/Lempert maneuver/barbecue roll maneuver; forced prolonged positioning

▶ **Precautions during physical therapy:** Close guarding and monitoring because the patient could have impaired postural control with nausea and vomiting; caution with patients who have hypomobility or hypermobility in the cervical spine

▶ **Complications interfering with physical therapy:** Use of vestibular suppressant medications; multiple semicircular canal involvement

Understanding the Health Condition

See Case 9 for understanding basic vestibular anatomy and BPPV.

Physical Therapy Patient/Client Management

The role of the physical therapist is to assist in accurate diagnosis of BPPV and to appropriately apply interventions that resolve BPPV symptoms that can greatly impact the patient's functional activities and participation roles within society. Lateral canal BPPV requires careful differential diagnosis on the part of the physical therapist.[1] Patient management begins with a careful history. If symptoms are consistent with BPPV, the posterior and anterior canals should be assessed using the Dix-Hallpike maneuver as described in Case 9. If these findings are negative, the BPPV assessment should continue with investigating for potential involvement of the lateral canals.[2-7] With respect to semicircular canal involvement, the lateral canal is the second most common type of BPPV (after the posterior canal).[8-10] More importantly, individuals who have been assessed and treated for posterior canal BPPV (with the Dix-Hallpike and Epley maneuvers, respectively) may present with lateral canal BPPV over time. This phenomenon is the so-called canal switch due to the otoconia moving from the posterior to the lateral canal.[11] Understanding a patient's vertigo symptoms and direction of nystagmus in the provoking position is critical for making an accurate differential diagnosis.[12]

Examination, Evaluation, and Diagnosis

The examination of a patient who reports vertigo involves careful history taking and assessment of past and current medical history, a review of medications, examination of postural control, and determination of provoking positions involved with everyday mobility. The physical therapist's examination includes position testing for the posterior and anterior canals as described in Case 9. If findings are negative, the therapist should assess the lateral canals using the supine roll test. Prior to initiating this test, the therapist should inform the patient of the possibility of provoking her vertigo symptoms. Additional precautions for this test include, but are not limited to, patients with cervical spine hypomobility (e.g., disorders such as scoliosis, stenosis) or hypermobility (e.g., Down syndrome, rheumatoid arthritis).[1] The **supine roll test** involves having the patient lie supine while the examiner flexes her head 20° (Fig. 10-1A) and then quickly rotates her head 90° to one side (Fig. 10-1B). The physical therapist assesses for nystagmus and the patient's complaints of vertigo. Once any provoked symptoms subside, the therapist rotates the patient's head back to the neutral position (maintaining the 20° of flexion) and waits again for any symptoms to subside (Fig. 10-1C). While maintaining 20° of cervical flexion, the therapist rotates the patient's head 90° to the opposite side and again assesses for nystagmus and/or vertigo symptoms (Fig. 10-1D). In contrast to the Dix-Hallpike assessment (Case 9) in which symptoms are more likely provoked by rotation toward one side, the supine roll test often provokes symptoms in

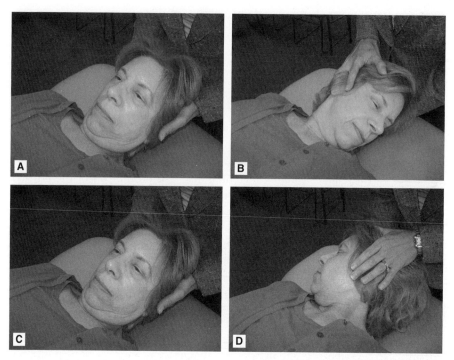

Figure 10-1. Supine roll test used to diagnose lateral canal BPPV. **A.** The physical therapist flexes patient's cervical spine 20°, and **B.** quickly rotates head 90° to one side while assessing for nystagmus and complaints of vertigo. **C.** The therapist rotates neck back to starting position, and **D.** rotates patient's head 90° to the opposite side and again assesses for nystagmus and/or vertigo symptoms.

both directions. Therefore, the physical therapist must carefully identify and compare the nystagmus responses when the head is rotated to the left and then to the right. The direction of the nystagmus during the supine roll test is either the more common geotropic (beating *toward* the ground as occurs in the canalithiasis form of BPPV) or the less common apogeotropic (beating *away* from the ground as occurs in the cupulolithiasis form of BPPV). In lateral canal BPPV, the direction of the nystagmus is typically direction changing, meaning that the nystagmus is geotropic (beating toward the undermost ear) in both head positions; however, the nystagmus is more intense when the patient is rolled toward the involved side. During the supine roll test, the involved ear is considered to be the ear toward which the head is rotated that provokes the *most intense* symptoms and nystagmus. Although the supine roll test is the preferred method for lateral canal examination, its specificity and sensitivity have yet to be reported. Even so, the supine roll test has been reported to be beneficial in efficiently diagnosing lateral canal BPPV.[11,13] The physical therapist may be able to prevent further unnecessary diagnostic testing by quickly and efficiently ruling out involvement of the posterior and anterior canals using the Dix-Hallpike maneuver, and then assessing the lateral canals with the supine roll test.

Standardized outcome measures should be used as an adjunct for a patient with BPPV. Potential measures to capture this patient's activity limitations and participation restrictions could include the **Functional Gait Assessment (FGA)** and the Dizziness Handicap Inventory. The FGA, which was established to assess the dynamic aspects of gait, can be used to assess this patient's activity limitations. This measure has 10 items that uniquely vary the dynamic aspects of gait. The patient is asked to walk at normal and fast speeds on a level surface, walk and make a pivot turn, walk with horizontal head movements and then vertical head movements, walk with eyes closed, walk backward, step over obstacles, walk with a narrow base of support, and step up and down stairs.[14] The FGA is scored on a four-point ordinal scale (0-3 points) with higher scores indicating fewer activity limitations. The FGA has been found to have good to excellent intra-rater and inter-rater reliability and has also been found to be a comprehensive measure that is sensitive to change when assessing gait and balance dysfunction in both community-dwelling elderly and individuals with vestibular dysfunction. An FGA score of $\leq 22/30$ is predictive of increased fall risk in the community-dwelling elderly population.[14-17]

The **Dizziness Handicap Inventory (DHI)** was established as a self-report measure of disability. This questionnaire has 25 items and can be subdivided into three categories that measure effects imposed by vestibular dysfunction: emotional, functional, and physical.[18] Each of the items is scored by having the patient select "yes" which equals 4 points, "sometimes" which equals 2 points, and "no" which equals 0 points. Total scores can range from 0 (no perceived disability) to 100 (maximal perceived disability). The DHI has been found to have high internal consistency and reliability.[18,19] For the current patient, the DHI could efficiently assess participation restrictions as well as the efficacy of physical therapy interventions.

Plan of Care and Interventions

Lateral canal BPPV is generally not responsive to the canalith repositioning procedure (CRP) described in Case 9. There are numerous repositioning techniques for both lateral canalithiasis and cupulolithiasis forms of BPPV. However, this case focuses on the maneuver used for treatment of left lateral canalithiasis BPPV.[20-22] In recalling the vestibular anatomy, the goal for lateral canal BPPV is to move the otoconia from the canal into the central vestibule.[23-25] The **roll maneuver** (also called the Lempert maneuver or barbecue roll maneuver) is the most widely accepted treatment for lateral canalithiasis BPPV.[11,24,26-28] The reported effectiveness varies considerably with an approximate value of 75% and a range from 50% to 100%.[11,26] In a recent prospective randomized study, a maximum of two roll maneuvers during a single treatment session resulted in better responses than a sham maneuver (69% vs. 35%) in patients with lateral canal BPPV.[20] The roll maneuver involves having the patient move a total of 360°. Each component of the maneuver involves a 90° head (and body) turn with an approximate 10 to 30-second hold in each position after the vertigo symptoms subside. This procedure continues until the patient's head returns to the starting position. The first position of the roll maneuver is a supine position with head rotated 90° toward the more involved ear (Fig. 10-2A). After holding this position for 10 to 30 seconds (or until the symptoms subside), the physical therapist moves the patient's head 90° away from the (more) involved ear so that she is in a nose-up, or neutral supine position looking at the ceiling (Fig. 10-2B). After holding this second position, the physical therapist then rolls the patient's head 90° from midline *away* from the more involved ear (Fig. 10-2C). The patient then moves to a prone or nose-down position (Fig. 10-2D) and finally moving back into the start position (Fig. 10-2A).[25,29-32]

Forced prolonged positioning (FPP) is another possible intervention for lateral canal BPPV. Numerous sources have found this treatment to be effective when used alone or in conjunction with the roll maneuver. In individual patient cases, the success rate has been documented to be between 75% and 90%.[1] For treating geotropic lateral canal BPPV, FPP involves having the patient lie supine and then roll onto the uninvolved/less involved side and remain in this position throughout the night. For treating apogeotropic lateral canal BPPV, the patient lies supine on her back and then rolls onto the more involved side and remains sidelying in this position throughout the night.[7,28,29,33]

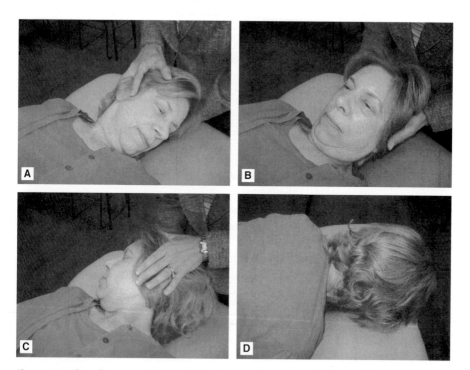

Figure 10-2. The roll maneuver (also called the Lempert maneuver or barbecue roll maneuver) used to treat left lateral canalithiasis BPPV. **A.** The patient is supine with head rotated 90° toward the more involved ear for 10 to 30 seconds, or until any nystagmus or vertigo subsides. **B.** The physical therapist moves the patient's head away from the (more) involved left ear so that she is in a nose-up supine position looking at the ceiling. **C.** The therapist rolls the patient's head 90° from midline *away* from the more involved ear. **D.** The therapist, along with assistance from the patient as appropriate, moves the patient's head into a nose-down position so the patient is prone. The therapist moves the patient's head toward her left side and the patient moves herself back to a supine position as in **A.**

Additional interventions for the individual with BPPV should include treatment within the body, structure, and function domain of the ICF model for loss of range of motion, declines in postural control, and muscle imbalance. In addition, impairments beyond the BPPV diagnosis can greatly impact the patient's activity limitations and participation restrictions, as measured by the FGA and DHI. All three domains of the ICF should be considered during interventions and careful consideration should be taken to understand how the contextual barriers and environment interact within the model to optimize patient-specific goals.

Evidence-Based Clinical Recommendations

SORT: Strength of Recommendation Taxonomy

A: Consistent, good-quality patient-oriented evidence
B: Inconsistent or limited-quality patient-oriented evidence
C: Consensus, disease-oriented evidence, usual practice, expert opinion, or case series

1. The preferred clinical test for diagnosis of lateral canal BPPV is the supine roll test. **Grade B**

2. The Functional Gait Assessment can be used by physical therapists to assess fall risk and activity limitations in patients with BPPV. **Grade B**

3. The Dizziness Handicap Inventory can be used by physical therapists to assess participation restrictions in patients with BPPV. **Grade C**

4. The roll maneuver (Lempert maneuver or barbecue roll maneuver) and forced prolonged positioning are effective treatments for lateral semicircular canal BPPV. **Grade B**

COMPREHENSION QUESTIONS

10.1 A physical therapist is evaluating a patient with BPPV involving the lateral semicircular canal. The maneuver with the best diagnostic accuracy for this condition is:

   A. Dix-Hallpike maneuver
   B. Supine roll test
   C. Epley maneuver
   D. Semont liberatory maneuver

10.2 Current evidence-based practice involves which maneuver(s) to treat lateral semicircular canal BPPV?

   A. Barbecue roll and/or forced prolonged positioning
   B. Dix-Hallpike maneuver
   C. Epley maneuver
   D. None of the above

10.3 Which standardized outcome measure is the most comprehensive and sensitive to change when assessing gait and balance dysfunction in a community-dwelling older adult with the vestibular pathology described in this case?

A. Functional Gait Assessment (FGA)

B. Dynamic Gait Index (DGI)

C. Berg Balance Scale

D. Performance Oriented Mobility Assessment (POMA)

ANSWERS

10.1 **B.** The supine roll test should be used by the physical therapist to diagnose lateral canal BPPV when the patient has symptoms of vertigo and nystagmus in the provoking test position. This test involves having the patient lie supine with her head in a neutral position. Next, the examiner quickly moves the patient's head 90° to the left (for testing left lateral canal) or right (for testing right lateral canal) while observing for nystagmus. Once the symptoms and any provoked nystagmus subside, the patient's head is moved back to the neutral position and this test is repeated to the opposite side.[4]

10.2 **A.** Both the barbecue roll and/or forced prolonged positioning are effective maneuvers to treat lateral semicircular canal (SCC) BPPV. The barbecue roll involves having the patient actually roll 360° in an effort to move or reposition the particles within the lateral SCC. Forced prolonged positioning (FPP) can be used alone and/or in conjunction with lateral SCC maneuvers. For treating *geotropic* lateral canal BPPV, FPP involves having the patient lie supine and then roll onto the uninvolved/less involved side and remain in this position throughout the night. For treating *apogeotropic* lateral canal BPPV, the patient lies supine on her back and then rolls onto the more involved side and remains sidelying in this position throughout the night.

10.3 **A.** Although moderate correlations exist between all the options listed, the FGA is the most comprehensive and sensitive to change when assessing gait and balance dysfunction in community-dwelling elderly and in individuals with vestibular dysfunction. An FGA score of ≤22/30 is predictive of increased fall risk.

REFERENCES

1. Bhattacharyya N, Baugh RF, Orvidas L, et al. Clinical practice guideline: benign paroxysmal positional vertigo. *Otolaryngol Head Neck Surg.* 2008;139:S47-S81.

2. Herdman SJ, Tusa RJ, Clendaniel RA. Eye movement signs in vertical canal benign paroxysmal positional vertigo. In: Fuch A, Brandt T, Buttner U, Zee D, eds. *Contemporary Ocular Motor and Vestibular Research: A Tribute to Dave A. Robinson.* Stuttgart, Germany: George Theime; 1994:385-387.3.

3. McClure JA. Horizontal canal BPV. *J Otolaryngol.* 1985;14:30-35.

4. Baloh RW, Jacobson K, Honrubia V. Horizontal semicircular canal variant of benign positional vertigo. *Neurology.*1993;43:2542-2549.

5. De la Meilleure G, Dehaene I, Depondt M, Damman W, Crevits L, Vanhooren G. Benign paroxysmal positional vertigo of the horizontal canal. *J Neurol Neurosurg Psychiatry.* 1996;60;68-71.

6. Nuti D, Vannucchi P, Pagnini P. Benign paroxysmal positional vertigo of the horizontal canal: a form of canalolithiasis with variable clinical features. *J Vestib Res.*1996;6;173-184.

7. Vannucchi P, Giannoni B, Pagnini P. Treatment of horizontal semicircular canal benign paroxysmal positional vertigo. *J Vestib Res.* 1997;7:1-6.

8. Imai T, Ito M, Takeda N, et al. Natural course of the remission of vertigo in patients with benign paroxysmal positional vertigo. *Neurology.* 2005;64:920-921.

9. Steenerson RL, Cronin GW, Marbach PM. Effectiveness of treatment techniques in 923 cases of benign paroxysmal positional vertigo. *Laryngoscope.* 2005;115:226-231.

10. Moon SY, Kim JS, Kim BK, et al. Clinical characteristics of benign paroxysmal positional vertigo in Korea: a multicenter study. *J Korean Med Sci.* 2006;21:539-543.

11. White JA, Coale KD, Catalano PJ, Oas JG. Diagnosis and management of lateral semicircular canal benign paroxysmal positional vertigo. *Otolaryngol Head Neck Surg.* 2005;133:278-284.

12. Herdman SJ. *Vestibular Rehabilitation.* 3rd ed. Philadelphia, PA: FA Davis; 2000.

13. Fife TD, Iverson DJ, Lempert T, et al. Practice parameter: therapies for benign paroxysmal positional vertigo (an evidence-based review): report of the Quality Standards Subcommittee of the American Academy of Neurology. *Neurology.* 2008;70;2067-2074.

14. Wrisley DM, Walker ML, Echternach JL, Strasnick B. Reliability of the dynamic gait index in people with vestibular disorders. *Arch Phys Med Rehabil.* 2003;84:1528-1533.

15. Wrisley DM, Marchetti GF, Kuharsky DK, Whitney SL. Reliability, internal consistency, and validity of data obtained with the functional gait assessment. *Phys Ther.* 2004;84:906-918.

16. Walker ML, Austin AG, Banke GM, et al. Reference group data for the functional gait assessment. *Phys Ther.* 2007;87:1468-1477.

17. Wrisley DM, Kumar NS. Functional gait assessment: concurrent discriminative, and predictive validity in community-dwelling older adults. *Phys Ther.* 2010;90:761-773.

18. Jacobson GP, Newman CW. The development of the Dizziness Handicap Inventory. *Arch Otolaryngeol Head Neck Surg.* 1990;116:424-427.

19. Jacobson GP, Newman CW, Hunter L, Baltzer GK. Balance function test correlates of the Dizziness Handicap Inventory. *J Am Acad Audiol.* 1991;2:253-260.

20. Kim JS, Oh SY, Lee SH, et al. Randomized clinical trial for geotropic horizontal canal benign paroxysmal positional vertigo. *Neurology.* 2012;79:700-707.

21. Kim SH, Jo SW, Chung WK, Byeon HK, Lee WS. A cupulolith repositioning maneuver in the treatment of horizontal canal cupulolithiasis. *Auris Nasus Larynx.* 2012;39:163-168.

22. Boleas-Aguirre MS, Perez N, Batuecas-Caletrio A. Bedside therapeutic experiences with horizontal canal benign paroxysmal positional vertigo (cupulolithiasis). *Acta Otolaryngol.* 2009;129:1217-1221.

23. Herdman SJ, Tusa RJ. Complications of the canalith repositioning procedure. *Arch Otolaryngol Head Neck Surg.*1996;122:281-286.

24. Fife TD. Recognition and management of horizontal canal benign positional vertigo. *Am J Otol.*1998;19:345-351.

25. Lempert T, Tiel-Wilck K. A positional maneuver for treatment of horizontal-canal benign positional vertigo. *Laryngoscope.* 1996;106:476-478.

26. Prokopakis EP, Chimona T, Tsagournisakis M, et al. Benign paroxysmal positional vertigo: 10-year experience in treating 592 patients with canalith repositioning procedure. *Laryngoscope.* 2005;115:1667-1671.

27. Nuti D, Agus G, Barbieri MT, Passali D. The management of horizontal-canal paroxysmal positional vertigo. *Acta Otolaryngol.* 1998;118:455-460.

28. Casani AP, Vannucchi G, Fattori B, Berrettini S. The treatment of horizontal canal positional vertigo: our experience in 66 cases. *Laryngoscope.* 2002;112:172-178.

29. Ciniglio Appiani G, Gagliardi M, Magliulo G. Physical treatment of horizontal canal benign positional vertigo. *Eur Arch Otorhinolaryngol.* 1997;254:326-328.

30. Asprella Libonati G. Diagnostic and treatment strategy of the lateral semicircular canal canalolithiasis. *Acta Otorhinolaryngol Ital.* 2005;25:277-283.

31. Tusa RJ, Herdman SJ. Canalith repositioning for benign paroxysmal positional vertigo. *American Academy of Neurology Publication 319*. St. Paul, MN: American Academy of Neurology; 1996.

32. Lempert T, Wolsley C, Davies R, Gresty MA, Bronstein AM. Three hundred sixty-degree rotation of the posterior semicircular canal for treatment of benign positional vertigo: a placebo-controlled trial. *Neurology.* 1997;49:729-733.

33. Chiou WY, Lee HL, Tsai SC, Yu TH, Lee XX. A single therapy for all subtypes of horizontal canal positional vertigo. *Laryngoscope.* 2005;115:1432-1435.

Vestibular Neuritis

Wendy Wood

A 37-year-old female construction worker at a high-rise building had an acute onset of spontaneous ongoing vertigo accompanied by nausea, vomiting, and severely impaired balance. She was unable to walk and had to crawl on the floor. After having 34 hours of continuous symptoms, she was taken to the emergency department (ED) by her sister. Her sister had to provide maximum assistance due to her significantly impaired mobility. The ED physician observed nystagmus during an ocular examination. He ordered diagnostic imaging of the brain, which demonstrated no abnormalities. The patient mentioned recently recovering from a flu virus. The physician administered intramuscular promethazine for the management of vertigo and nausea. He prescribed an oral antivertiginous drug (meclizine [Antivert]) to be taken up to three times per day for the next 30 days. Since her vertigo was eliminated within an hour after the intramuscular injection, he discharged her home with a recommendation to follow-up with her primary care physician. The ED physician suggested "relative bed rest" for the next 2 to 3 days. The patient saw her primary care physician on the fifth day after the initial event. At this stage, she was experiencing vague dizziness and oscillopsia with quick motions but no further vertigo or nausea. She was avoiding moving her head because this exacerbated her dizziness and caused loss of balance. The primary care physician diagnosed the patient with a severe sinus infection for which he prescribed an antihistamine (loratadine [Claritin]). After 2 weeks, she had no change in her symptoms of dizziness, motion intolerance, and imbalance. The primary care physician referred her to an ear, nose, and throat (ENT) physician who requested the audiologist in his office to perform a hearing test (which was normal) and a videonystagmography test, which indicated a 42% left caloric weakness. Based on these tests, the ENT physician diagnosed the patient with vestibular neuritis. She has not been able to work at her construction job for a month and is concerned about her finances. She also does not feel confident in driving. She lives in a two-story home with her domestic partner who works full-time. The ENT physician instructed the patient to stop taking meclizine and referred her to an outpatient balance and vestibular physical therapy clinic due to her persistent symptoms.

► What are the most appropriate examination tests?
► What are the critical elements of the clinical examination of the patient?
► What are the most appropriate physical therapy interventions?
► What is her rehabilitation prognosis?

KEY DEFINITIONS

ALEXANDER'S LAW: Looking in the direction of the fast component of the nystagmus increases its amplitude and frequency while looking in the reverse direction has the opposite effect

COMPUTERIZED DYNAMIC POSTUROGRAPHY (CDP): Laboratory tests that measure balance or center of gravity sway

DYNAMIC GAIT INDEX (DGI): Gait and fall risk assessment developed for patients with vestibular dysfunction

DYNAMIC VISUAL ACUITY TEST (DVAT): Clinical test of vestibular function that measures visual acuity with the head in motion compared to visual acuity with the head held statically

FRENZEL GOGGLES OR LENSES: Goggles that magnify and illuminate the patient's eyes with lenses that block the ability to fixate the eyes; they are useful in vestibular evaluation because the examiner is able to clearly see eye motions such as nystagmus

HEAD IMPULSE OR THRUST TEST: Clinical test that requires the individual to fixate her gaze on a stationary target while the clinician moves the individual's head quickly in a horizontal direction; if the clinician observes a corrective saccade at the end of the head motion, the test is positive for vestibular hypofunction and is suggestive of a decrease in the gain of the vestibulo-ocular reflex

NYSTAGMUS: Involuntary jerk or back-and-forth eye movements; movements may be rotary, horizontal, or vertical

OSCILLOPSIA: False illusion of movement of objects in the environment

UNILATERAL PERIPHERAL VESTIBULAR DYSFUNCTION: Disorders such as vestibular neuritis, Meniere's disease, benign paroxysmal positional vertigo, and acoustic neuroma that affect one side of the vestibular labyrinth; the origin of the pathology is not in the brain.

VERTIGO: Illusion of movement; a sense of spinning

VIDEONYSTAGMOGRAPHY (VNG): Recording of eye movements in response to vestibular stimuli

Objectives

1. Describe the function of the vestibular system.
2. Describe the pathophysiology of vestibular neuritis and the signs and symptoms of this condition.
3. Describe the vestibular function tests used for differential diagnosis of vestibular disorders.
4. Identify and describe appropriate physical therapy interventions for vestibular neuritis.

Physical Therapy Considerations

PT considerations during management of the individual with complaints of dizziness and imbalance due to vestibular neuritis:

▶ **General physical therapy plan of care/goals:** Decrease symptoms of motion sensitivity and dizziness; improve dynamic visual acuity, improve balance, balance confidence, and gait; reduce risk of falls; return to work

▶ **Physical therapy interventions:** Balance and vestibular training including dynamic visual acuity and gaze stabilization training; habituation exercises to decrease motion sensitivity and dizziness; postural control exercises; dynamic gait training; patient education on the disorder; home exercise program

▶ **Precautions during physical therapy:** Fall prevention and safety awareness; close supervision and/or guarding of the patient due to impairments with balance and dizziness; performance of vestibular exercises may cause some dizziness

▶ **Complications interfering with physical therapy:** Overuse or continued use of antivertiginous medications that may interfere with compensation and recovery

Understanding the Health Condition

Vestibular neuritis (also known as vestibular neuronitis) affects the peripheral vestibular system, specifically the vestibular portion of the vestibulocochlear nerve (CN VIII). When the cochlear or hearing portion of the nerve is also affected, the condition is known as labyrinthitis. The vestibular system has both sensory and motor functions. It is one of the three main sensory systems for balance (vestibular, vision, proprioception). The vestibular system senses angular and linear acceleration of the head. This information is utilized to accurately estimate head and body position. The motor functions of the vestibular system coordinate head and eye motion for gaze stability, maintenance of postural control, and stabilization of the head over the neck. There are two primary motor reflexes of the vestibular system: the vestibulo-ocular reflex (VOR) and the vestibulospinal reflex (VSR). The VOR coordinates eye motion with head motion. As the head moves in one direction, the eyes move in the opposite direction by an equal number of degrees. This reflex ensures that the image being viewed is stabilized on the fovea of the retina for clear visual acuity. The afferent pathway begins with information about head motion from the vestibular labyrinths (within the inner ears) transmitted via the vestibulocochlear nerve to the vestibular nuclei in the brain. Projections from the nuclei relay information to the extraocular eye muscles. An eye movement is then generated that counteracts the head motion. With the VSR, neural connections from vestibular nuclei travel to antigravity muscles for balance and postural control.

The brain integrates information from the right and left peripheral vestibular systems. Typically, there is a tonic resting firing rate of the afferent nerves on each side. Vestibular neuritis causes a hypofunction on the involved side, and thus a neural imbalance. In the acute phase, the clinical presentation includes vertigo, nystagmus, oscillopsia, nausea, vomiting, the *absence* of hearing loss or tinnitus (which would indicate cochlear involvement), and the absence of other neurological signs or symptoms such as hemiplegia, dysarthria, and other stroke-related signs. Acutely, a mixed horizontal and torsional nystagmus can be observed in the direction of the intact nerve. Nystagmus, an involuntary jerk motion of the eyes involving a quick motion or saccade and then a re-setting or slow movement, is named according to the direction of the fast phase. A vestibular lesion drives the slow phase of the nystagmus so that a left-sided vestibular neuritis (hypofunction of the left vestibulocochlear nerve) causes a right-beating nystagmus.[1-4] This pathological eye motion causes the patient to be very disoriented, dizzy, imbalanced, and quite often nauseated. The patient has a tendency to fall or veer toward the lesioned side. The nystagmus is more readily observed with visual fixation blocked, such as with Frenzel or infrared video goggles. It may be suppressed in room light. The intensity of the nystagmus also increases when the individual looks in the direction of the quick phases (Alexander's law). Nystagmus typically resolves in room light within 1 to 3 days.[1,2] However, the patient can experience dizziness and imbalance for weeks or months, and nystagmus can be observed weeks later if visual fixation is blocked.[1-4]

Vestibular neuritis is the second[1,2] or third[3,5] most common cause of vertigo, and occurs more frequently in adults between 20 and 60 years of age.[5-8] There are many causes of vestibular neuritis. A virus in the herpes family is considered to be one of the primary causes of the condition.[1,2] Frequently, the patient reports a recent history of an upper respiratory infection.[6-9] Vestibular neuritis is a benign disorder, but several differential diagnoses must be considered: vertebrobasilar insufficiency, Meniere's disease, and benign paroxysmal positional vertigo (BPPV). Vertebrobasilar insufficiency (VBI) is a type of cerebrovascular accident (CVA) that often presents with sudden vertigo. It is usually associated with other neurological findings such as diplopia, dysarthria, hemiparesis, and facial or tongue numbness. If VBI is suspected, computed tomography (CT) imaging is warranted. Meniere's disease is also a unilateral peripheral vestibular disorder. In contrast to the long-lasting vertigo (1-3 days) experienced by patients with vestibular neuritis, patients with Meniere's disease experience spontaneous attacks of vertigo lasting hours. Meniere's disease is also associated with hearing loss and tinnitus. In BPPV, vertigo is related to positional changes, but vertiginous spells last only seconds. BPPV does not result in hearing loss. Physicians involved in the differential diagnosis of the "dizzy" patient may include specialists such as otologists, neurologists, or otolaryngologists (ENTs). A CT or MRI scan may be ordered if the physician believes these tests are warranted to rule out involvement of the central nervous system. Blood tests may be ordered to rule out otic syphilis or vasculitis. An audiologist may conduct hearing and vestibular function tests. With vestibular neuritis, there should not be any associated hearing impairment. Videonystagmography (VNG) measures eye motion in response to visual or vestibular stimulation. It can help distinguish whether there is *peripheral* inner ear or *central* nervous system dysfunction. There are four parts to the test: ocular mobility, optokinetic nystagmus, positional, and calorics. During the caloric test, warm water and then cold water is irrigated into the ear. Alternately, air may be used. The response of the eyes (*i.e.*, nystagmus) to the vestibular stimulus of water or air is observed, and each side is compared. A difference of >25% between sides is typically considered clinically significant to indicate a unilateral peripheral vestibular hypofunction. In the acute stage of many of these "dizzy" conditions, physicians may prescribe medications to alleviate symptoms; these should only be used for 1 week or less.[1,2,10] These medications include vestibular suppressants such as meclizine (Bonine or Antivert) and promethazine.[2,11] Prednisone (a glucocorticoid) and acyclovir (an antiviral) are medications that may be prescribed during the first 10 days after onset of the symptoms.[2,10,11] Vestibular rehabilitation exercises are very important for recovery.[12]

Physical Therapy Patient/Client Management

Physical therapists play a significant role in the treatment of vestibular disorders. The symptoms of these disorders are dizziness, motion sensitivity, fear of falling, imbalance, and impaired gait. The physical therapist collaborates with other members of the healthcare team such as the ENT physician or audiologist to confirm a diagnosis. If the physical therapist suspects a more serious cause of dizziness such as a brain lesion, cardiovascular problem, or other undiagnosed vestibular deficit, clear and rapid communication with the physician is required. The therapist may also make patients aware of recommendations against the long-term use of vestibular suppressant medications that may interfere with the patient's ability to effectively recover from the injury to the vestibular system.[2] These pharmacological agents also have adverse effects such as dizziness, incoordination, and lethargy that can increase the patient's risk of falling.

Examination, Evaluation, and Diagnosis

The examination of a patient reporting vertigo should always begin with a thorough history. In the case of a patient reporting dizziness and imbalance, the physical therapist should determine the onset of the patient's symptoms, the provoking factors, and an accurate description and clarification of the type and timeframe of the dizziness experienced.[1,2,13] Vertigo—a key symptom of vestibular neuritis—refers to a true spinning or rotational sensation. However, this term is often misused and the therapist should give the patient enough time to clearly describe her symptoms to determine whether she is truly experiencing vertigo. Vestibular neuritis causes spontaneous and acute onset of vertigo lasting 1 to 3 days. Once the vertigo resolves, the patient commonly reports imbalance and dizziness associated with quick movements, especially those of the head.

The Dizziness Handicap Inventory (DHI) is a subjective outcome measure that is helpful to identify and quantify the impact of dizziness and unsteadiness on a person's quality of life. It is a 25-item questionnaire covering three primary domains: physical, emotional, and functional. The questions were derived from case histories of patients reporting dizziness.[14] The DHI has been shown to have high internal consistency. Higher scores on the DHI have been associated with a greater frequency of dizziness and greater functional impairment.[15] Concurrent validity has also been established.[16-18] Jacobson and Newman[14] examined this instrument and demonstrated satisfactory test-retest reliability and determined that an 18-point change indicated a minimal clinically important difference (MCID). The **Activities-Specific Balance Confidence (ABC) Scale** is another subjective outcome measure developed for patients with dizziness and/or balance deficits. This measure quantifies balance confidence and identifies potential fear of falling.[19] The questionnaire contains 16 different items related to daily function. The individual is requested to rate her percent confidence on each item. Powell and Myers[19] compared the ABC scale with the Falls Efficacy Scale (FES), finding that the ABC Scale had high internal consistency, and high test-retest reliability. The ABC scores had a moderate correlation with Physical Self-Efficacy Scale scores and FES scores. Lower scores on the ABC Scale were associated with lower levels of mobility and a higher occurrence of falls. Talley et al.[20] compared the psychometric properties of the ABC scale and the Survey of Activities and Fear of Falling in the Elderly (SAFE). Both scales demonstrated strong internal consistency (Cronbach's $\alpha = 0.95$ for the ABC and 0.82 for the SAFE). Both scales are also strongly correlated with physical performance measures of the Berg Balance Scale, Timed Up and Go, gait speed, and the self-report measure of the Medical Outcomes Measure 36-item Short Form Survey.[20] Similarly, Huang and Wang[21] found the ABC had high internal consistency and strong concurrent validity when compared to the FES. Lajoi and Gallagher[22] determined that a cut-off score on the ABC scale of 67% resulted in 87.5% specificity and 84.4% sensitivity in identifying fallers. In 2011, Moore et al.[23] established a correlation of the ABC Scale with five other fall-related psychological instruments (the FES, modified Survey of Activities and Fear of Falling in the Elderly [mSAFFE], Consequences of Falling [CoF], Physical Activity Scale for the Elderly [PASE], and the 36-item Short-Form Health Survey) and with mobility. The ABC Scale was helpful in differentiating fallers and non-fallers and in predicting fall risk.[21] Scores on the ABC Scale improved after patients participated in a balance exercise program.[24] Though the ABC Scale is related to balance confidence and fear of falling, it has been found to be a valid outcome measure to assess patients with vestibular dysfunction and associated dizziness.[15,25,26] The DHI and ABC Scales are important subjective outcome measures that can help identify activity and participations limitations.

The physical therapist should also administer appropriate objective measures. A comprehensive clinical examination is necessary for a patient with dizziness. Elements of the examination include oculomotor and vestibulo-ocular testing (including dynamic visual acuity), sensory examination, and tests of gait, balance, and postural control. The clinical examination usually begins with ocular motor testing. It is critical to rule out central causes of dizziness as these are more serious and warrant immediate medical attention. Nystagmus can be seen more readily when visual fixation is blocked such as with the use of Frenzel lenses or infrared video goggles (Fig. 11-1). Nystagmus caused by a peripheral disorder such as a vestibular neuritis can be suppressed with fixation in room light. In the case of a peripheral vestibular lesion, nystagmus increases in intensity when the subject gazes toward the direction of the fast phase of the nystagmus. In contrast, nystagmus from central vestibular disorders is not decreased with fixation, and it may increase when the patient looks

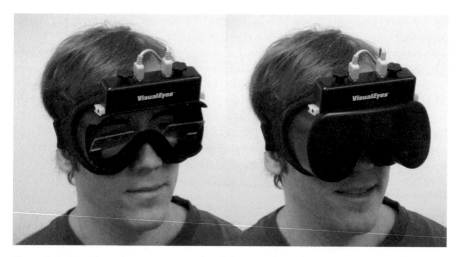

Figure 11-1. Frenzel goggles worn to magnify and illuminate the patient's eyes while blocking the ability of the patient to fixate his eyes. The Frenzel goggles allow the examiner to clearly see eye motions such as nystagmus. (Image furnished by Micromedical Technologies, 10 Kemp Drive, Chatham, IL 62629.)

in any direction. Saccades or abnormal eye motions with smooth pursuits may also indicate a central lesion. Although the physician conducted an MRI of the brain that was normal, more serious conditions affecting the brain are sometimes transient and can be missed.[27-29] A CT scan may be warranted to visualize the vestibular basilar artery system. The physical therapist can also assess the integrity and accuracy of the patient's VOR with the **head thrust or head impulse test**. The therapist conducts the head thrust test by having the patient fixate on an easily viewed target. The eyes are observed after the therapist turns the patient's head quickly 30° and in a direction that is unpredictable to the patient. If a refixation saccade is observed, the head thrust test is considered positive. This indicates a decreased VOR gain and confirms a peripheral lesion consistent with a vestibular hypofunction. Reported diagnostic accuracy of the head thrust test varies. When compared to bithermal caloric testing, specificity has been reported as 100%, but sensitivity was only 34%.[30] In the case of *severe* vestibular neural paresis, the head thrust test was very sensitive (87.5%), but the test was not useful in accurately detecting mild or moderate weakness.[30] Strategies have been employed to enhance the diagnostic accuracy of the head thrust test. When the test was performed with random amplitudes of head thrust, saccades were better detected.[31] Similarly, performing the test at higher accelerations improved results.[32] The authors of the latter study recommended repetition of the test to avoid false negatives. Sensitivity was improved to 71% and specificity to 82% when the head was pitched 30° downward and the timing and direction of the thrust were unpredictable.[33] As may be expected, the accuracy of the head thrust test was decreased when the patient performed a voluntary head movement during the test.[34]

It is essential to test the patient's dynamic visual acuity (DVA), balance, and gait. The DVA test is a functional test of the VOR. Dynamic visual acuity may be tested by utilizing an eye chart or by using a computer program. Computerized dynamic visual acuity is more accurate. When an eye chart is used, the difference between static visual acuity when the patient reads the chart with her head still is compared to when the therapist moves the patient's head at a frequency of 2 Hz. A difference of more than two lines on the eye chart between the static visual acuity and dynamic visual acuity is considered abnormal. The baseline static visual acuity test is also an assessment of visual integrity, which is another component of balance. The other major component of balance is somatosensation. Intact sensation of the feet and lower legs is especially important for balance. Vibration, proprioception, and light touch should be tested. There are numerous balance and gait tests. These include static tests of balance such as the Romberg and functional tests such as the Berg Balance Scale, Dynamic Gait Index, and Functional Gait Assessment. Because this patient had a previously high level of function, the Dynamic Gait Index or the Functional Gait Assessment was appropriate. This patient was also tested with computerized dynamic posturography. Coordination testing with the finger-to-nose test was negative, ruling out cerebellar involvement.

Plan of Care and Interventions

The goals of vestibular rehabilitation are to decrease dizziness, improve balance and gait, decrease or eliminate fear of falling, prevent falls, and improve dynamic visual acuity. The types of exercises used vary depending on the individual's subjective complaints and the results of the objective examination. However, typical interventions include adaptation exercises to improve dynamic visual acuity and balance, habituation exercises to decrease dizziness, gait training on variable surfaces and with head motions, patient and caregiver education regarding the vestibular disorder and its prognosis, and a home exercise program.

A common dynamic visual acuity or gaze stabilization exercise involves instructing the patient to turn her head rapidly for 30 seconds to 1 minute while fixating her gaze on an object that is a few feet away. The patient should be instructed to turn her head at a speed that she can see the image clearly. The patient is typically instructed to perform this exercise for 30 seconds to 1 minute, 5 to 10 times per day. Exercise progression includes focusing on targets that are further away and then performing the exercise during ambulation. The goal of this exercise is to promote adaptation of the vestibulo-ocular system.

There are numerous balance exercises appropriate for a patient with balance impairments due to vestibular neuritis. The therapist may ask the patient to progressively narrow her base of support while maintaining postural control. Single limb, tandem, and Romberg stance are examples. The therapist may manipulate the environment by having the patient stand on a compliant surface such as foam. Head or body turns can then be added to increase the challenge. Gait should be progressively challenged on level and uneven surfaces and slopes.

Habituation exercises are frequently prescribed for individuals with peripheral vestibular impairments. These exercises involve asking the patient to repeat movements that may elicit some dizziness in an effort to train the central nervous system to be "less dizzy." Because the experience of a vestibular disorder can be very frightening and can feel life-threatening, the patient may be fearful of movements that elicit dizziness. Patients often need reassurance of the potential benefits of these exercises. They should be educated that these movements may ultimately help decrease symptoms and improve function. The progression of the exercises should be tailored to the specific needs of the patient.

Various forms of **vestibular rehabilitation (VR) exercises** have been shown to facilitate recovery from vestibular disorders. In a retrospective analysis of 20 patients diagnosed with either central or peripheral dysfunction, Badke et al.[35] reported significant improvements in balance, visual acuity, and gait stability after participation in individualized VR programs. Scores on the Dynamic Gait Index improved in 95% of the subjects; 58% demonstrated improvements in dynamic visual acuity. In 53 adults with *chronic* vertigo complaints for at least 2 months (that was not due to Meniere's disease, BPPV, acute vestibular neuronitis or labyrinthitis, or history of head trauma), Cohen and Kimball[36] showed that even a simple home exercise program of VR exercises (designed to take 5-10 minutes and performed 5 times per day) resulted in greater independence and decreased vertigo within 30 to 45 days. In a study with more comprehensive VR and objective outcome measures, Horak et al.[37] randomly assigned patients with chronic unilateral vestibular hypofunction to one of three groups: (1) a customized program of VR including gaze stability, habituation, and balance exercises; (2) general conditioning exercises, or (3) vestibular suppressant medications. These authors found that only the VR group reported significantly decreased dizziness and improved postural stability as measured by postural sway and single limb stance. The other two groups showed no improvement. In a prospective, randomized controlled study, Herdman et al.[38] compared the effect of vestibular exercises involving head motions to placebo exercises on changes in dynamic visual acuity in 21 adults with unilateral vestibular hypofunction. Only the group that performed exercises in which they turned their head rapidly and stabilized their gaze significantly improved visual acuity in both predictable and unpredictable motions.

A 2011 Cochrane review by Hillier and McDonnell[39] concluded that there is moderate to strong evidence supporting the efficacy of VR for the symptoms of unilateral peripheral vestibular dysfunction (UPVD). The review summarized the results of 27 trials including 1668 subjects. The included trials compared VR to control or placebo treatment or to other treatment (*e.g.*, pharmacological), or comparisons of different types of VR. VR included any combination of habituation exercises, eye and head coordination motions, balance training, gait training, and patient education on their disorders. The authors concluded that moderate evidence supports that VR can result in symptom resolution and improvements on subjective and objective outcomes measures of gait, balance, vision, and activities of daily living that were maintained for 3 to 12 months after VR in studies with follow-up assessments. There were no reported adverse effects of VR. Since the studies were a heterogeneous mix of trials, there is no clear evidence to support the ideal frequency, timing, intensity, or specific VR exercises. However, even a minimal home exercise program was shown to be effective.

Evidence-Based Clinical Recommendations

SORT: Strength of Recommendation Taxonomy
A: Consistent, good-quality patient-oriented evidence
B: Inconsistent or limited-quality patient-oriented evidence
C: Consensus, disease-oriented evidence, usual practice, expert opinion, or case series

1. The Activities-Specific Balance Confidence (ABC) scale has good intra- and inter-rater reliability and has been validated for use in patients with vestibular disorders. **Grade B**

2. The head thrust test has high specificity, allowing a physical therapist to confidently *rule in* a diagnosis of peripheral vestibular hypofunction. **Grade B**

3. Vestibular rehabilitation is effective for the management of unilateral peripheral disorders such as vestibular neuritis. **Grade A**

COMPREHENSION QUESTIONS

11.1 Which of the following descriptions of nystagmus is most consistent with an acute (4 days) left unilateral peripheral disorder?

A. Nystagmus that is purely vertical, observable in room light but not with fixation blocked, and that increases in intensity when the patient looks upward

B. Nystagmus that is likely not observable in room light, but may be seen with fixation blocked, that is mixed horizontal and torsional right nystagmus, and increases in intensity when the patient looks to the right

C. Nystagmus that is observable in either room light or with fixation blocked, torsional left beating, and does not increase in intensity in any direction that patient looks

D. No nystagmus observed with the patient in the Dix-Hallpike position

11.2 Which option *best* describes the psychometric properties of the head thrust or impulse test?

A. Low sensitivity for mild to moderate vestibular hypofunction

B. High sensitivity for severe vestibular lesions

C. Moderate to high sensitivity and specificity when the head is flexed 30° and thrust rapidly and in a direction unpredictable to the patient

D. All of the above

11.3   Habituation exercises are a component of vestibular rehabilitation. The premise behind these exercises is to:

A.   Avoid head motion until dizziness completely goes away.

B.   Perform rapid and repeated head motions to induce severe vertigo to the point of extreme nausea and loss of balance.

C.   Gradually perform head and body movements that induce dizziness until symptoms are alleviated.

D.   Take vestibular suppressants to desensitize the nervous system over time.

ANSWERS

11.1   **B.** With a unilateral peripheral vestibular disorder (UPVD), the patient may be able to suppress the nystagmus in room light, especially after the third day since the onset of symptoms. The patient will likely not be able to suppress the nystagmus if visual fixation is blocked by Frenzel goggles. With a UPVD, nystagmus will be mixed horizontal and torsional and occur in the direction of the intact ear—in this case, the right ear, since the person has left UPVD. According to Alexander's law, nystagmus will also increase when the patient looks toward the fast phase (left in this case).

11.2   **D.** The head thrust test has been reported to have a sensitivity of 34% and a specificity of 100% for detecting unilateral vestibular hypofunction when compared to bithermal caloric testing. The sensitivity of the test was improved with the head flexed 30° and when the thrust was random in amplitude and direction.

11.3   **B.** Habituation exercises involve repeated, gradual, and graded performance of exercises that induce dizziness with the goal of getting the nervous system accustomed to not being dizzy.

REFERENCES

1.   Herdman SJ. *Vestibular Rehabilitation*. 3rd ed. Philadelphia, PA: FA Davis; 2000.

2.   Herdman SJ, Clendaniel RA. *Vestibular Rehabilitation: A Competency Based Course*. Atlanta, GA: Emory School of Medicine and American Physical Therapy Association; 2006.

3.   Strupp M, Brandt T. Vestibular neuritis. *Semin Neurol*. 2009;29:509-519.

4.   Schubert MC, Minor LB. Vestibulo-ocular physiology underlying vestibular hypofunction. *Phys Ther*. 2004;84:273-284.

5.   Hain TC. Vestibular neuritis and labyrinthitis. http://www.tchain.com/otoneurology/disorders/unilat/vneurit.html. Accessed February 4, 2013.

6.   Dix MR, Hallpike CS. The pathology, symptomatology, and diagnosis of certain common disorders of the vestibular system. *Ann Otol Rhinol Laryngol*. 1952;61:987-1017.

7.   Lumio JS, Aho J. Vestibular neuronitis. *Ann Otol Rhino Laryngol*. 1965;74:264-270.

8.   Sperling H, Lesoine W. Neuronitis vestibularis. *HNO*. 1968;16:264-265.

9.   Aschan G, Stahle J. Vestibular neuritis: a nystagmographical study. *J Laryngol Otol*. 1956;70:497-511.

10. Hain TC, Uddin M. Pharmacological treatment of vertigo. *CNS Drugs*. 2003;17:85-100.

11. Cesarani A, Alpini D, Monti B, Raponi G. The treatment of acute vertigo. *Neurol Sci*. 2004;25: S26-S30.

12. Hiller SL, McDonnell M. Vestibular rehabilitation for unilateral peripheral dysfunction. *Cochrane Database Syst Rev*. 2011 Feb 16;2:CD0005397.

13. Lopez-Escamez JA, Lopez-Nevot A, Gamiz MJ, et al. Diagnosis of common causes of vertigo using a structured clinical history. *Acta Otorrinolaringol Esp*. 2000;51:25-30.

14. Jacobson GP, Newman CW. The development of the Dizziness Handicap Inventory. *Arch Otolaryngol Head Neck Surg*. 1990;116:424-427.

15. Whitney SL, Wrisley DM, Brown KE, Furman JM. Is perception of handicap related to functional performance in persons with vestibular dysfunction? *Otol Neurotol*. 2004;25:139-143.

16. Jacobson GP, Newman CW, Hunter L, Balzer GK. Balance function tests correlates of the Dizziness Handicap Inventory. *J Am Acad Audiol*. 1991;2:253-260.

17. Fielder H, Denholm SW, Lyons RA, Fielder CP. Measurement of health status in patients with vertigo. *Clin Otolaryngol Allied Sci*. 1996;21:124-126.

18. Enloe LJ, Shields RK. Evaluation of health-related quality of life measures in individuals with vestibular disease using disease-specific and general outcome measures. *Phys Ther*. 1997;77:890-903.

19. Powell LE, Myers AM. The Activities-specific Balance Confidence (ABC) scale. *J Gerontol A Biol Sci*. 1995;50:M28-M34.

20. Talley KM, Wyman JF, Gross CR. Psychometric properties of the activities-specific balance confidence scale and the survey of activities and fear of falling in older women. *J Am Geriatr Soc*. 2008;56:328-333.

21. Huang TT, Wang WS. Comparison of the three established measures of fear of falling in community-dwelling older adults: psychometric testing. *Int J Nurs Stud*. 2009;46:1313-1319.

22. Lajoie Y, Gallagher SP. Predicting falls within the elderly community: comparison of postural sway, reaction time, the Berg Balance Scale and the activities-specific balance confidence scale for comparing fallers and non-fallers. *Arch Gerontol Geriatr*. 2004;38:11-226.

23. Moore DS, Ellis R, Kosma M, Fabre JM, McCarter KS, Wood RH. Comparison of the validity of four fall-related psychological measures in a community-based falls risk screening. *Res Q Exerc Sport*. 2011;82:545-554.

24. Myers AM, Fletcher PC, Myers AH, Sherk W. Discriminative and evaluative properties of the activities-specific balance confidence (ABC) scale. *J Gerontol A Biol Sci*. 1998;53:M287-M294.

25. Whitney SL, Hudak MT, Marchetti GF. The activities-specific balance confidence scale and the dizziness handicap inventory: a comparison. *J Vestib Res*. 1999;9:253-259.

26. Legters K, Whitney SL, Porter R, Buczek F. The relationship between the activities-specific balance confidence scale and the dynamic gait index in peripheral vestibular dysfunction. *Physiother Res Int*. 2005;10:10-22.

27. Braun EM, Tomazic PV, Ropposch T, Nemetz U, Lackner A, Walsh C. Misdiagnosis of acute peripheral vestibulopathy in central nervous system ischemic infarction. *Otol Neurotol*. 2011;32:1518-1521.

28. Chen L, Lee W, Chambers BR, Dewey HM. Diagnostic accuracy of acute vestibular syndrome at the bedside in a stroke unit. *J Neurotol*. 2011;258:855-561.

29. Newman-Toker DE, Kattah JC, Alvernia JE, Wang DZ. Normal head impulse test differentiates acute cerebellar strokes from vestibular neuritis. *Neurology*. 2008;70(24 pt 2):2378-2385.

30. Beynon CG, Jani P, Beguley DM. A clinical evaluation of the head impulse test. *Clin Otolaryngol Allied Sci*. 1998;2:117-122.

31. Tjernstrom F, Nystrom A, Magnusson M. How to uncover the covert saccade during the head impulse test. *Otol Neurotol*. 2012;33:1583-1585.

32. Weber KP, Aw ST, Todd MJ, McGarvie LA, Curthoys IS, Halmagyi GM. Head impulse test in unilateral vestibular loss: vestibulo-ocular reflex and catch-up saccades. *Neurology*. 2008;70:454-463.

33. Schubert MC, Tusa RJ, Grine LE, Herdman SJ. Optimizing the sensitivity of the head thrust test for identifying vestibular dysfunction. *Phys Ther.* 2004;84:151-158.

34. Della Santina CC, Cremer PD, Carey JP, Minor LB. Comparison of the head thrust test with head autorotation test reveals that the vestibule-ocular reflex is enhanced during voluntary head movements. *Ach Otolaryngol Head Neck Surg.* 2002;128:1044-1054.

35. Badke MB, Shea TA, Miedaner JA, Grove CR. Outcomes after rehabilitation for adults with balance dysfunction. *Arch Phys Med Rehabil.* 2004;5:227-233.

36. Cohen HS, Kimball HT. Increased independence and decreased vertigo after vestibular rehabilitation. *Otolaryngol Head Neck Surg.* 2003;128:60-70.

37. Horak FB, Jones-Rycewicz C, Black FO, Shumway-Cook A. Effects of vestibular rehabilitation on dizziness and imbalance. *Otolaryngol Head Neck Surg.* 1992;106:175-180.

38. Herdman SJ, Schubert MC, Das VE, Tusa RJ. Recovery of dynamic visual acuity in unilateral vestibular hypofunction. *Ach Otolaryngol Head Neck Surg.* 2003;129:819-824.

39. Hillier SL, McDonnell M. Vestibular rehabilitation for unilateral peripheral dysfunction *Cochrane Database Syst Rev.* 2011 Feb 16;2:CD005397.

Bell's Palsy

Michael Furtado

A 64-year-old male presented to the emergency department after waking with acute facial nerve palsy. His main complaints were of right-sided facial drooping, difficulty keeping food or drink in his mouth, pain, and inability to blink or close his right eye. During the intake examination, he could not identify a precipitating event that led to the weakness, citing good health in the 3 months prior to onset. His past medical history was remarkable for hypertension, hypercholesterolemia, and shingles 10 years ago. Neurologic examination revealed slight movement of the muscles of the right side of face with an inability to close the right eye, raise the right eyebrow, sniffle, smile, pucker, or frown. The rest of the neurologic examination was within normal limits including light touch sensation to the right side of the face, intact jaw reflex, and intact ability to see and distinguish smells. The patient was not admitted to the hospital and was discharged with no specific laboratory testing or imaging studies performed. A diagnosis of Bell's palsy was made because of the idiopathic onset of signs and symptoms and the absence of other neurologic deficits. He was prescribed ibuprofen and prednisone to reduce pain and inflammation associated with facial nerve swelling, and was advised to visit his primary care physician (PCP). At the time of his follow-up visit with his PCP 10 days later, the patient reported no improvement in function and a worsening of facial weakness that continued for about 5 days after the initial onset. An electromyography (EMG) test was performed which demonstrated a motor response that was 25% of the amplitude of the left side. The physician decided to refer the patient to physical therapy. The physical therapist is evaluating the patient in an outpatient clinic 2 weeks after onset of the facial palsy. The patient is a retired engineer who is active in his community. He lives in a three-story home with his wife.

▶ What examination signs may be associated with this diagnosis?
▶ What are the most appropriate physical therapy interventions?
▶ Describe a physical therapy plan of care based on each stage of the diagnosis.
▶ What is his rehabilitation prognosis?
▶ Identify possible psychological/psychosocial factors apparent in this case.

KEY DEFINITIONS

BELL'S PALSY: Temporary facial paralysis (complete loss of movement) or paresis (weakness) resulting from damage or trauma to one (in some occurrences both) of the facial nerves; synonyms include: acute peripheral facial nerve palsy, idiopathic nerve palsy

BELL'S PHENOMENON: Rolling of the eyeball upward and outward when an attempt is made to close the eye on the affected side of the face

HYPERACUSIS: Increased sensitivity to sound in certain frequency ranges

PREDNISONE: Glucocorticoid given to decrease inflammation and suppress the immune system

SYNKINESIS: Abnormal regeneration of the facial nerve that results in a cross-wiring in the muscle motor end plates (e.g., when the patient smiles, the eyelid closes on the affected side)

Objectives

1. Describe Bell's palsy including the clinical presentation, differential diagnosis, diagnostic assessment, and medical intervention.

2. Discuss appropriate components of the physical therapy examination including the difference in grading schemes for facial muscle strength testing.

3. Identify key findings in the history of present illness, prior level of function, physical therapy examination, and/or psychosocial factors that may impact the prognosis.

4. Describe appropriate physical therapy interventions to treat a patient in varying stages of the condition.

5. Identify an outcome tool to measure function of the facial nerve.

6. Discuss the role of members of the healthcare team: neurologist, primary care physician, ear nose and throat physician, and speech language pathologist.

Physical Therapy Considerations

PT considerations during management of the individual with facial paralysis/paresis status/post onset of Bell's palsy:

▶ **General physical therapy plan of care/goals:** Prevent or minimize loss of flexibility in facial musculature; improve range of motion (ROM) of the temporomandibular joint; improve strength, functional capacity, and coordination of muscles responsible for facial movement; maximize functional independence in the management of paresis or paralysis while minimizing secondary impairments; improve quality of life and participation in life and societal roles

▶ **Physical therapy interventions**: Manual therapy (joint mobilizations, myofascial release); therapeutic exercise (stretching, strengthening, endurance training); modalities (neuromuscular electrical stimulation and/or biofeedback); neuromuscular re-education for improved coordination and timing; prescription of a home exercise program; patient education on progression of condition; adaptive devices to improve quality of life

▶ **Precautions during physical therapy**: Monitor vital signs and neurological status

▶ **Complications interfering with physical therapy**: Progressive or worsening paralysis, adverse drug reactions (ADRs) of glucocorticoids, hearing loss, severe pain, sudden change in neurological status (*e.g.*, extremity weakness, visual loss, change in sensation)

Understanding the Health Condition

Bell's palsy (also called idiopathic facial palsy), is an acute disorder of the facial nerve which may begin with pain in the mastoid region and partial or full paralysis on one side of the face.[1] Increasing evidence suggests that the main etiology of Bell's palsy is reactivation of latent herpes simplex virus type 1 in the cranial nerve ganglia.[2] However, the exact cause is not fully understood. Most cases of Bell's palsy are thought to be secondary to inflammatory or immune responses to viruses such as herpes zoster, adenovirus, rubella, or mumps.[3] Older literature describes Bell's palsy as a diagnosis of exclusion. That is, other conditions that can lead to facial palsy or paralysis must be ruled out: Lyme disease, human immunodeficiency virus (HIV), Ramsay Hunt syndrome, parotid gland tumors, meningeal processes, stroke, and intracranial tumors.[3-4] Therefore, the term *Bell's palsy* should be reserved for cases of facial paralysis in which signs and symptoms are consistent with the condition and in which a diligent search fails to identify another cause for the clinical findings.[4] Sixty years ago, Taverner[5] outlined the minimum diagnostic criteria to emphasize the diagnosis of Bell's palsy on the basis of specific clinical features. These include: (1) paralysis or paresis of all muscle groups on one side of the face; (2) sudden onset; (3) absence of signs of central nervous system (CNS) disease; (4) absence of signs of ear or cerebellopontine angle disease.

The estimated annual incidence of Bell's palsy is 20 to 30 patients per 100,000. The peak incidence appears to be in individuals over 70 years old and pregnant females (especially during the third trimester and/or 1 week postpartum). Older age, pregnancy, and diabetes mellitus appear to be risk factors for the development of Bell's palsy.[4] The male-to-female ratio for Bell's palsy is approximately equal, except for predominance in women younger than 20 years of age and a slight predominance in men older than 40 years. In both sexes, 40 years is the median age of onset.[3,6] The left and right sides of the face appear to be equally affected; 30% of patients have incomplete unilateral paralysis on presentation, and bilateral paralysis occurs in 0.3% of patients.[7] It has been estimated that 9% of patients with Bell's palsy have a history of at least one episode of previous facial paralysis, and a family history of Bell's palsy has been linked in 8% of patients.[6]

The onset of Bell's palsy is typically sudden and signs and symptoms tend to peak in less than 48 hours. The most common clinical presentation includes acute onset of unilateral upper and lower facial paralysis/paresis, posterior auricular pain, decreased tearing, hyperacusis, taste disturbances, and/or otalgia.[8] The paralysis/paresis *must* include the forehead and lower aspect of the face. If the paralysis/paresis involves only the lower portion of the face, a central cause is typically suspected.[8] The degree of injury to the facial nerve depends on how proximally the nerve is affected and the extent of involvement of its associated branches.[3] Progression of the paralysis/ paresis is possible, but it usually does not progress beyond 7 to 10 days after onset.[8] Maximal weakness can last up to 3 weeks after onset. Patients frequently report an inability to close the eye or to smile on the affected side as well as numbness on the side of the paralysis. Some authors believe numbness is secondary to involvement of the trigeminal nerve, whereas others argue that this symptom is probably due to lack of mobility of the facial muscles and not due to a direct impairment of sensory innervation.[8]

The natural course of Bell's palsy varies from early complete recovery to substantial nerve injury with permanent sequelae such as persistent paralysis and synkinesis. Prognostically, patients fall into three groups.[8] In Group 1, individuals have complete recovery of facial motor function without sequelae. In Group 2, there is incomplete recovery of facial motor function, but no cosmetic defects are apparent to the untrained eye. In Group 3, individuals have permanent neurologic sequelae that are cosmetically and clinically apparent. The prognosis for most patients with Bell's palsy is excellent: 80% to 90% recover completely within 6 weeks to 3 months.[9] The most important prognostic factor is whether the paralysis is incomplete or complete. The prognosis for affected persons in whom complete facial paralysis never develops is excellent: 95% to 100% with no identifiable sequelae.[9] Factors associated with a poor outcome include: hyperacusis, decreased tearing, age older than 60 years, diabetes mellitus, hypertension, and severe aural, anterior facial, or radicular pain.[10] Individuals aged 60 years or older have an approximately 40% chance of complete recovery and have a higher rate of sequelae. In contrast, younger individuals (< 30 years of age) have an 85% to 90% chance of a complete recovery without long-term sequelae.[8] Of those who do not recover completely, about 23% are left with either moderate to severe symptoms, partial motor recovery, tears upon salivation, contracture, or synkinesis.[1,8] The prognosis also depends to a great extent on the time at which recovery begins with early recovery predicting a good prognosis and late recovery predicting a bad prognosis. If recovery begins within 1 week after onset, 88% obtain full recovery. With recovery within 1 to 2 weeks, 83% obtain full recovery, and in those who experience recovery within 2 to 3 weeks, 61% obtain full recovery.[11] It has been noted that patients can achieve partial to full recovery 2 to 3 months after onset, although it is much less likely.

A complete medical diagnostic work-up is not indicated for most cases of Bell's palsy because the diagnosis depends on the history and physical examination. However, if the clinical findings are doubtful or if paralysis lasts longer than 6 to 8 weeks, further investigations are recommended.[3,8] Recommended laboratory tests depend on the patient's symptoms, but may include serum glucose level, complete blood cell count, cerebrospinal fluid analysis, and testing for HIV and antibodies to the bacterium that causes Lyme disease. Electrodiagnostic tests of the motor branches of the facial nerve have been used to assess function and predict outcome. However, testing should be delayed because abnormalities will not be evident until nerve degeneration has reached the site of stimulation, which is usually 4 to 5 days after onset of signs and symptoms of Bell's palsy. Initially, facial motor response is normal and then rapidly decreases depending on the severity of the lesion. Facial motor function is compared to the contralateral (unaffected) side; a motor response that is 10% of the amplitude of the unaffected side has been defined as a critical value in which recovery was poor.[3,12] Imaging studies are not usually indicated unless there is fracture of the skull such as in a trauma, or if there is suspicion of other CNS involvement. If so, a computerized tomography (CT) scan of the temporal bone or magnetic resonance image (MRI) of the brain is recommended.

Management of Bell's palsy has evolved over time. Currently, there are no clinical practice guidelines that are regularly followed. The spontaneous recovery and excellent prognosis that the majority of individuals encounter make it difficult for clinicians to determine best practice guidelines. Medical treatments currently advocated include glucocorticoids, surgical decompression, and/or antiviral agents.[12] Nonpharmacological interventions include observation ("wait and see"), physical therapy, and/or acupuncture. Reviews suggest that physical therapy may result in faster recovery and reduced sequelae when compared to no intervention, but further randomized controlled trials are needed to confirm any benefit.[13] Initially, the focus of management is on protecting the cornea from drying and abrasions due to impaired eye closure and tear production. Eye drops, ointment, and/or an eye patch are often recommended to protect the eye. The main goals of treatment then become to improve facial nerve function and reduce the potential for further facial nerve damage.

In 2001, the American Academy of Neurology published a practice parameter stating that glucocorticoids are *probably* effective and the addition of an antiviral agent such as acyclovir (with prednisone) is only possibly effective for treatment of Bell's palsy.[14] Thus, glucocorticoid therapy has become the most common approach to the management of Bell's palsy.[15] In a meta-analysis, Ramsey and colleagues[16] concluded that patients treated with glucocorticoids had a 17% better chance of complete recovery than patients who did not receive glucocorticoids. Further, they concluded that the odds of recovery with glucocorticoid treatment ranged from 49% to 97% versus 23% to 64% for untreated patients. Thus, the emerging consensus is that recovery time is shorter when individuals are treated with glucocorticoids, and that antivirals do not provide much improvement compared to placebo. This has led to most treatment guidelines recommending prednisone (although dosage and frequency are not agreed upon). However, some authors still recommend treatment with antivirals, especially if a viral etiology is suspected.[3] Surgical intervention, which may include facial nerve decompression, subocularis oculi fat (SOOF) lift, implantable devices placed into the eyelid, transposition of the temporalis muscle, facial nerve grafting, and direct brow lift, is controversial and typically only considered when patients have not responded to medical therapy and have > 90% axonal degeneration on electrodiagnostic testing. Surgical decompression of the facial nerve appears promising, but it has been difficult to assemble a large enough series of patients to definitively establish its value. In addition, it is associated with the possibility of significant additional injury. Individuals with a poor prognosis identified by facial nerve testing or persistent paralysis appear to benefit the most from surgical intervention such as facial nerve decompression. However, results from studies have been mixed as far as how much benefit or recovery is gained.[14]

Physical Therapy Patient/Client Management

Individuals with Bell's palsy can present to physical therapy in different stages of the condition. Most often, a patient presents to an outpatient neurorehabilitation facility. The typical course of treatment is that of emergency management in the hospital upon onset of the facial paralysis. After excluding more serious pathologies, the patient is discharged home. Then, the patient usually meets with a primary care physician or neurologist for medical management. Depending on the course of action selected, the patient may be referred to physical therapy, provided medication, and/or instructed to continue to monitor and observe symptoms. Some patients may be seen acutely in physical therapy while others may be seen 2 months or more after initial onset if other treatments have failed or signs/symptoms have not completely resolved. A patient may also be referred to speech therapy for management of swallowing difficulties or speech deficits. A psychologist or psychiatrist may be involved to handle emotional stress experienced by the patient. The physical therapist must be empathetic and sensitive to the patient's frustration as this disorder potentially has a negative impact on self-esteem. Patients may avoid social situations and may not view themselves positively because their cosmetic appearance has changed. Overall, their participation and activity in social, personal, and professional roles may be diminished. Since there is an overall excellent prognosis for Bell's palsy, the physical therapist can be optimistic yet realistic about prognosis, citing that some signs and symptoms may persist over time. The role of the physical therapist is to create a plan of care that optimizes functional recovery and minimizes loss of movement. Other specific roles are to provide patient education and reassurance. These include, but are not limited to, advising the patient to be compliant with the prescribed medication regimen, decrease exposure to lighting, and use eye drops/eye patch, if the eye is involved. The therapist should assess ROM, strength, and functional movement while also considering postural imbalance, provide interventions for pain and neuromuscular re-education, facilitate improved muscle contraction and facial symmetry, design a home exercise program, and prevent secondary complications that may occur.

Examination, Evaluation, and Diagnosis

The patient examination begins with an interview that should include the following information: (1) present history (date of onset, progression of condition); (2) course of treatment (physicians seen, medical recommendations, results of imaging and/or diagnostic tests); (3) past medical history (relevant medical problems/comorbidities); (4) social history (occupation and current status, hobbies, marital status, living situation); (5) psychological impact (emotional status); (6) patient's goals; and (7) medication list. Since glucocorticoids are often prescribed, it is important to ask the dosage and how the physician is weaning the patient from the medication. This is important because of the ADRs associated with long-term glucocorticoid use which include hyperglycemia, increased risk of infections, osteoporosis, suppressed adrenal gland hormone production, slower wound healing, and easy bruising.[17] The patient may also be taking an antiviral medication; it is prudent for the physical therapist to investigate the ADRs of the specific antiviral. Following a thorough history taking, a systems review should be performed. Priority should be given to the neurological system focusing on screening of cranial nerve function and postural control. Performing a screen of extremity strength, sensation, and muscle tone should be included, especially if the patient complains of secondary complications. This is crucial to determine if the patient is experiencing idiopathic facial nerve palsy or if he has an undiagnosed CNS or medical disorder. If the physical therapist is suspicious of a concomitant disorder or observes signs and symptoms that do not match facial nerve paralysis, immediate referral to the primary care physician and/or neurologist is warranted.

During the history and systems review, the physical therapist should observe facial symmetry and movement. Many clinicians take videos or photographs to document baseline symmetry as well as subsequent progression. The following should be observed and documented: facial symmetry (*i.e.*, eyebrow lift on the involved side, drawing of the lips to the uninvolved side), facial movement, synkinesis, lacrimation, and/or Bell's phenomenon. Sensation testing will depend on the specific modality being tested. It is typically advisable to test any exteroceptive sensation that the patient complains of lacking (*e.g.*, light touch, temperature, pain discrimination, taste). However, a true Bell's palsy affecting the facial nerve should only present with loss of taste on the anterior two-thirds of the tongue. The information regarding taste can be obtained via history taking, but the clinician should test overall sensation as a screen for other CNS signs and symptoms.

For individuals with Bell's palsy, the most frequent locations of pain are over the mastoid, at the exit point of the facial nerve at the internal auditory meatus, and the cervical spine (due to compensatory posture following onset). Although not studied for reliability or validity in this patient population, the visual analog scale (VAS) and the numeric pain rating scale (NPRS) are frequently used. The VAS has been used in a randomized controlled trial looking at the effectiveness of prednisone on pain.[18] The VAS has excellent test-retest reliability[19] and the NPRS has good convergent validity with the VAS.[20] Therefore, either scale could be used in this patient population.

In terms of ROM, it is prudent to assess the temporomandibular joint. Although the muscles of mastication are primarily innervated by the trigeminal nerve, the decreased facial movement (due to involvement of the buccinator muscle) can make chewing difficult. Thus, decreased movement at this joint can lead to hypomobility. There are standardized testing procedures to measure depression, protrusion, and lateral deviation of the mandible. Normative values for adults are 43 cm of depression, 7 cm of protrusion, and 9 cm of lateral deviation.[21] While measuring ROM, the physical therapist can also assess mobility of the temporomandibular joint and the myofascial tightness of the musculature surrounding it (*e.g.*, pterygoids, masseter).

Facial muscle strength is tested in a systematic way to assess the functional movement of the face. Muscles innervated by the cranial nerves are not scored in the same manner as other muscles (*e.g.*, by manual muscle tests) because they do not have a bony lever. Instead, strength can be measured as described by Daniels and Worthingham's Muscle Testing Examination that classifies the muscles of the face as functional (F), weak functional (WF), nonfunctional (NF), or absent (0).[22] Typically, a muscle that is classified as "F" can perform a specific action and hold against resistance. A muscle that is classified as "WF" can almost go through the full specific action and functional task. A muscle that is classified as "NF" is one that likely only has a quiver or flicker of contraction that does not perform the specific action or task the therapist is looking for. A muscle classified as "0" means the muscle has no movement. Table 12-1 lists the most common facial muscles tested and the specific action or functional task the intact muscle should be able to perform. When grading, the therapist should also note synkinesis, lack of coordination (*e.g.*, inability to perform left and right when asked), and speed (*e.g.*, number of repetitions in 10 seconds).

Measurement of facial nerve function in a consistent, reliable way has been a challenge for many years. The difficulty stems from the inherent complexity of the facial nerve itself since it controls multiple regions of the face as well as lacrimation, salivation, and taste. Any composite measure of overall facial nerve function therefore must attempt to qualify or quantify these different types of functions into one common scale.[23] There are a few scales that have been created and used in the rehabilitation setting that include: (1) House-Brackmann Scale (HBS), (2) Burres-Fisch system, (3) Nottingham system, (4) Sunnybrook scale. Due to the inherent subjectivity of descriptions of facial expression, there is inter-observer variation when assessing a patient with *any* of these scales. The House-Brackmann Scale was introduced in 1983 and was endorsed by the Facial Nerve Disorders Committee of the American Academy of Otolaryngology.[24] Ever since the HBS was adopted into clinical practice, several of its shortcomings have been identified. For example, the HBS cannot distinguish finer differences in facial function well because it is a gross

Table 12-1 FACIAL MUSCLE STRENGTH TESTING	
Muscle	Functional Action
Frontalis	Raising the eyebrow
Corrugator	Frowning, draw eyebrows in
Orbicularis oculi	Closing the eye
Procerus	Wrinkle the nose
Dilator nasalis	Flare nostrils
Risorius	Smile without teeth
Zygomaticus major	Smile with teeth, laughing
Orbicularis oris	Purse lips/pucker
Levator anguli oris	Smile with teeth; unilateral = sneering

scale. As new surgical procedures for facial nerve repair and reanimation emerge, the HBS is not sensitive enough to quantify small changes. The subjectivity in the middle scores of the HBS lead to inter-observer error.[25] Last, throughout the grading scale there is ambiguity regarding secondary defects such as synkinesis, contracture, and spasm. These shortcomings of the HBS led to the development of additional grading scales. However, they have been studied less and have not been widely adopted for reasons such as time and expensive equipment requirements. Therefore, the use of the HBS is acceptable in a clinical setting. When documenting the progress of a patient with Bell's palsy, it is important to note observed subtle changes and secondary defects while considering improvement in function. Table 12-2 describes the classification of facial function for the HBS.

Up to this point in the assessment, many of the tests and measures have focused on body function and structure or impairments. Since disorders of the facial neuromuscular system can result in marked disfigurement of the face and difficulties in activities of daily living such as eating, drinking, and communicating, an individual with Bell's palsy often has deficits in his activity or participation in multiple roles. Clinical researchers from the Facial Nerve Center at the University of Pittsburgh Medical Center recognized the lack of disability measures in the management of

Table 12-2 HOUSE-BRACKMANN SCALE FOR CLASSIFICATION OF FACIAL FUNCTION[26]

Grade	Degree	Gross	At Rest	In Motion
		Description		
		Gross	At Rest	In Motion
1	Normal	Normal facial function in all nerve branches	Normal facial function in all nerve branches	Normal facial function in all nerve branches
2	Slight	Slight weakness on close inspection, slight asymmetry	Normal tone and symmetry	Forehead: good to moderate movement; eye: complete closure with minimum effort; mouth: slight asymmetry
3	Moderate	Obvious but not disfiguring facial asymmetry. Synkinesis is noticeable but not severe, may have hemi-facial spasm or contracture	Normal tone and symmetry	Forehead: slight to moderate movement; eye: complete closure with effort; mouth: slight weakness with maximum effort
4	Moderately severe	Asymmetry is disfiguring and/or obvious facial weakness	Normal tone and symmetry	Forehead: no movement; eye: incomplete closure; mouth: asymmetrical with maximum effort
5	Severe	Only slight, barely noticeable movement	Asymmetrical facial appearance	Forehead: no movement; eye: incomplete closure; mouth: slight movement
6	Total paralysis	No facial function	No facial function	No facial function

Reproduced with permission from House JW, Brackmann DE. Facial nerve grading system. Otolaryngol Head Neck Surg. 1985;93;146-147.

individuals with Bell's palsy. In 1996, they introduced the **Facial Disability Index (FDI)**. It is a disease-specific measure for disorders of the face that is a brief, self-report questionnaire of physical disability and psychosocial factors related to facial neuromuscular function.[27] It is subdivided into two domains: physical function and social/well-being function. A score of 100 on each domain demonstrates that the individual has no difficulty in physical functioning and has not experienced any social/well-being dysfunction any time in his daily living. The tool is quick, easy to administer, and simple to score. VanSwearingen and Brach[27] demonstrated that the FDI is reliable with a good internal consistency score for both domains. In the physical functioning subscale, construct validity was demonstrated by correlation with a clinician's physical examination of facial movement; in the social/well-being subscale, construct validity was demonstrated by correlation with psychosocial status on the 36-Item Short-Form Health Survey. In a physical therapy clinic, the FDI is recommended to determine the impact of Bell's palsy on activity limitations and participation restrictions.

Plan of Care and Interventions

The frequency of treatment sessions and specific interventions selected differ according to the severity and prognosis of each patient. Electrodiagnostic testing performed by the physician can identify the type of facial nerve injury, which can guide the physical therapist in selecting a particular type of intervention. Different types of nerve injuries include conduction block (neuropraxia), axonal degeneration, and neurotmesis. A conduction block such as a neuropraxia typically recovers quickly. Axonal degeneration takes longer to recover because nerve regeneration needs to occur prior to muscle reinnervation. Neurotmesis is a complete disruption of the nerve in which regenerating axons may not reconnect with the original target muscle. This most severe nerve injury results in an incomplete recovery. It is recommended that individuals with Bell's palsy receive physical therapy interventions: 3 times per week for individuals with severe deficits in the acute stage of Bell's palsy; twice per week for individuals with moderate deficits or in the subacute stage; and, once per week for individuals with minimal deficits or in the chronic stage.[28] Individuals should be referred to the physician for further evaluation if no progress is noticed upon re-examination. Recovery rates vary from rapid to over 1 year.[28]

If an individual is experiencing severe deficits such as severe resting asymmetry, minimal to no voluntary movement, and impaired function (but without synkinesis), "**initiation exercises**" are recommended. These exercises may include mobility exercises of the temporomandibular joint, muscle flexibility exercises (with taping to help reduce droop or muscle lengthening), and active assisted range of motion (AAROM) exercises. For AAROM exercises, the patient should be in a gravity-reduced position (supine) and taught to use his hand to place a muscle at a position specific to a motion (e.g., pucker, close eye, smile) and then slowly remove his hand and try to maintain the position. In this stage, it is common for the eye to be significantly impaired. An exercise that appears to allow the patient to control the Bell's phenomenon can be performed. The patient focuses both eyes on an object positioned down and in front of the patient while trying to close both eyes. Focusing the eyes downward theoretically helps initiate lowering of the upper eyelid, preventing the Bell's phenomenon.[28,29] Since the patient is susceptible to fatigue in this stage, a prescription of low-intensity, high-frequency exercise is beneficial. In most clinical practice and in a case report, the exercise prescription includes less than 10 repetitions of a particular motion the patient is lacking, up to 3 to 4 times per day.[28] In this phase, the patient should also be educated on the process of recovery and/or the use of a sleep aid such as an eye patch.

Once the patient has increased voluntary movement with no synkinesis, it is appropriate to begin "**facilitation exercises.**" These exercises may include tasks to increase movement that is emerging and manual therapy to improve mobility and flexibility of joint and muscle (joint mobilizations, facial stretching exercises). Facilitation exercises also involve symmetrical active facial movements without allowing the uninvolved side to take over the specific action required (*e.g.*, if left side is involved, right side pulls cheek up too high in a smile with teeth). Placing the uninvolved side in a shortened position will impact the length of the muscles on the involved side. If the patient is not experiencing signs of synkinesis and the muscle strength grade is at least weak functional (WF), introducing resistance exercises with manual holds using the patient's hand is appropriate as long as there is neither overcontraction of the uninvolved side nor synkinesis. Fatigue is not a concern at this stage and increasing repetitions is important to improve endurance. The therapist can adjust the exercise prescription to 3 sets of 10 repetitions performed twice per day (or until the patient demonstrates fatigue or poor form).[28] Functional exercises should be introduced to keep the activities meaningful: drinking from a straw of wide diameter and progressing to small diameter, blowing kisses, closing eyes, etc. In this time period, the patient may continue to need additional equipment to manage daily tasks such as sleeping (eye patch) or eating (larger straws to prevent drooling) and continued education on the recovery process.

At some point within the recovery phase, it is likely that inappropriate muscle activity such as abnormal, overcompensated movement will be apparent with or without synkinesis. Once this occurs, it is important to introduce relaxation techniques while working on movement control. Exercises can still focus on facilitating normal movement on the involved side, but now the patient is cautioned to control or inhibit the abnormal movement. Typically, it is helpful to provide the patient feedback using biofeedback or a mirror for self-correction. The patient is instructed to perform a specific action as much as possible without eliciting synkinesis. For example, the patient may work on keeping the eye open while smiling without showing his teeth. If his eye closes while smiling, he is instructed to let the eye open and smile while maintaining the eye open. The exercise can be progressed as long as there is no impaired or synkinetic movement. In this phase, it is best to focus on the *quality* of each movement and not quantity. Asking the patient to perform as many repetitions as possible with good form several times per day is generally indicated.[28] Strengthening may continue until the patient has functional strength without synkinesis.

There are few high-quality randomized controlled trials supporting physical therapy interventions in patients with Bell's palsy. Due to the overall excellent recovery rate, difficulty with classifying the stage of Bell's palsy, and the unique presentation of each patient, evidence supporting physical therapy interventions is generally lacking. In a study by Manikandan[30] in 2007, 59 patients were randomly divided into two groups: one received "conventional exercise" and the other received individualized **facial neuromuscular re-education** 3 times per day for 2 weeks. Both groups statistically improved function based on the Facial Grading Scale, but the neuromuscular re-education group improved significantly more. In 2004, Beurskens and Heymans[31] looked at archived data of over 155 patients with Bell's palsy who received mime therapy (described as facial exercises that the patient mimics) with significant observed improvements in facial symmetry and functioning. Similar studies had findings that support exercise in the treatment of Bell's palsy, but the description of the type of exercise is limited.[28,31] Through clinical experience, individualized therapeutic exercise is an excellent form of rehabilitation for patients with Bell's palsy. Modalities are commonly used in the clinical setting and should be considered in the plan of care, including electrical stimulation, electromyography biofeedback, short-wave diathermy, ultrasound, and laser. Electrotherapy has been used clinically to improve the function of an intact facial nerve. In general, electrotherapy is still lacking strong evidence to support its use due to inappropriate research methodology, small sample size, undefined treatment parameters, and inconsistent follow-up.[32] There is currently no evidence to support electrical stimulation in the acute stage of Bell's palsy (defined as the first 10 days), but it appears to be effective in a more subacute or chronic stage.[32] Caution must also be undertaken with a regenerating nerve because electrical stimulation can be a contraindication.[32] Therefore, it is best to discuss with the referring physician *prior* to eliciting this modality. Biofeedback has been found to be therapeutically effective when muscle activity is present; this can be used for facilitation or relaxation.[28,32,33] No evidence supports any benefit of using continuous mode short-wave diathermy, but pulse mode may facilitate healing in acute Bell's palsy. Ultrasound may be beneficial for acute Bell's palsy, but research has not investigated its long-term effect.[28]

Evidence-Based Clinical Recommendations

SORT: Strength of Recommendation Taxonomy
A: Consistent, good-quality patient-oriented evidence
B: Inconsistent or limited-quality patient-oriented evidence
C: Consensus, disease-oriented evidence, usual practice, expert opinion, or case series

1. A patient with Bell's palsy can be assessed with the Facial Disability Index to quantify restrictions in physical functioning and social/well-being functioning. **Grade C**

2. Initiation and facilitation exercises targeting specific facial muscles decrease the presence of motor synkinesis and contracture and improve function in individuals with Bell's palsy. **Grade B**

3. Facial neuromuscular re-education facilitates symmetrical movement and controls undesired gross motor activity (*e.g.*, synkinesis) in individuals with Bell's palsy. **Grade B**

COMPREHENSION QUESTIONS

12.1 If a patient with Bell's palsy presents with weak functional strength of the frontalis, orbicularis oculi, and orbicularis oris with some facial drooping on the right side and eyelid closure noted with smiling, which of the following House-Brackmann grades would the patient be classified as?

A. Grade 1

B. Grade 2

C. Grade 3

D. Grade 4

12.2 A physical therapist is working with a patient with Bell's palsy whose onset of symptoms was 3 weeks ago. The patient presents with severe resting facial droop, minimal to no voluntary movement on the right side of the face, and difficulty closing the right eye to sleep. Which of the following intervention strategies would *best* improve the patient's impairments and functional limitations at this time?

A. Electrical stimulation

B. Active assisted facial exercises

C. Ultrasound

D. Biofeedback

ANSWERS

12.1 **C.** The muscle scores indicate that this patient has movement of the forehead, eye, and mouth that is functional, but weak. The facial drooping and movement of the eyelid with smiling indicates asymmetry and synkinesis. Therefore, the best grade for this patient in the House-Brackmann scale is a grade of 3.

12.2 **B.** This patient appears to be in the acute stage of Bell's palsy. Evidence supports the use of exercise more than modalities in the acute stage of Bell's palsy. Ultrasound may be beneficial in the acute stage, but this patient requires active assisted exercises to improve the ability to close the eye for sleep, and improve facial droop (option C). Without further information about the quality and injury to the facial nerve, electrical stimulation would not be indicated (option A). Biofeedback would also not be indicated because the patient does not have facial movement at this time (option D).

REFERENCES

1. Valenca MM, Valenca LP, Lima MC. Idiopathic facial paralysis (Bell's palsy): a study of 180 patients. *Arq Neuro Psiquiatr.* 2001;59:733-739.

2. Holland NJ, Weiner GM. Recent developments in Bell's palsy. *BMJ.* 2004;329:553-557.

3. Sladky J. Bell's Palsy: Diseases and Disorders. www.expertconsult.com. Accessed December 31, 2011.

4. Flint PW, Haughey BH, Lund VJ, Mattox DE. *Clinical Disorders of the Facial Nerve in Cummings Otolaryngology: Head and Neck Surgery.* 5th ed. Philadelphia, PA: Mosby Elsevier; 2010.

5. Taverner D. The prognosis and treatment of spontaneous facial palsy. *Proc R Soc Med.* 1959;52:1077.

6. Adour KK, Byl FM, Hilsinger RL, Jr, Kahn ZM, Sheldon MI. The true nature of Bell's palsy: analysis of 1000 consecutive patients. *Laryngoscope.* 1978;88:787-801.

7. Peitersen E. Natural history of Bell's palsy. *Acta Otolaryngol Suppl.* 1992;492:122-124.

8. Taylor DC, Keegan M. Bell palsy. http://emedicine.medscape.com/article/1146903-overview. Accessed December 31, 2011.

9. Katusic SK, Beard CM, Wiederholt WC, et al. Incidence, clinical features, and prognosis in Bell's palsy: Rochester, Minnesota, 1968-1982. *Ann Neurol.* 1986;20:622-627.

10. Adour KK, Wingerd J, Bell DN, Manning JJ, Hurley JP. Prednisone treatment for idiopathic facial paralysis (Bell's palsy). *N Engl J Med.* 1972;287:1268-1272.

11. Teixeira LJ, Soares BG, Vieria VP, Prado GF. Physical therapy for Bell's palsy (idiopathic facial paralysis). *Cochrane Database Syst Rev.* 2008;Jul 16(3):CD006283.

12. Manni JJ, Stennert E. Diagnostic methods in facial nerve pathology. *Adv Otorhinolaryngol.* 1984;34:202-213.

13. Cardoso JR, Teixeira EC, Moreira MD, et al. Effects of exercises on Bell's palsy: systematic review of randomized controlled trials. *Otol Neurotol.* 2008;29:557-560.

14. Grogan PM, Gronseth GS. Practice parameter: steroids, acyclovir, and surgery for Bell's palsy (an evidence-based review). Report of the Quality Standards Subcommittee of the American Academy of Neurology. *Neurology.* 2001;56:830-836.

15. American Academy of Otolaryngology—Head and Neck Surgery, Committee on Drugs and Devices. 1981 Drug survey. *AAO Bull.* 1982;1:1.

16. Ramsey MH, DerSimonian R, Holtel MR, Burgess LP. Corticosteroid treatment for idiopathic facial nerve paralysis: a meta-analysis. *Laryngoscope.* 2000;110:335-341.

17. Prednisone and other corticosteroids: balance the risks and benefits. http://www.mayoclinic.com/health/steroids/HQ01431. Accessed December 6, 2011.

18. Berg T, Axelsson S, Engström M, et al. The course of pain in Bell's palsy: treatment with prednisolone and valacyclovir. *Otol Neurotol.* 2009;30:842-846.

19. Scott J, Huskisson EC. Vertical or horizontal visual analogue scales. *Ann Rheum Dis.* 1979;38:560.

20. Stratford PW, Spadoni G. The reliability, consistency, and clinical application of a numeric pain rating scale. *Physiother Can.* 2001;53:88-91.

21. Walker N, Bohannon RW, Cameron D. Discriminant validity of temporomandibular joint range of motion measurements obtained with a rule. *J Orthop Sports Phys Ther.* 2000;30:484-492.

22. Hislop HJ, Montgomery J. *Daniels and Worthingham's Muscle Testing: Techniques of Manual Examination.* 7th ed. Philadelphia, PA: Saunders; 2002.

23. Kang TS, Vrabec JT, Giddings N, Terris DJ. Facial nerve grading systems (1985-2002): beyond the House-Brackmann Scale. *Otol Neurotol.* 2002;23:767-771.

24. House JW. Facial nerve grading systems. *Laryngoscope.* 1993;93:1056-1069.

25. Lewis BI, Ardour KK. An analysis of the Adour-Swanson and House-Brackmann grading systems for facial nerve recovery. *Eur Arch Otorhinolaryngol.* 1995;252:265-269.

26. House JW, Brackmann DE. Facial nerve grading system. *Otolaryngol Head Neck Surg.* 1985;93: 146-147.

27. VanSwearingen JM, Brach JS. The Facial Disability Index: reliability and validity of a disability assessment instrument for disorders of the facial neuromuscular system. *Phys Ther.* 1996;76: 1288-1300.

28. Brach JS, VanSwearingen JM. Physical therapy for facial paralysis: a tailored treatment approach. *Phys Ther.* 1999;79:397-404.

29. Jelks GW, Smith B, Bosniak S. The evaluation and management of the eye in facial palsy. *Clin Plast Surg.* 1979;6:397-419.

30. Manikandan N. Effect of facial neuromuscular re-education on facial symmetry in patients with Bell's palsy: a randomized controlled trial. *Clin Rehabil.* 2007;21:338-343.

31. Beurskens CH, Heymans PG. Physiotherapy in patients with facial nerve paresis: description of outcomes. *Am J Otolaryngol.* 2004;2:394-400.

32. Quinn R, Cramp F. The efficacy of electrotherapy for Bell's palsy: a systematic review. *Phys Ther Reviews.* 2003;8:151-164.

33. Targan RS, Alon G, Kay SL. Effect of long-term electrical stimulation and improvement of clinical residuals in patients with unresolved facial nerve palsy. *Otolaryngol Head Neck Surg.* 2000;122:246-252.

Cervical Radiculopathy

Annie Burke-Doe

A 49-year-old right-hand dominant female presents to an outpatient physical therapy clinic with a 3-week history of moderate neck pain radiating into her right shoulder and arm distally to the elbow. She reports having pain that began after an episode of sneezing. Recently, she rearranged her computer workstation, which she felt was contributing to her symptoms. Her past medical history is significant for cervical disc compression resulting from a figure skating accident at 18 years of age. In the examination room, the patient was seated and leaning back against the wall, holding her right arm on top of her head, with her head tilted forward and toward the left side. She reports that this position is how she has been sleeping in a reclining chair at home.

▶ Based on the case presented, what are the key signs and symptoms present?
▶ What are the best provocation tests to assist with the diagnosis?
▶ What is her rehabilitation prognosis?
▶ What are the most appropriate physical therapy functional assessments for cervical spine dysfunction?

KEY DEFINITIONS

CERVICAL RADICULOPATHY: Neurologic condition characterized by dysfunction of a cervical spinal nerve, its roots, or both; usually presents with unilateral neck and arm pain with paresthesia, weakness, or reflex changes in the affected nerve root distribution

NECK DISTRACTION TEST: Clinical provocative test that attempts to unload a compressed nerve and lessen radicular symptoms in patients with suspected cervical radiculopathy; the patient lies supine and the therapist grasps under the chin and occiput, flexes the patient's neck comfortably, and gradually applies a distraction force; a positive test is the reduction or elimination of symptoms during neck distraction

SPURLING'S A TEST: Clinical provocative test used on patients with suspected cervical spondylosis or acute cervical radiculopathy; the patient is seated, the neck is passively laterally flexed toward the symptomatic side, and overpressure (~7 kg) is applied to the patient's head;[1] a positive test is reproduction of the patient's symptoms

UPPER LIMB TENSION TEST A: Clinical provocative test that positions patient's neck and arm to relieve or aggravate arm symptoms; used in patients with suspected cervical radiculopathy

Objectives

1. Describe cervical radiculopathy.
2. Identify key questions to assist in the diagnosis of cervical radiculopathy.
3. Identify the presence of red flags that would indicate the patient's problem is not musculoskeletal in origin.
4. Identify reliable and valid outcome tools to measure cervical dysfunction.
5. Discuss appropriate components of the examination.

Physical Therapy Considerations

PT considerations during management of the individual with cervical radiculopathy:

▶ **General physical therapy plan of care/goals:** Relieve pain, improve neurologic function, prevent recurrence

▶ **Physical therapy interventions:** Manual therapy; modalities (including cervical traction); postural re-education; neck muscle strengthening and stretching; ergonomic modifications, if necessary

▶ **Precautions during physical therapy:** Constant or progressive pain that does not change with movement or position[2]; dizziness, vertigo, tinnitus, nausea, dysphagia; visual disturbances that occur with cervical rotation and extension

Understanding the Health Condition

Cervical radiculopathy is a neurologic condition characterized by dysfunction of a cervical spinal nerve, the roots of the nerve, or both.[2,3] It usually presents with pain in the neck and one arm, with a combination of sensory loss, loss of motor function, and/or reflex changes in the affected nerve root distribution.[2,4] Cervical radiculopathy has an annual incidence of approximately 107 per 100,000 for men and 64 per 100,000 for women with a peak at 50 to 54 years of age.[5] In the younger population, cervical radiculopathy is often the result of a disc herniation (20%-25% of cases) or an acute injury causing foraminal impingement of an exiting nerve.[6] In the older population, common causes include foraminal encroachment from osteophyte formation (70%-75% of cases), decreased disc height, degenerative changes of uncovertebral joints anteriorly and facet joints posteriorly.[3,6]

Contributing causes for radicular symptoms include heavy lifting, driving a vehicle or operating vibrating equipment (*e.g.*, jackhammer), nerve root compression and hypoxia, and disc herniation. Uncommon causes include tumor, expanding cervical synovial cyst, synovial chondromatosis in the cervical facet joint, giant cell arteritis, and spinal infection.[7-9] Common clinical features of cervical radiculopathy include muscle wasting, motor weakness, depressed deep tendon reflexes, and sensory changes in the involved nerve root (root signs).[2] The pain is described as sharp, stabbing, and exacerbated by coughing; it often radiates over the shoulder and down the arm. Frequently, numbness, tingling, and pain follow a dermatomal distribution. The associated motor reflex and motor and sensory distribution affected by involvement at each neurologic level is shown in Table 13-1.

Although there is no gold standard, magnetic resonance imaging has become the diagnostic test of choice to distinguish cervical radiculopathy from disc and bone disease.[10] Electromyography (EMG) studies may be helpful when the patient's history and physical examination are inadequate to distinguish cervical radiculopathy from other neurologic causes of neck and arm pain.[3] In addition, EMG may sometimes be used to rule out other disease processes.[11]

Table 13-1 MUSCLE, SENSORY, AND REFLEX TESTING TO DETERMINE NERVE ROOT LEVEL INVOLVEMENT IN CERVICAL RADICULOPATHY			
Neurologic Level	**Motor**	**Reflex**	**Sensory**
C4	Trapezius, rhomboids	None	Top of shoulder
C5	Deltoids, biceps, brachioradialis	Biceps tendon	Lateral arm from summit of shoulder to the elbow
C6	Biceps, extensor carpi radialis longus and brevis	Brachioradialis	Lateral forearm, thumb index finger
C7	Triceps, pronator teres	Triceps	Middle finger
C8	Interossei, flexor digitorum profundus		Medial forearm, little and ring finger

Physical Therapy Patient/Client Management

A patient with cervical radiculopathy typically presents with unilateral neck and arm pain, with any combination of paresthesia, weakness, or reflex changes in the affected nerve root distribution. Identification of impairments, dysfunction, and functional limitations such as presence of headache, impairments of strength, range of motion (ROM), endurance, posture, and gait as well as decreased independence helps the therapist determine goals and interventions. The primary physical therapy goals are to relieve pain, improve neurologic function, and prevent recurrences. Physical therapy interventions may include manipulation and mobilization, cervical traction, postural re-education, specific neck muscle strengthening and stretching exercises, modalities for pain, and ergonomic changes, as needed. Continued care by the general practitioner (including prescription of anti-inflammatory and analgesic medications) may assist in recovery.

Examination, Evaluation, and Diagnosis

Prior to seeing the patient, the physical therapist needs to acquire pertinent information from the patient, including history, prior diagnostic testing, medications, and prior level of function. Examples of questions may include: "What is your chief complaint (e.g., pain, numbness, weakness)?" and "Where are these symptoms?" A visual analog scale can be used to determine the patient's level of pain. Anatomic pain drawings can also be helpful in giving the therapist a quick review of the patient's pain pattern. Further questioning may include: "What activities and head positions decrease or increase symptoms?" and "When did the injury occur, what was the mechanism of the injury, and what was done to relieve the symptoms at that time?" The patient's responses assist the therapist in determining appropriate tests and measures to administer. To rule out vertebral artery involvement, the therapist should ask if the patient experiences dizziness, tinnitus, vertigo, nausea, or blurred vision.[12] The presence of red flags must be determined during the medical history. Red flags include fever, chills, unexplained weight loss, unremitting night pain, previous cancer, and/or immunosuppression. The presence of any red flags should alert the clinician to the possibility of a more serious disease such as tumor or infection[3] and merits referral to the primary healthcare provider. The therapist should also ask about the presence of symptoms indicative of myelopathy, a pathological change in the spinal cord. Symptoms may occasionally be subtle or attributed to other causes.[3] For example, diffuse hand numbness and clumsiness are often attributed to peripheral neuropathy or carpal tunnel syndrome. Other signs of myelopathy include balance impairments and sphincter disturbances.[3]

Chronic pain is commonly associated with cervical radiculopathy. Some authors have proposed that psychosocial, cognitive, and behavioral factors such as fear, avoidance, or believing that spinal pain is harmful or potentially disabling may increase the risk of developing chronic pain.[13-15] Patients with these risk factors may benefit from referral to psychosocial health professionals.

To determine the diagnosis of cervical radiculopathy and level of cervical nerve root involvement, the physical therapist assesses posture, ROM, muscle tenderness, strength, and reflex integrity. Clinical provocation tests also assist in the diagnosis of cervical radiculopathy. The therapist should observe head and neck posture from the front, side, and rear. Deviations from normal alignment are frequently seen in spinal disorders.[16] Often, a patient holds her neck stiffly and positions her head *away* from the side of injury. Neck active ROM is usually reduced[9] and pain is usually triggered or intensified with cervical extension, rotation, and lateral flexion, either toward or away from the affected nerve root. Increased pain with lateral flexion *away from* the symptomatic side may be due to increased displacement of a herniated disc onto a nerve root, whereas increased pain with lateral flexion *toward* the symptomatic side suggests impingement of a nerve root because this position further closes an already narrowed foramen.[1,16]

On palpation, tenderness along the cervical paraspinal muscles may be particularly pronounced on the ipsilateral side of the affected nerve root. Muscles in which symptoms are referred (*e.g.*, in the medial scapula, proximal arm, lateral epicondyle) may also be tender. Associated hypertonicity or spasm on palpation in these tender muscles may occur. Letchuman et al.[17] showed that cervical radiculopathy is associated with increased tender spots (both trigger and tender points) on the side of the radiculopathy, with a predilection toward the muscles innervated by the involved nerve root.

Muscle, sensory, and reflex testing should be performed to determine the nerve root level involvement in cervical radiculopathy (Table 13-1). Manual muscle testing may detect subtle weakness in a myotomal distribution. The sensory examination (usually light touch) assists in determining whether altered or lost sensation is present in a dermatomal distribution. In addition, patients with radiculopathy may demonstrate hyperesthesia to light touch and pinprick stimuli. Upper extremity deep tendon reflexes should be assessed. Any reflex grade can be normal, but *asymmetry* of the reflexes is a helpful diagnostic finding in patients who present with limb symptoms suggestive of a radiculopathy.

Clinical provocative tests of the neck that specifically position the patient's neck and/or arm to relieve or aggravate arm symptoms can be used in patients with suspected cervical radiculopathy. Three common provocation tests include the Upper Limb Tension Test A (ULTT-A), the cervical distraction test, and Spurling's A test. For the ULTT-A, the patient lies supine and the therapist *sequentially* positions the patient's upper extremity and neck in the following series: (1) scapular depression, (2) shoulder abduction, (3) forearm supination, wrist and finger extension, (4) shoulder lateral rotation, (5) elbow extension, and (6) contralateral, then ipsilateral cervical lateral flexion. The patient is questioned regarding symptom reproduction throughout the test.[18] The ULTT-A is considered positive if the patient's symptoms are reproduced, if there is a side-to-side difference of > 10° in elbow extension, or if symptoms are increased with contralateral cervical lateral rotation or decreased with ipsilateral cervical lateral flexion.[19-21] Wainner et al.[21] assessed the reliability and diagnostic accuracy of clinical examination (including three provocation tests) and self-report measures for cervical radiculopathy. In 82 adults with suspected cervical radiculopathy or carpal tunnel syndrome, the ULTT-A had high sensitivity (97%), but low specificity (22%). Thus, this test has been shown to be better at ruling out cervical radiculopathy as a probable diagnosis than ruling it in.[21] The manual cervical distraction test (Neck Distraction Test) is a provocative test in which the patient lies supine and the therapist provides gentle manual distraction of the neck. In this test, a positive sign is if the patient's symptoms decrease during the distraction. This provocative test was more specific (90%) than sensitive (44%).[21] The Spurling's A test is a foraminal compression test. With the patient in a seated position, the therapist passively laterally flexes the patient's neck toward the symptomatic side and provides several kilograms of overpressure. The test is considered positive if the patient's pain is reproduced. In this way, it is analogous to sciatica produced by straight leg raise in the patient with a herniated lumber disc. The Spurling's A test was found to be very specific (86%), but not sensitive (50%), in diagnosing acute cervical radiculopathy.[21] Therefore, it is not useful as a screening test, but it can be clinically useful in confirming the diagnosis of cervical radiculopathy.[22] Wainner et al.[21] found that the **presence of ≥ 3 of 4 specific variables more accurately diagnosed cervical radiculopathy than any single test of the clinical examination.** These four predictor variables include: positive ULTT-A, active cervical rotation *toward* the involved side < 60°, positive cervical distraction test, and positive Spurling's A test.

There are several reliable and valid outcome measures that can assist the clinician in determining the effectiveness and efficiency of treatment in cervical radiculopathy. Outcome measures for patients with cervical spine disorders should be completed before, during, and after a period of treatment to assist the therapist in determining the patient's progress. The **Neck Disability Index (NDI)** is a self-report instrument that contains 10 items related to how neck pain affects the ability to manage in everyday life. Seven items are related to activities of daily living, two are related to pain, and one item is related to concentration. The NDI is a revision of the Oswestry Disability Questionnaire; it is designed to measure the level of reduction in activities of daily living in patients with neck pain. The NDI has been widely researched and validated.[23] It has a test-retest reliability of 0.89.[23] The **Northwick Park Neck Pain Questionnaire** contains nine sections that cover activities likely to affect neck pain.[24] Each section contains five statements related to the patient's perceived level of difficulty performing the activity described in each section. Scores on the questionnaire range from 0% to 100%, with 0% being associated with no disability and 100% being associated with severe disability. The questionnaire has good short-term repeatability and internal consistency.[25]

Plan of Care and Interventions

Specific physical therapy goals are set after the evaluation. Goals should be based on the individual's current status and history of functional abilities. Interventions most commonly used for treating individuals with cervical radiculopathy include modalities for pain and inflammation, neck mobilization and/or manipulation, neck muscle re-education and energy techniques, therapeutic exercise, and education. In the absence of red flags, patients who present with acute neck and arm pain suggestive of cervical radiculopathy are typically treated with analgesics, anti-inflammatory drugs, and physical therapy.

In two case series, the majority of patients exhibited improved outcomes (as measured by the NDI and numerical pain rating scale) with **manual therapy, strengthening exercises, and cervical traction.**[26,27] Cleland et al.[27] found that the combination of mobilization, cervical traction, and deep neck flexor strengthening was associated with a greater occurrence of clinically important outcomes in this population. In a prospective cohort study of 96 adults, Cleland et al.[28] provided a model to predict which patients with cervical radiculopathy would substantially benefit from short-term (~28 days) physical therapy. Treatment success was defined by exceeding the minimal clinically important differences (MCIDs) on the NDI, Patient-Specific Functional Scale (PSFS), numeric pain rating scale, and Global Rating of Change (GROC). Their analysis yielded a combination of four variables that accurately predicted a successful outcome with physical therapy. These variables were < 54 years of age, dominant arm unaffected, looking down does not worsen symptoms, and multimodal treatment (*i.e.*, cervical traction, manual therapy, and deep neck flexor training) at a minimum of 50% of visits. While the overall success rate for patients receiving nonstandardized individualized physical therapy was 53%, the post-test probability of a successful outcome increased to 85% or 90% when three or four of the criteria were met, respectively.

Surgery is reserved for patients who have persisting and disabling pain after at least 6 to 12 weeks of nonsurgical management, progression of neurological deficits, or signs of moderate to severe myelopathy.[3]

Evidence-Based Clinical Recommendations

SORT: Strength of Recommendation Taxonomy

A. Consistent, good-quality patient-oriented evidence
B. Inconsistent or limited-quality patient-oriented evidence
C. Consensus, disease-oriented evidence, usual practice, expert opinion, or case series

1. The presence of ≥ 3 of the following increase the likelihood of the diagnosis of cervical radiculopathy: positive Upper Limb Tension Test A, active cervical rotation toward the involved side < 60°, positive cervical distraction test, positive Spurling's A test. **Grade B**

2. Physical therapists can use the Neck Disability Index and Northwick Park Neck Pain Questionnaire to reliably measure changes in neck pain and disability. **Grade A**

3. Use of a multimodal treatment program including intermittent cervical traction, manual therapy, and strengthening of deep neck flexors decreases pain and increases function in patients with cervical radiculopathy. **Grade B**

COMPREHENSION QUESTIONS

13.1 A physical therapist is working with a 55-year-old female 3 weeks after a motor vehicle accident that resulted in whiplash injury. The patient complains of left shoulder pain and numbness that radiates down to the thumb and increases with neck extension. Motor examination reveals decreased shoulder abduction strength (4/5) and decreased sharp/dull sensation at the left shoulder. What is the most likely cervical level of involvement?
   A. C4
   B. C5
   C. C6
   D. C7

13.2 Which outcome measure would be *most* appropriate to determine whether neck pain decreases the ability of a person to perform his/her activities of daily living?
   A. Northwick Park Neck Pain Questionnaire
   B. Standardized electrophysiological examination
   C. Neck Disability Index
   D. Numeric pain rating scale

ANSWERS

13.1 **B.** The C5 nerve root supplies sensation to the shoulder. Motor innervation to the deltoid muscle is supplied by the axillary nerve, which gets its predominant supply from the C5 nerve root.

13.2 **C.** The Neck Disability Index (NDI) is a self-report instrument that contains 10 items related to how neck pain affects the ability to manage in everyday life. Seven items are related to activities of daily living, two are related to pain, and one item is related to concentration. The NDI is a revision of the Oswestry Disability Questionnaire and was designed to measure the level of reduction in activities of daily living in patients with neck pain.

REFERENCES

1. Spurling RG, Scoville WB. Lateral rupture of the cervical intervertebral discs: a common cause of shoulder and arm pain. *Surg Gynecol Obstet.* 1944;78:350-358.

2. Waddell G. *The Back Pain Revolution.* 2nd ed. New York: Churchill Livingstone; 2004.

3. Carette S, Fehlings MG. Clinical practice. Cervical radiculopathy. *New Engl J Med.* 2005;353: 392-399.

4. Bogduk N. The anatomy and pathophysiology of neck pain. *Phys Med Rehabil Clin N Am.* 2003;14:455-472.

5. Radhakrishnan K, Litchy WJ, O'Fallon WM, Kurland LT. Epidemiology of cervical radiculopathy. A population-based study from Rochester, Minnesota, 1976 through 1990. *Brain*. 1994;117:325-335.

6. Murphey F, Simmons JC, Brunson B. Chapter 2. Ruptured cervical discs, 1939 to 1972. *Clin Neurosurg*. 1973;20:9-17.

7. Shelerud RA, Paynter KS. Rarer causes of radiculopathy: spinal tumors, infections, and other unusual causes. *Phys Med Rehabil Clin N Am*. 2002;13:645-696.

8. Soubrier M, Dubost JJ, Tournadre A, Deffond D, Clavelou P, Ristori JM. Cervical radiculopathy as a manifestation of giant cell arteritis. *Joint Bone Spine*. 2002;69:316-318.

9. Malanga GA, Romello MA. Cervical radiculopathy. *Medscape*. 2011. http://emedicine.medscape.com/article/94118-overview. Accessed: December 30, 2012.

10. Brown BM, Schwartz RH, Frank E, Blank NK. Preoperative evaluation of cervical radiculopathy and myelopathy by surface-coil MR imaging. *AJR Am J Roentgenol*. 1988;151:1205-1212.

11. Knoop KJ, Stack LB, Storrow AB, Thurman RJ. Extremity conditions. In: Tubbs RJ, Savitt DL, Suner S, eds. *The Atlas of Emergency Medicine*. 3rd ed. Access Medicine: McGraw Hill; 2010.

12. Grant R. Vertebral artery concerns: premanipulative testing of the cervical spine. In: Grant R, ed. *Physical Therapy of the Cervical and Thoracic Spine*. 2nd ed. New York: Churchill Livingstone; 1994:145-166.

13. Sions JM, Hicks GE. Fear-avoidance beliefs are associated with disability in older American adults with low back pain. *Phys Ther*. 2011;91:525-534.

14. Guez M, Hildingsson C, Stegmayr B, Toolanen G. Chronic neck pain of traumatic and non-traumatic origin: a population-based study. *Acta Orthop Scand*. 2003;74:576-579.

15. Cibulka MT. Understanding sacroiliac joint movement as a guide to the management of a patient with unilateral low back pain. *Man Ther*. 2002;7:215-221.

16. Chiarello C. Spinal disorders. In: Cameron MH, Monroe LG, eds. *Physical Rehabilitation Evidence-Based Examination, Evaluation and Interventions*. St. Louis, MO: Saunders Elsevier; 2007.

17. Letchuman R, Gay RE, Shelerud RA, VanOstrand LA. Are tender points associated with cervical radiculopathy? *Arch Phys Med Rehabil*. 2005;86:1333-1337.

18. Elvey RL. The investigation of arm pain: signs of adverse responses to the physical examination of the brachial plexus and related tissues. In: Boyling JD, Grieve GP, Jull GA, eds. *Grieve's Modern Manual Therapy*. 2nd ed. New York: Churchill Livingston; 1994:577-585.

19. Butler DA. *Mobilization of the Nervous System*. Melbourne, Australia: Churchill Livingstone; 1991.

20. Butler D, Gifford L. The concept of adverse mechanical tension in nervous system. Part 1: Testing for dural tension. *Physiotherapy*. 1989;75:622-628.

21. Wainner RS, Fritz JM, Irrgang JJ, Boninger ML, Delitto A, Allison S. Reliability and diagnostic accuracy of the clinical examination and patient self-report measures for cervical radiculopathy. *Spine*. 2003;28:52-62.

22. Nordin M, Carragee EJ, Hogg-Johnson S, et al. Assessment of neck pain and its associated disorders: results of the Bone and Joint Decade 2000-2010 Task Force on Neck Pain and Its Associated Disorders. *Spine*. 2008;33:S101-S122.

23. Vernon H, Mior S. The Neck Disability Index: a study of reliability and validity. *J Manipulative Physiol Ther*. 1991;14:409-415.

24. Leak AM, Cooper J, Dyer S, Williams KA, Turner-Stokes L, Frank AO. The Northwick Park Neck Pain Questionnaire, devised to measure neck pain and disability. *Br J Rheumatol*. 1994;33:469-474.

25. Hoving JL, O'Leary EF, Niere KR, Green S, Buchbinder R. Validity of the neck disability index, Northwick Park neck pain questionnaire, and problem elicitation technique for measuring disability associated with whiplash-associated disorders. *Pain*. 2003;102:273-281.

26. Waldrop MA. Diagnosis and treatment of cervical radiculopathy using a clinical prediction rule and a multimodal intervention approach: a case series. *J Orthop Sports Phys Ther*. 2006;36:152-159.

27. Cleland JA, Whitman JM, Fritz JM, Palmer JA. Manual physical therapy, cervical traction, and strengthening exercises in patients with cervical radiculopathy: a case series. *J Orthop Sports Phys Ther*. 2005;35:802-811.

28. Cleland JA, Fritz JM, Whitman JM, Heath R. Predictors of short-term outcome in people with a clinical diagnosis of cervical radiculopathy. *Phys Ther*. 2007;87:1619-1632.

Spinal Cord Injury—Intensive Care Unit

Heather David

One week ago, a 24-year-old female suffered a complete spinal cord injury at the neurological level of C7 as a result of a motor vehicle accident (MVA). Surgical interventions immediately following the MVA included a laminectomy and fusion of the C6 to T1 vertebral levels. Four days after surgery, she developed a deep vein thrombosis in her calf and had an inferior vena cava filter placed to prevent pulmonary embolism. She is currently in the intensive care unit (ICU). Her impairments include paralysis and sensory loss in bilateral lower extremities, trunk, and upper extremities. Spinal shock is resolving and she now presents with lower extremity spasticity, hyperreflexia, reflexive bowel and bladder, and difficulty clearing secretions from her lungs. She is an elementary school teacher and lives with her husband in a single story home. She enjoys playing basketball, surfing, and playing with her dogs. She does not have children, but she and her husband planned on starting a family in a few years. The physical therapist is asked to evaluate and treat the patient in the ICU.

► Based on her health condition, what do you anticipate will be the contributors to activity limitations?
► What precautions should be taken during physical therapy examination?
► What are the examination priorities?
► What are the most appropriate physical therapy outcome measures?
► What are possible complications interfering with physical therapy?

KEY DEFINITIONS

DEEP VEIN THROMBOSIS (DVT): Partial or complete occlusion of a deep vein by a thrombus (clot) usually caused by venous stasis, hypercoagulability, and/or injury to the wall of the vein

INFERIOR VENA CAVA FILTER: Vascular filter placed in the inferior vena cava to prevent pulmonary embolism

PULMONARY EMBOLISM: Blood clot that becomes lodged in a pulmonary artery and obstructs blood supply to the lung, and can result in death; most common cause is a DVT that has become dislodged

SPINAL SHOCK: Flaccid muscle paralysis and absence of reflexes below the level of a spinal cord injury; can last for hours to weeks

Objectives

1. Describe the etiology, incidence, and prevalence of spinal cord injuries.
2. Use the American Spinal Injury Association (ASIA) classification guidelines of spinal cord injury to determine motor levels, sensory levels, a single neurologic level, and the zone of partial preservation, if appropriate.
3. Describe clinical syndromes related to incomplete spinal cord injuries.
4. Describe primary and secondary impairments common in individuals with spinal cord injuries.
5. Describe the physical therapy evaluation and potential need for referral to other healthcare professionals for individuals with spinal cord injury.

Physical Therapy Considerations

PT considerations during management of the individual with loss of muscle activation and sensation, decreased functional mobility, and multiple medical complications due to spinal cord injury:

▶ **General physical therapy plan of care/goals:** Improve functional mobility including bed mobility, transfers, and locomotion (wheelchair propulsion); improve sitting tolerance and balance

▶ **Physical therapy tests and measures:** Assessment of range of motion (ROM) and strength; reliable and valid tools for functional mobility, balance, and participation restrictions

▶ **Precautions during physical therapy:** Orthostatic hypotension, autonomic dysreflexia, DVT, spinal instability, skin breakdown

▶ **Complications interfering with physical therapy:** Pain, spasticity, orthostatic hypotension, autonomic dysreflexia, spinal precautions, ROM restrictions, bowel and bladder management

Understanding the Health Condition

Spinal cord injuries are caused by neurologic disruption of the spinal cord potentially resulting in paralysis/paresis, sensory loss, changes in autonomic activity, and changes in reflexive responses.[1] Spinal cord injuries are most commonly caused by trauma, but may also occur as a result of disease, congenital malformations, vascular damage, tumors, infections, and neurological diseases.[1-3] In the United States, the annual incidence of spinal cord injuries is approximately 12,000 cases, not including those who die at the accident scene.[4] In 2010, approximately 265,000 individuals with a spinal cord injury (SCI) were living in the United States. Approximately half of individuals with spinal cord injuries are between the ages of 16 and 30 years of age.[5] Males comprise roughly 80% of reported spinal cord injuries,[5] and these are most prevalent among young males. The three leading causes are the same for males and females: motor vehicle accidents, falls, and gunshot wounds. Direct trauma to spinal cord tissue that occurs at the time of injury is referred to as the primary injury. This initial trauma rarely results in complete transection of the spinal cord regardless of the completeness of neurological injury. Secondary neurologic tissue damage occurs after the initial injury and can be caused by ischemia, edema, demyelination of axons, necrosis of the spinal cord, and scar tissue formation.[1] This secondary tissue damage is responsible for additional loss of motor and sensory function beyond the initial injury.[1] Approximately 30 to 60 minutes after trauma to the spinal cord, the individual experiences a period of spinal shock that is characterized by flaccid muscle paralysis and absence of reflexes *below* the level of spinal cord injury. Spinal shock can last for hours to weeks and an individual's completeness of injury cannot be determined until spinal shock has resolved.[2]

The spinal cord extends from the brain stem down to the level of the L1 or L2 vertebra. The caudal end of the spinal cord is called the conus medullaris. Spinal nerve roots from C1 to C7 exit *above* the corresponding vertebral body, whereas nerve roots from C8 and below exit *below* the corresponding vertebral level. During fetal development, the spinal cord runs the length of the spinal column and the spinal nerves exit horizontally. As an individual grows, the vertebrae grow in length but the spinal cord does not. Due to the shortened spinal cord relative to the vertebral column, the spinal nerve roots travel down the spinal canal before exiting. Due to this anatomical relationship between the vertebrae and the spinal cord, the spinal level of skeletal damage is often *different* from the spinal level of neurologic damage. The spinal nerve roots caudal to the conus medullaris are called the cauda equina. Tetraplegia (or, quadriplegia) is caused by damage to the spinal cord in the cervical spine, resulting in disruption of motor and/or sensory function in the upper and lower extremities, trunk, and pelvic organs. Paraplegia is caused by damage to nervous tissue within the spinal canal in the thoracic, lumbar, or sacral regions of the spinal column. Paraplegia results in disruption of motor and/or sensory function in the lower extremities, trunk, and pelvic organs. From 2005 to 2010, the most frequent neurologic category for SCI at hospital discharge was incomplete tetraplegia (39.5%), followed by complete paraplegia (22.1%), incomplete paraplegia (21.7%), and complete tetraplegia (16.3%).[4]

An individual's neurological level of injury is determined using the **American Spinal Injury Association (ASIA) Classification Scale.**[1,6,7] A systematic review to examine the psychometric properties of the ASIA Classification Scale to assess motor and sensory function was performed in 2006. Of the 39 studies initially identified, 18 studies fulfilled the inclusion and exclusion criteria set by the authors. The authors found that the 2000 version of the ASIA Classification Scale was more reliable than earlier versions. Although criterion validity could not be established due to lack of a gold standard for assessing individuals with SCI, construct validity was strong in several studies that compared ASIA motor scores with functional task performance, walking parameters, imaging, and electrophysiological evaluation. Based on their findings, the authors recommended using the ASIA at 72 hours after SCI for comparison with other neurological evaluations. The authors also supported reporting ASIA upper and lower extremity motor subscores instead of a single ASIA motor score. Further research is needed to determine the minimal clinically important difference of ASIA Classification.[6]

Figure 14-1 is the ASIA Classification of SCI and the ASIA Impairment Scale. To determine an individual's neurological level of injury, the clinician must perform a sensory examination and a motor examination. The sensory examination includes distinguishing sharp, dull, and light touch stimuli at *key* points determined to represent specific dermatomal levels. The examiner enters a 0, 1, or 2 at each tested site to represent absent, impaired, or normal sensory function, respectively. The motor examination includes manual muscle testing of *key* muscles determined to represent specific myotome levels. The examiner uses a 0 to 5 scale with 0 representing no muscle contraction and 5 representing normal muscle strength. A key muscle with a motor grade of 3 to 5 is considered to be neurologically intact if all the key muscles above that level have a grade of 5/5. For spinal levels that are represented by myotomes that cannot be specifically tested with a manual muscle test (*i.e.*, C2-C4 and T2-L1), the sensory level is presumed to be the same as the motor level. The ASIA examination also includes digital examination of the rectum to determine if there is voluntary motor function at the anal sphincter or deep anal sensation.[7] Using the ASIA classification system, the clinician obtains information regarding motor levels for the right and left sides of the body and sensory levels for the right and left sides of the body. This results in four spinal levels representing the most caudal area of normal function for each. The single neurological level is the most caudal level where all motor and sensory testing demonstrate normal innervation.[7] In addition to determining an individual's single neurological level, the examiner determines one of five categories (A-E) on the ASIA Impairment Scale (AIS). Steps to determine classification of spinal cord injuries can be found on the ASIA worksheet in Fig. 14-1. An individual is classified AIS A if the injury is complete, indicating the absence of motor and sensory function in the lowest sacral segments of the spinal cord (S4-S5) determined by digital examination as described above.[7] An individual with sensory and/or motor function in the lowest sacral segments is said to have an incomplete injury and is classified with an AIS level B to D. An individual without sensory or motor impairment is considered normal on the ASIA scale and is classified as AIS E. An individual with a complete injury (*i.e.*, AIS A) may have some sparing of motor or sensory function caudal to the single neurological level; this

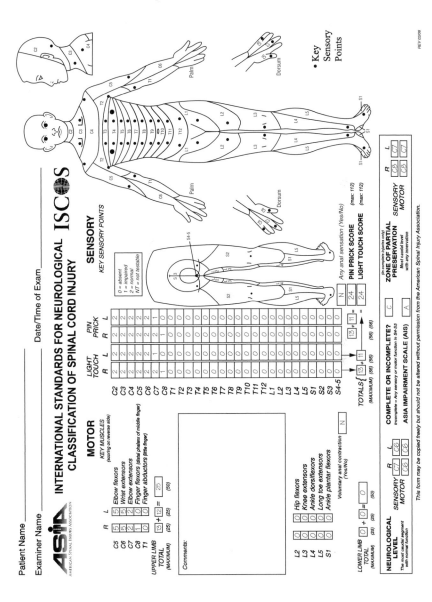

Figure 14-1. American Spinal Injury Association Neurological Classification of Spinal Cord Injury form for the case patient. (Reproduced with permission from American Spinal Injury Association: International Standards for Neurological Classification of Spinal Cord Injury, revised 2011; Atlanta, GA. Reprinted 2011.)

Muscle Function Grading

0 = total paralysis

1 = palpable or visible contraction

2 = active movement, full range of motion (ROM) with gravity eliminated

3 = active movement, full ROM against gravity

4 = active movement, full ROM against gravity and moderate resistance in a muscle specific position.

5 = (normal) active movement, full ROM against gravity and full resistance in a muscle specific position expected from an otherwise unimpaired person.

5* = (normal) active movement, full ROM against gravity and sufficient resistance to be considered normal if identified inhibiting factors (i.e. pain, disuse) were not present.

NT = not testable (i.e. due to immobilization, severe pain such that the patient cannot be graded, amputation of limb, or contracture of >50% of the range of motion).

ASIA Impairment (AIS) Scale

☐ **A = Complete.** No sensory or motor function is preserved in the sacral segments S4-S5.

☐ **B = Sensory Incomplete.** Sensory but not motor function is preserved below the neurological level and includes the sacral segments S4-S5 (light touch, pin prick at S4-S5: or deep anal pressure (DAP)), AND no motor function is preserved more than three levels below the motor level on either side of the body.

☐ **C = Motor Incomplete.** Motor function is preserved below the neurological level**, and more than half of key muscle functions below the single neurological level of injury (NLI) have a muscle grade less than 3 (Grades 0-2).

☐ **D = Motor Incomplete.** Motor function is preserved below the neurological level**, and at least half (half or more) of key muscle functions below the NLI have a muscle grade ≥ 3.

☐ **E = Normal.** If sensation and motor function as tested with the ISNCSCI are graded as normal in all segments, and the patient had prior deficits, then the AIS grade is E. Someone without an initial SCI does not receive an AIS grade.

**For an individual to receive a grade of C or D, i.e. motor incomplete status, they must have either (1) voluntary anal sphincter contraction or (2) sacral sensory sparing with sparing of motor function more than three levels below the motor level for that side of the body. The Standards at this time allows even non-key muscle function more than 3 levels below the motor level to be used in determining motor incomplete status (AIS B versus C).

NOTE: When assessing the extent of motor sparing below the level for distinguishing between AIS B and C, the *motor level* on each side is used; whereas to differentiate between AIS C and D (based on proportion of key muscle functions with strength grade 3 or greater) the *single neurological level* is used.

Steps in Classification

The following order is recommended in determining the classification of individuals with SCI.

1. Determine sensory levels for right and left sides.

2. Determine motor levels for right and left sides.
   Note: in regions where there is no myotome to test, the motor level is presumed to be the same as the sensory level, if testable motor function above that level is also normal.

3. Determine the single neurological level.
   This is the lowest segment where motor and sensory function is normal on both sides, and is the most cephalad of the sensory and motor levels determined in steps 1 and 2.

4. Determine whether the injury is Complete or Incomplete.
   (i.e. absence or presence of sacral sparing)
   If voluntary anal contraction = **No** AND all S4-5 sensory scores = **0** AND deep anal pressure = **No**, then injury is COMPLETE. Otherwise, injury is incomplete.

5. Determine ASIA Impairment Scale (AIS) Grade:
   Is injury Complete?   If YES, AIS=A and can record ZPP
   (lowest dermatome or myotome on each side with some preservation)

   NO

   Is injury motor Incomplete?   If NO, AIS = B
   (Yes=voluntary anal contraction OR motor function more than three levels below the motor level on a given side, if the patient has sensory incomplete classification)

   YES

   Are at least half of the key muscles below the single neurological level graded 3 or better?

   NO   **YES**

   AIS = C   AIS = D

   If sensation and motor function is normal in all segments, AIS = E
   Note: AIS E is used in follow-up testing when an individual with a documented SCI has recovered normal function. If at initial testing no deficits are found, the individual is neurologically intact; the ASIA Impairment Scale does not apply.

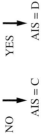

Figure 14-1. (Continued)

area of preservation is called the zone of partial preservation and this term is used only with complete SCI.[7] ASIA examination is performed repeatedly throughout an individual's recovery process. ASIA testing is often performed in the acute care setting after spinal shock has resolved and at admission to each progressive level of care, including inpatient rehabilitation and outpatient therapy settings.

Some incomplete spinal cord injuries have distinct patterns of sensory and motor loss determined by the location of spinal cord damage due to the somatotopic organization of the spinal cord and the location of ascending and descending spinal tracts.[1,2] These spinal cord injuries are described as clinical syndromes known as Brown-Séquard, central cord, anterior cord, posterior cord, conus medullaris, and cauda equina. Table 14-1 reviews incomplete SCI clinical syndromes.

Spinal cord injuries can result in primary and secondary impairments. Primary impairments can include loss or alterations in motor function, muscle tone, sensation, respiratory function, voluntary bowel and bladder function, genital function, cardiovascular function, and thermoregulation.[1] Muscle paralysis is caused by damage to descending motor tracts, anterior horn cells, and/or spinal nerve roots. Damage located peripheral to or at the anterior horn cell results in a lower motor neuron (LMN) lesion with *flaccid* paralysis below the level of injury. SCI affecting the descending motor tracts results in an upper motor neuron (UMN) lesion with *spastic* paralysis below the level of injury. Most spinal cord injuries result in combined damage to motor tracts, anterior horn cells, and spinal nerves, resulting in a combination of UMN and LMN lesions. The location of damage will determine

Table 14-1 INCOMPLETE SPINAL CORD INJURY CLINICAL SYNDROMES		
	Area of Spinal Damage	**Clinical Presentation**
Brown-Séquard syndrome	Hemisection of the spinal cord	Ipsilateral weakness and loss of proprioception and vibratory sense Contralateral loss of pain and temperature
Central cord syndrome	Central region of the cervical spinal cord	Loss of upper extremity function greater than lower extremity and sparing of sacral functioning
Anterior cord syndrome	Anterior and anterolateral portions of the spinal cord	Loss of motor function, pain and temperature bilaterally and preservation of proprioception bilaterally
Posterior cord syndrome	Posterior aspects of the spinal cord	Bilateral loss of proprioception, stereognosis, two-point discrimination, and vibration sense below the level of injury with preservation of motor, pain, and light touch
Conus medullaris syndrome	Conus medullaris and damage to the lumbar and sacral nerve roots	Bilateral flaccid lower extremity paralysis, loss of sensation, and areflexive bowel and bladder
Cauda equina syndrome	Cauda equina with injuries to the lumbar and sacral nerve roots	Typically incomplete bilateral flaccid paralysis of the lower extremities, loss of sensation, and areflexive bowel and bladder function

the type of muscle tone alterations experienced as a result of SCI.[1] Spasticity, the velocity-dependent resistance to passive muscle elongation, is also associated with hyperreflexia and clonus.[1,3] As a result of UMN damage, spasticity may become present in individuals with cervical and upper thoracic spinal cord injuries (after a period of flaccidity during spinal shock). LMN damage related to conus medullaris or cauda equina injuries can result in flaccidity in paralyzed muscles. Flaccid muscle paralysis results in decreased or absent deep tendon reflexes and decreased or absent resistance to passive muscle elongation. A combination of UMN and LMN damage can occur with higher level injuries and may lead to a mixed presentation with some flaccid muscle groups and some spastic muscle groups.[1,3] Sensory dysfunction occurs with SCI because of damage to ascending sensory spinal tracts. Mixed sensory deficits may be seen as a result of an incomplete SCI as described in the clinical syndromes of incomplete SCI.

The ability to breathe and cough is often altered in individuals with spinal cord injuries. Since the diaphragm is innervated by the C3 to C5 spinal cord segments, individuals with complete spinal cord injuries at C3 or above will require mechanical ventilation for breathing. Many individuals with a C4 neurological level will also require mechanical ventilation. The ability to produce an efficient cough requires the coordination of the diaphragm, abdominal, and accessory muscles. An efficient cough is impaired in individuals without innervation of this musculature (C1-T12).[1]

Bowel and bladder function is commonly impaired in individuals with spinal cord injuries due to a loss of sacral spinal cord function. Bowel and bladder function will differ depending on the type and location of spinal cord or nerve damage. A reflexive bladder (as presented by the current patient) occurs in individuals with spinal cord injuries *above* the conus medullaris (*i.e.*, an UMN lesion). A reflexive bladder is characterized by filling and reflexive emptying at a particular filling level. This reflexive emptying can be manually stimulated.[1,3,8] An areflexive bladder may result from injuries at or below T12. The areflexive bladder is characterized by a loss of detrusor and external sphincter function that results in small amounts of overflow incontinence when the bladder becomes full; the remaining urine retained in the bladder can cause bladder distention if not drained artificially. Individuals with SCI will likely require the use of intermittent or indwelling catheterization for bladder management. Individuals with SCI can lose voluntary bowel control and sensation of bowel fullness. Similar to the bladder dysfunctions, SCI can result in a reflexive bowel in higher level SCI resulting from UMN damage or an areflexive bowel resulting from LMN damage. A reflexive bowel results in maintenance of resting internal anal sphincter tone with reflexive relaxation upon rectum filling. An areflexive bowel results in decreased tone or flaccidity of the internal and external anal sphincter, which results in incontinence.[1] Genital function and sexual responses are often altered or lost in individuals with SCI. Fertility in males is often decreased, while fertility in women is likely not affected.[1]

SCI can affect cardiovascular function due to an imbalance between sympathetic stimulation (from spinal segments T1-L2/L3) and parasympathetic stimulation (from the vagus nerve, CN X). This imbalance is especially apparent in individuals with injuries at T6 and above. These individuals commonly experience bradycardia, bradyarrhythmias, hypotension, and orthostatic hypotension. Impairments in thermoregulation vary depending on the SCI level, with higher level injuries caus-ing greater impairment in thermoregulation. The ability to sweat is typically absent *below* the level of injury.[1]

Secondary impairments due to SCI include skin breakdown, respiratory compli-cations, orthostatic hypotension, autonomic dysreflexia, loss of ROM and contrac-ture development, osteoporosis, heterotopic ossification, DVT, pain, bladder and urinary tract infections, and cardiovascular disease.[1,9] Due to the lack of normal sensory function and limited physical mobility, individuals with SCI are at high risk for skin breakdown. The development of pressure ulcers is the most common secondary complication in an individual with SCI.[1,10] Respiratory complications result from decreased ventilation and coughing ability, which can lead to respiratory insufficiency and pneumonia.[1,11] Orthostatic hypotension can result from the lack of sympathetic reflexes to regulate blood pressure with postural changes. In addition, prolonged bedrest and decreased venous return due to abdominal and lower extrem-ity paralysis increase the risk of orthostatic hypotension.[9] Symptoms of orthostatic hypotension include dizziness, loss of vision, nausea, ringing in the ears, and loss of consciousness. If symptoms occur, individuals with SCI should be assisted into a supine position or reclined back in a wheelchair with legs raised up to promote a more reclined position. Gradual transitions from supine to sitting, lower extremity compression stockings, and an abdominal binder help decrease the risk of ortho-static hypotension.[1]

Autonomic dysreflexia is a potentially life-threatening condition that can occur in individuals with spinal cord injuries above the T6 level in response to a noxious stimulus occurring *below* the level of injury that triggers a sympathetic response. It is characterized by hypertension, bradycardia, severe headache, sweating *above* the level of injury, and blurred vision. Bowel and bladder distension are the most com-mon causes of autonomic dysreflexia. Autonomic dysreflexia is considered a medical emergency due to the sudden sustained increase in blood pressure that can put the individual at risk for stroke or death.[12,13] In response to an episode of autonomic dysreflexia, the clinician or caregiver should sit the individual upright with the legs dependent to help decrease the elevated blood pressure, obtain medical assistance, monitor blood pressure, and work to identify and remove the noxious stimulus.[1,13]

Immobility, paralysis, and prolonged positioning in a bed or wheelchair increases the risk of developing contractures due to decreased active and passive ROM.[1] Osteoporosis is also common in individuals with SCI likely due to a combination of decreased weightbearing in the lower extremities, loss of muscular contraction on bones, and circulatory changes. The presence of osteoporosis increases the risk of fracture.[1] Heterotopic ossification (HO) is the formation of new bone in soft tis-sue; individuals with SCI are at increased risk of developing HO below the level of injury, most often in the hips, knees, and elbows. The cause of HO is unknown and usually appears 1 to 6 months after SCI.[1]

After SCI, deep vein thromboses are common, especially in the acute phase, due to lack of venous muscle pump from lower extremity muscle paralysis and a tem-porary increase in blood coagulation following traumatic injury.[14] This is a serious medical concern and must be monitored carefully for prevention and early identifi-cation to prevent a pulmonary embolism (PE), caused when a DVT breaks free and travels to the lungs.[14,15] Pulmonary embolism is the most common cause of death in the first year following SCI.[1] Prophylaxis against thrombus formation is initiated within hours of injury and includes anti-coagulation medications, compression stockings, intermittent pneumatic compression devices, early mobilization and ROM exercises, and sometimes inferior vena cava filter placement.[1,9,16]

Patients with SCI often experience pain from multiple causes including orthopaedic trauma or overuse, visceral, or neuropathic pain. Pain can be above, below, and/or at the transitional level of injury. Pain can negatively influence the individual's quality of life.[1,3] Urinary tract infections are another common secondary complication to SCI due to urinary retention and chronic use of catheters.[1]

Physical Therapy Patient/Client Management

Immediate medical management at the scene of the accident for a patient with a traumatic SCI involves stabilization of the spine, ventilation and circulation assistance as needed, and emergency transport to a hospital. Level I trauma centers, especially those with specialized SCI centers, are the preferred settings for the immediate care of patients with traumatic SCI.[1,9] Medical management at the hospital includes monitoring and assisting with ventilation and circulation as necessary, spinal protection, radiographic imaging, traction or surgical spinal stabilization, stabilization of extraspinal fractures, and potential administration of glucocorticoids to minimize secondary tissue damage.[9] Spinal orthoses (braces) are often prescribed following surgical or nonsurgical stabilization of individuals with spinal fractures. The type of orthosis will depend on the spinal restrictions required for the specific injury.[1]

Rehabilitation for individuals with SCI occurs in a broad spectrum of facilities including the acute hospital, inpatient rehabilitation hospital, skilled nursing facility, outpatient day program, outpatient clinic, and within the individual's home. Physical therapy management for a patient with SCI includes teaching the individual functional mobility skills, self-care activities, and prevention of secondary complications. The physical therapist often works as part of a medical team including primary care physicians, neurologists, physiatrists, nurses, occupational therapists, speech therapists, mental health professionals, and other allied health professionals. It may be necessary to refer the individual to mental health professionals to help with disability-related adjustment issues; assistive technology professionals for adaptive equipment including wheelchairs; and other physicians for pain relief, spasticity management, and bowel or bladder management.

Examination, Evaluation, and Diagnosis

A physical therapy examination is comprised of specific screening and testing procedures leading to a physical therapy diagnosis and referral to other members of the healthcare team when appropriate. The physical therapist has multiple tools to evaluate impairments and loss of functional mobility in an individual with SCI.

Physical therapy evaluation of the individual with SCI should focus on examining vital signs, respiration function, skin integrity, sensation, ROM, strength, muscle tone, and functional mobility limitations. It is essential to monitor vital signs including blood pressure, heart rate, and respiratory rate. It is especially important in the acute stages to monitor for orthostatic hypotension while increasing the individual's tolerance for upright posture. Examination of respiratory function includes assessing the strength of the respiratory muscles: diaphragm, abdominals, intercostal muscles, sternocleidomastoids, and scalenes. Chest expansion can be quantified with circumferential measurement at the axilla and xiphoid process. Measurements should be taken at the end of maximal exhalation and at the end of maximal inhalation. For adults, normal chest expansion at the xiphoid process is approximately 2.5 to 3.0 inches.[3] Assessment of vital capacity can be done using a handheld spirometer. In addition to respiration measurement, assessment of cough effectiveness is imperative.[3] Every member of the healthcare team must frequently evaluate skin integrity, especially in the acute stages of injury when functional mobility is severely limited and the individual is reliant upon others to perform pressure reliefs.

Sensory testing, including sharp/dull and light touch assessment, is performed as part of the ASIA examination. The physical therapist should also assess proprioception to ascertain information regarding the patient's ability to know where her limbs are in space, which will affect her ability to perform functional mobility skills. Muscle tone should be reassessed frequently for the presence of spasticity or flaccidity, especially in the acute stages during and following spinal shock.[1] Muscle tone assessment is performed with slow passive ROM through a joint's available range, followed by fast passive elongation of the same muscles. Spasticity is a type of hypertonicity that occurs in response to *fast* passive elongation of a muscle group. Spasticity can be graded using the Modified Ashworth Scale[17] (Table 14-2). Hypertonicity can lead to pain, contracture formation, pressure ulcers, and may limit functional activities.[1] The Patient Reported Impact of Spasticity Management (PRISM) is a standardized self-report questionnaire that can be used to assess the impact of spasticity on an individual's quality of life.[18] Passive ROM assessment must be done to determine muscle length and any joint ROM restrictions that may negatively affect functional mobility training.[1] Manual muscle testing of key muscle groups is performed as a part of the ASIA examination, but additional muscle testing beyond

Table 14-2	MODIFIED ASHWORTH SCALE FOR GRADING SPASTICITY[17]
0	No increase in muscle tone
1	Slight increase in muscle tone, marked by a catch and release or by minimal resistance at the end of the range of motion when the affected part(s) is moved in flexion or extension
1+	Slight increase in muscle tone, marked by a catch, followed by minimal resistance throughout the remainder (less than half) of the ROM
2	More marked increase in muscle tone through most of the ROM, but affected part(s) easily moved
3	Considerable increase in muscle tone, passive movement difficult
4	Affected part(s) rigid in flexion or extension

Reproduced with permission from Bohannon RW, Smith MB. Interrater reliability of a modified Ashworth scale of muscle spasticity. Phys Ther. 1987;67:206-207.

the key muscle groups can be beneficial to develop a plan of care for the individual. ROM and muscle testing should be performed carefully to prevent stress on areas of spinal instability, especially during upper extremity testing in individuals with tetraplegia and lower extremity testing in individuals with paraplegia.[1] Due to increased demands on the upper extremities for mobility, individuals with chronic SCI should be assessed for overuse injuries of the upper extremities.

Functional mobility assessment is an extremely important part of the physical therapy examination and will be assessed frequently throughout the plan of care and across rehabilitation settings. Assessment includes what mobility skills the individual is able to perform, what level of assistance is needed to perform the skill, and what adaptive equipment is necessary for successful completion of the skill. In the hospital setting where this patient is currently located, the initial functional mobility evaluation includes bed mobility skills, transfer skills, and locomotor ability (wheelchair skills in this patient case).[1] In the ICU and acute care setting, the individual requires a high level of assistance with these types of tasks and not all mobility will be appropriate to test. Expected functional outcomes for an individual with SCI at the C7 neurological level are discussed in Case 15.

Plan of Care and Interventions

In the ICU and acute hospital setting, the physical therapy plan of care focuses on prevention of secondary complications, increasing the individual's tolerance to upright positions, early functional mobility, and patient/family education. Prevention of secondary complications includes performing ROM and proper patient positioning in bed to prevent contracture and pressure ulcer development.[1,3,9] Daily ROM throughout the entire range of all four extremities should be performed. Exceptions include joints limited by movement contraindications or joints and tissues in which tightness provides function—such as tight finger flexors that promote tenodesis in individuals without active finger flexion and tight low back extensors that promote trunk control and mobility. A tenodesis grasp is accomplished by extending the wrist (using extensor carpi radialis longus and brevis), which results in passive tension in the finger flexors (flexor digitorum profundus, flexor digitorum superficialis, flexor pollicis longus). This causes the fingers to flex and the thumb to form a lateral pinch with the index finger.[1,19] Preservation of tightness in the finger flexors is critical for individuals with C7 and higher tetraplegia (like the current case patient) to allow the individual to grasp and manipulate objects using active wrist extension. Although individuals with C5 and above tetraplegia do not have active wrist extension, the finger flexors in these patients should still be allowed to tighten to allow use of the hand as a hook and because of the possibility for the return of voluntary motor function caudal to the neurological level of injury in the months and years following injury. Overstretching the long finger flexors will prevent the use of a tenodesis grasp. Once the finger flexors are overstretched, it is very difficult to regain this tightness and the individual can lose the ability to use a tenodesis grasp in the future. The physical therapist is responsible for educating patients, families, and other members of the healthcare team about the importance of preserving tightness in the finger flexors. The hand should be positioned with the wrists in extension and the fingers should be allowed to relax in a flexed position. Passive splints may be appropriate to help promote shortening of the finger flexors and active splints can help the individual develop the skill of using a tenodesis grasp.[1,3] It is also important for individuals with tetraplegia and paraplegia to maintain mild tightness in the low back to help with trunk control and mobility skills that the individual develops throughout her rehabilitation. In the ICU and acute setting, the physical therapist can work to maximize the individual's hamstring length (as long as this type of mobility is not contraindicated due to surgical stabilization or other factors). Improving hamstring length in the ICU and acute care setting will prepare the individual for bed and mat mobility skills that will begin in the inpatient rehabilitation setting. Bed and mat mobility skills require progressively longer periods of time in the long sitting position, which requires adequate hamstring length to prevent overstretching low back extensors. Positioning ankle boots or splints may be used to prevent shortening of the plantarflexors due to the unopposed force of gravity and the potential for spasticity of the plantarflexors. These boots or splints position the individual's ankles in a neutral position and often unload ("float") the heels to prevent skin breakdown.[3,10]

The physical therapist works with the healthcare team to prevent pressure ulcers with the use of specialized equipment to minimize pressure on the individual's skin (*e.g.*, alternating-pressure mattresses or overlays, active support surfaces, specialized wheelchair cushions, boots and splints), compliance with pressure relief schedules, and frequent checks that the individual's skin remains clean and dry.[1,10] The risk of pressure ulcers is greatest over bony prominences and varies depending on the individual's positioning. In supine, areas at risk of pressure ulcers include the occiput, scapulae, iliac crests, sacrum, and heels. In sidelying, areas of risk include the greater trochanters, knees, and ankles. In sitting, areas of risk include the ischial tuberosities, sacrum, and coccyx. **Prevention of pressure ulcer formation** in bed requires a turning schedule in which the individual's position is changed *at least* every 2 hours. While this is the traditional positioning schedule, some individuals with more risk factors for skin breakdown require a more frequent turning schedule to avoid skin breakdown.[1,10] The individual's skin should be assessed each time she is turned. During position changes, it is important to avoid sliding the individual across the surface she is sitting or lying on due to shear forces that increase the risk of skin breakdown. In sitting, the individual should be seated on a specialized wheelchair cushion (*e.g.*, Roho, Jay) and she should perform pressure reliefs every 15 to 20 minutes.[10,20] A pressure relief is simply a change in position or shift in weight off the surfaces that have been weightbearing. The amount of time that an individual should perform a pressure relief while seated in a wheelchair is unclear. A study in the *Journal of Spinal Cord Medicine* found that the amount of time required for tissue perfusion recovery during a pressure relief is 200 to 300 seconds (roughly 3.5 to 5 minutes). The average amount of time pressure reliefs were performed in this study was 49 seconds.[20] The method of performing a pressure relief may determine the duration of each pressure relief. In a manual wheelchair, the pressure relief can initially be performed with the assistance of another person to lift the buttocks, shift the trunk laterally or anteriorly, or by tilting the individual back in the wheelchair.[1,10,20] Caution should be taken when reclining an individual back in a wheelchair because this can cause a shearing force at the sacrum. In a power wheelchair, even an individual with very limited mobility can perform her own pressure reliefs using the power tilt feature of the wheelchair.[1,10]

The physical therapist in the ICU or acute care setting begins working on improving the individual's tolerance to upright positions. Individuals with SCI need to develop a tolerance to sitting upright without a drop in blood pressure that could cause nausea, vomiting, or loss of consciousness. The physical therapist works with the patient to gradually accommodate to elevation of the head above horizontal. The use of lower extremity compression stockings and an abdominal binder can assist with venous return and should be used while the individual is developing a tolerance to sitting upright. A reclining wheelchair can be used to progressively raise the individual to a fully vertical position. With the wheelchair in the fully reclined position, the individual is almost completely horizontal with her legs elevated in footrests. The physical therapist can raise the chair vertically and lower the legs in small increments while monitoring for signs and symptoms of orthostatic hypotension. If or when the individual becomes symptomatic with reports of dizziness, changes in vision, changes in hearing, nausea, or if she begins to lose consciousness, the therapist can tip the wheelchair back into a more reclined position and/or the legs can be elevated.[1,3]

The physical therapy plan of care, goal setting, and interventions for the current patient with a complete SCI at the C7 neurological level is presented as she moves to an inpatient rehabilitation facility (Case 15) and to an outpatient physical therapy department (Case 16).

Evidence-Based Clinical Recommendations

SORT: Strength of Recommendation Taxonomy

A: Consistent, good-quality patient-oriented evidence
B: Inconsistent or limited-quality patient-oriented evidence
C: Consensus, disease-oriented evidence, usual practice, expert opinion, or case series

1. The American Spinal Injury Association (ASIA) classification guidelines of spinal cord injury have good concurrent validity between motor and sensory scores and an individual's functional abilities. **Grade A**

2. To decrease the risk of pressure ulcer formation, individuals with spinal cord injury in acute and rehabilitation settings should be turned or repositioned every 2 hours in supine and should perform pressure reliefs every 15 minutes in sitting. **Grade C**

COMPREHENSION QUESTIONS

14.1 A physical therapist has evaluated a 35-year-old male with SCI in an acute care setting. The therapist has worked with nursing staff to complete ASIA examination testing. What is the ASIA classification including neurological level of injury for this patient?

Motor			Sensory				
				Light Touch		Pin Prick	
	R	L		R	L	R	L
			C2-C4	2	2	2	2
C5 Elbow Flexors	5	5	C5	2	2	2	2
C6 Wrist Extensors	5	5	C6	2	2	2	2
C7 Triceps	5	5	C7	2	2	2	2
C8 Long Finger Flexors	3	3	C8	2	2	2	2
T1 Finger abductors	0	0	T1	2	1	1	1
L2-S1 (lower extremities)	0	0	T2-S5	0	0	0	0
Voluntary Anal Contraction?	No		Any Anal Sensation?		Yes		

A. AIS B; single neurological level C8; zone of partial preservation T1

B. AIS B; single neurological level C7

C. AIS A; single neurological level C6; zone of partial preservation T1

D. AIS B; single neurological level C8

14.2 In the ICU, a physical therapist is evaluating a patient with SCI who has no motor or sensory function in her trunk or bilateral lower extremities. The patient has received medical clearance to get out of bed and into a wheelchair. Upon sitting at the edge of the bed, the patient reports dizziness, nausea, and loss of vision. What is the *most* likely cause of these symptoms and signs and what should the physical therapist do immediately?

A. Autonomic dysreflexia; sit the patient upright with her legs dependent

B. Autonomic dysreflexia; lie the patient down with her legs elevated

C. Orthostatic hypotension; sit the patient upright with her legs dependent

D. Orthostatic hypotension; lie the patient down with her legs elevated

14.3 A physical therapist is evaluating a patient who has suffered a complete SCI with a C7 neurological level. The physical therapist is asking the patient about her home environment while she is reclined in her wheelchair. The patient's face begins to turn red and sweaty; she begins complaining of a pounding headache. What is the *most* likely cause of the headache and sweating, and what should the physical therapist do immediately?

A. Autonomic dysreflexia; sit the patient upright with her legs dependent

B. Autonomic dysreflexia; recline the patient further with her legs elevated

C. Orthostatic hypotension; sit the patient upright with her legs dependent

D. Orthostatic hypotension; lie the patient down with her legs elevated

14.4 In the ICU, a physical therapist has evaluated a patient with SCI. The therapist found strength and sensory function losses greater in the upper extremities than the lower extremities. What clinical syndrome related to incomplete spinal cord injuries describes this patient's presentation *best*?

A. Brown-Séquard

B. Central cord

C. Anterior cord

D. Posterior cord

ANSWERS

14.1 **D.** The single neurological level is C8 because this is the last level at which motor function and sensory function as tested by light touch and sharp/dull are all intact. Motor function at C8 was reported to be 3/5 bilaterally because all the key muscles above this motor level are considered neurologically intact. The AIS B classification denotes that this is a sensory incomplete injury; there *is* sensory but there is *no* motor function in the lowest sacral segments as tested by deep anal pressure and voluntary anal contraction. The zone of partial preservation is a term reserved for use with complete injuries; therefore, there is no zone of partial preservation for this patient case (options A and C).

14.2 **D.** Common symptoms of orthostatic hypotension are dizziness, nausea, ringing in the ears, decreased vision, and syncope. It is important to be able to recognize these symptoms because orthostatic hypotension is very common in the early stages after spinal cord injury. The correct response is to lie the patient down (or recline her with her legs elevated if she is seated in a wheelchair) to promote an increase in blood pressure.

14.3 **A.** Autonomic dysreflexia is common in individuals with SCI at the T6 level and higher. This is a life-threatening condition and must be recognized by healthcare professionals to allow for immediate action. The individual's elevated blood pressure is what contributes to the serious risk of heart attack or stroke; therefore, it is advised to sit the individual up to help decrease blood pressure.

14.4 B. Central cord syndrome is caused by damage to the central aspects of the cervical spinal cord with preservation of the peripheral aspects of the spinal cord. Due to the somatotopic organization of the spinal cord, individuals with central cord syndrome present with a greater loss of upper extremity function than lower extremity and sacral function.

REFERENCES

1. Somers MF. *Spinal Cord Injury Functional Rehabilitation*. 3rd ed. New Jersey, NJ: Pearson; 2010.

2. Umphred DA. *Neurological Rehabilitation*. 5th ed. St. Louis, MO: Mosby Elsevier; 2007.

3. O'Sullivan SB, Schmitz TJ. *Physical Rehabilitation*. Philadelphia, PA: FA Davis; 2007.

4. Spinal Cord Injury Facts and Figures at a Glance. Birmingham, Alabama: National Spinal Cord Injury Statistical Center; 2011. https://www.nscisc.uab.edu/PublicDocuments/nscisc_home/pdf/Facts%202011%20Feb%20Final.pdf. Accessed January 31, 2013.

5. Spinal Cord Injury Statistical Center. Annual Report for the Spinal Cord Injury Model Systems 2012. https://www.nscisc.uab.edu/PublicDocuments/reports/pdf/2010%20NSCISC%20Annual%20Statistical%20Report%20-%20Complete%20Public%20Version.pdf. Accessed February 4, 2013.

6. Furlan JC, Fehlings MG, Tator CH, Davis AM. Motor and sensory assessment of patients in clinical trials for pharmacological therapy of acute spinal cord injury: psychometric properties of the ASIA Standards. *J Neurotrauma*. 2008;25:1273-1301.

7. American Spinal Injury Association. *American Spinal Injury Association: International Standards for Neurological Classification of Spinal Cord Injury*. Chicago, IL: American Spinal Injury Association; 2003.

8. Consortium for Spinal Cord Medicine, Paralyzed Veterans of America. *Bladder Management for Adults with Spinal Cord Injury: A Clinical Practice Guideline for Health-Care Providers*. Washington, DC; Consortium for Spinal Cord Medicine; 2006. www.pva.org. Accessed January 31, 2013.

9. Consortium for Spinal Cord Medicine, Paralyzed Veterans of America. *Early Acute Management for Adults with Spinal Cord Injury: A Clinical Practice Guideline for Health-Care Providers*. Washington, DC: Consortium for Spinal Cord Medicine; 2008. www.pva.org. Accessed January 31, 2013.

10. Consortium for Spinal Cord Medicine, Paralyzed Veterans of America. *Pressure Ulcer Prevention and Treatment Following Spinal Cord Injury: A Clinical Practice Guideline for Health-Care Providers*. Washington, DC: Consortium for Spinal Cord Medicine; 2000. www.pva.org. Accessed June 12, 2012.

11. Consortium for Spinal Cord Medicine, Paralyzed Veterans of America. *Respiratory Management Following Spinal Cord Injury: A Clinical Practice Guideline for Health-Care Providers*. Washington, DC: Consortium for Spinal Cord Medicine; 2005. www.pva.org. Accessed June 12, 2012.

12. Consortium for Spinal Cord Medicine, Paralyzed Veterans of America. *Acute Management of Autonomic Dysreflexia: Individuals with Spinal Cord Injury Presenting to Health-Care Facilities*. Washington, DC: Consortium for Spinal Cord Medicine; 2001. www.pva.org. Accessed January 31, 2013.

13. Krassioukov A, Warburton DE, Teasell R, Eng JJ. A systematic review of the management of autonomic dysreflexia after spinal cord injury. *Arch Phys Med Rehabil*. 2009;90:682-695.

14. Consortium for Spinal Cord Medicine, Paralyzed Veterans of America. *Prevention of Thromboembolism in Spinal Cord Injury: A Clinical Practice Guideline for Health-Care Providers*. Washington, DC: Consortium for Spinal Cord Medicine; 1999. www.pva.org. Accessed January 31, 2013.

15. Goodman CC, Fuller KS. *Pathology: Implications for the Physical Therapist*. 3rd ed. Philadelphia, PA: Saunders; 2008.

16. Roberts A, Young W. Prophylactic retrievable inferior vena cava filters in spinal cord injured patients. *Surg Neurol Int*. 2010;1:68.

17. Bohannon RW, Smith MB. Interrater reliability of a modified Ashworth scale of muscle spasticity. *Phys Ther*. 1987;67:206-207.

18. Cook KF, Teal CR, Engebretson JC, et al. Development and validation of Patient Reported Impact of Spasticity Measure (PRISM). *J Rehabil Res Dev.* 2007;44:363-372.

19. Harvey L. Principles of conservative management for a non-orthotic tenodesis grip in tetraplegics. *J Hand Ther.* 1996;9:238-342.

20. Makhsous M, Priebe M, Bankard J, et al. Measuring tissue perfusion during pressure relief maneuvers: insights into preventing pressure ulcers. *J Spinal Cord Med.* 2007;30:497-507.

Spinal Cord Injury—Inpatient Rehabilitation Facility

Heather David

CASE 15

A 24-year-old female suffered a complete (AIS A) spinal cord injury (SCI) at the neurological level of C7 as a result of a motor vehicle accident (MVA). The patient was determined to be medically stable 2 weeks after her accident and was transferred to an inpatient rehabilitation facility where she has been evaluated by the rehabilitation team. She currently requires total assistance for bed mobility, transfers, bowel and bladder management, wheelchair propulsion, and pressure relief. She and her husband have many questions related to expectations for her recovery, the amount of assistance she will need, as well as the type of equipment and home modifications that will be necessary. She is eager to work with physical therapy to increase her tolerance to sitting upright, improve her bed mobility, initiate transfer training, and learn to propel a wheelchair.

► What are possible complications interfering with physical therapy?
► Identify her functional limitations and assets.
► What is her rehabilitation prognosis?

Objectives

1. Identify appropriate outcome measures to assess functional mobility in individuals with spinal cord injury.
2. Describe appropriate functional goals and a plan of care specific to a patient's neurologic level and completeness of spinal cord injury within the inpatient rehabilitation setting.
3. Describe adaptive equipment that may be required based on an individual's level and completeness of injury.

Physical Therapy Considerations

PT considerations in the inpatient rehabilitation setting for management of the individual with loss of muscle activation and sensation, decreased functional mobility, and multiple medical complications due to spinal cord injury:

▶ **General physical therapy plan of care/goals:** Improve functional mobility including bed mobility, transfers, and locomotion (wheelchair propulsion); improve sitting tolerance and balance

▶ **Physical therapy tests and measures:** Assessment of range of motion (ROM) and strength; reliable and valid tools for functional mobility, balance, and participation restrictions

▶ **Precautions during physical therapy:** Orthostatic hypotension, autonomic dysreflexia, deep vein thrombosis, spinal instability, skin breakdown

▶ **Complications interfering with physical therapy:** Pain, spasticity, orthostatic hypotension, autonomic dysreflexia, spinal precautions, ROM restrictions, bowel and bladder management

Understanding the Health Condition

See Case 14 for understanding spinal cord injury.

Physical Therapy Patient/Client Management

Individuals with SCI are treated in a broad spectrum of facilities, including acute hospitals, inpatient rehabilitation centers, skilled nursing facilities, outpatient day programs, outpatient clinics, and within individuals' homes. Physical therapy management includes teaching the individual functional mobility skills, self-care activities, and prevention of secondary complications. Typically, patients spend 1 to 2 weeks in the acute hospital after a traumatic SCI. This patient has just been transferred to an inpatient rehabilitation hospital (sometimes referred to as "acute rehab" or "inpatient rehab") after spending 2 weeks in the acute hospital. An inpatient rehabilitation program consists of coordinated medical and rehabilitation services provided 24 h/d, which encourages active patient and caregiver participation. Each individual's rehabilitation program is designed in collaboration with interprofessional team members to achieve predicted outcomes and discharge to the appropriate setting. The intensity of the inpatient rehabilitation program is dependent on the individual's medical stability and acuity. However, for individuals to be admitted to inpatient rehabilitation, typically they must be able to tolerate 3 hours of combined therapy sessions over an 8- to 10-hour day.[1] In acute rehab, physical therapy management is focused on functional goal setting with consideration of the level and completeness of the SCI, discharge planning, improving functional mobility, educating patients on the use of assistive devices, and improving wheelchair mobility.

Examination, Evaluation, and Diagnosis

A physical therapy examination is comprised of specific screening and testing procedures leading to a physical therapy diagnosis and referral to other members of the healthcare team when appropriate. The physical therapist has multiple tools to evaluate impairments and loss of functional mobility in an individual with SCI. Physical therapy evaluation of the individual with SCI focuses on examining vital signs, respiration function, skin integrity, sensation, ROM, strength, muscle tone, and functional mobility skills and limitations.

A tool frequently used in rehabilitation hospitals to document the level of assistance needed to perform functional mobility skills is the Functional Independence Measure (FIM®). The FIM® is an 18-item standardized outcome measure to grade an individual's functional abilities related to self-care activities, bowel and bladder management, transfer ability, locomotion, cognition, and communication. Outcomes are sometimes reported separately for motor and cognitive functioning. Motor items include self-care activities, sphincter control, and mobility, while cognitive items include communication and social cognition. Table 15-1 shows the scoring used on the FIM® from complete independence (7) to total assistance (1). Scoring for the

Table 15-1 FIM® INSTRUMENT LEVELS OF ASSISTANCE [2]	
FIM® Rating Levels	
No Helper	7 Complete Independence (Timely, Safety)
	6 Modified Independence (Device)
Helper- Modified Dependence	5 Supervision (Subject = 100%)
	4 Minimal Assistance (Subject = 75% or more)
	3 Moderate Assistance (Subject = 50% or more)
Helper- Complete Dependence	2 Maximal Assistance (Subject = 25% or more)
	1 Total Assistance or not testable (Subject less than 25%)

FIM® is typically done at admission to inpatient rehabilitation and at discharge.[2] The **motor scoring in the FIM®** has been found to be valid (correlations ranging from 0.58 to 0.92) in detecting changes in mobility in individuals with SCI. The cognitive scoring, however, was not found to be valid in detecting subtle changes in cognition in persons with SCI.[3]

The FIM® is used widely in rehabilitation settings with a variety of patient populations. However, it is *not* designed specifically for use with individuals with SCI. The **Spinal Cord Injury Independence Measure (SCIM)** is a functional mobility tool designed specifically for use with individuals with SCI. The third version of the SCIM (SCIM III) has demonstrated reliability and validity and is more sensitive than the FIM® in demonstrating changes in persons with SCI.[4] The SCIM III consists of three subscales: (1) self-care, which consists of six tasks ranging in score from 0 to 20; (2) respiration and sphincter management, which consists of four tasks with a scoring range from 0 to 40; and, (3) mobility, which includes nine tasks with a score ranging from 0 to 40. Total scores on the SCIM III range between 0 and 100.[4] In a multisite study of 425 patients, inter-rater reliability ranged between 0.63 and 0.82 (Kappa coefficient) for all items on the SCIM III with all items demonstrating statistical significance. Validity between the SCIM III and FIM® was also statistically significant (Pearson correlation coefficient 0.79). The SCIM III demonstrated better responsiveness than the FIM® in the areas of respiration, sphincter management, and mobility indoors and outdoors subscales. In the subscales of self-care and mobility in the room and toilet, there were no statistically significant differences between the SCIM III and the FIM®.[4]

Functional mobility assessments help the therapist set goals and create a plan of care specific to the individual's needs and abilities. In addition, knowledge regarding anticipated functional potential for individuals with SCI at various neurological levels helps the therapist set realistic goals. Evaluation of an individual's home environment is important early in the rehabilitation process for functional mobility training, adaptive devices, and to make any necessary home modifications that would allow the individual to return home, if possible.

Plan of Care and Interventions

Guidelines that have been set forth by the Consortium for Spinal Cord Medicine can assist the clinician with functional goal setting based on an individual's level of injury. The Consortium for Spinal Cord Medicine developed guidelines based on a 12-step process including choosing a panel of experts, reviewing literature, preparing evidence tables, grading and ranking the quality of evidence, and conducting statistical meta-analyses. Through this process, the panel compiled data from the Uniform Data Systems and the National Spinal Cord Injury Statistical Center to develop **expectations for functional outcome based on level of complete SCI.**[5] These data were compiled as guidelines that allow a clinician to have a global understanding for the potential for functional mobility independence, adaptive equipment needs, and personal attendant needs. It is important to understand that each individual has assets that may allow her to surpass goals or liabilities that inhibit reaching potential goals outlined for the specific level of injury.[5] Setting goals for individuals with SCI should include long-term functional goals that direct the individual's rehabilitation toward an *optimal* outcome based on the individual's level of injury, comorbidities, secondary complications, cognitive abilities, fitness level, age, body type, psychological factors, social support, financial resources, and cultural factors. Short-term goals should be set as measureable, functional, and progressive in order to achieve the long-term goals.[5] Table 15-2 outlines the major muscles and innervation levels and the active movements possible based on SCI level.

Table 15-3 includes the expected functional outcomes for the current patient, based on her C7 neurological level of injury. These outcomes can serve as guidelines related to an expected level of independence based on complete SCI under optimal circumstances.[5] Assistance levels stated are consistent with those from the FIM®.[2]

Table 15-2 AVAILABLE MUSCLE INNERVATION FOR PATIENTS WITH SCI BASED ON NEUROLOGICAL LEVEL[5-8]		
Distal Nerve Root Innervation	**Major Muscle Innervation**	**Available Movements**
C1-C3	Facial muscles, sternocleidomastoid, cervical paraspinals, neck accessories	Talking, chewing, sipping, blowing, cervical flexion, extension, rotation
C4	Diaphragm Upper trapezius Cervical paraspinals	Inspiration Scapular elevation Cervical flexion, extension, rotation
C5	Deltoids, biceps, brachialis, brachioradialis, rhomboids	Shoulder: flexion (limited), abduction (to 90°), extension, external rotation Elbow: flexion, supination
C6	Extensor carpi radialis longus, serratus anterior, clavicular portion of pectoralis major, infraspinatus, latissimus dorsi, teres minor, pronator teres	Scapula: abduction, upward rotation Shoulder: flexion, extension, internal rotation, adduction Elbow: forearm pronation Wrist: extension (tenodesis grasp)
C7	Triceps, extensor pollicis longus and brevis, extrinsic finger extensors, flexor carpi radialis	Shoulder: as above Elbow: elbow extension Wrist: flexion Finger: extension
C8	Extrinsic finger flexors, flexor carpi ulnaris, flexor pollicis longus and brevis	Full upper extremity movements
T1	Intrinsic finger flexors	Full upper extremity movements
T2-T9	Full upper extremity innervation	Full upper extremity movements
T10-L1	Intercostals, external obliques, rectus abdominis	Trunk stability
L2-S5	Intact trunk musculature; depending on level, possible hip flexors, extensors, abductors, adductors; knee flexors, extensors; ankle dorsiflexors, plantar flexors	Trunk stability; some lower extremity function possible

Table 15-3 EXPECTED FUNCTIONAL OUTCOMES FOR THE INDIVIDUAL WITH SCI AT THE C7 NEUROLOGICAL LEVEL[5-8]			
Distal Nerve Root Innervation and Major Muscles	Available Movements	Expected Functional Outcomes	Equipment and Assistance Required
C7 Triceps, extensor pollicis longus and brevis, extrinsic finger extensors, flexor carpi radialis	Shoulder: • Full shoulder movements possible Elbow: • Flexion and extension Forearm: • Pronation and supination Wrist: • Extension and flexion	Respiratory: decreased vital capacity, may require assistance to clear secretions Modified Independent to total assistance for: • Bowel management • Bladder management • Bathing • Lower body dressing • Homemaking • Transportation • Standing (with equipment) Modified Independent to moderate assistance: • Bed mobility *Rolling*: modified independent *Supine to sitting*: modified independent *LE management*: moderate assistance to modified independent • Transfers (level and uneven surfaces; with or without transfer board) Modified Independent to minimal assistance: • Eating • Grooming • Skin inspection • Pressure reliefs • Manual wheelchair propulsion on level and incline/declined surfaces • Upper body dressing Unable to functionally ambulate	Adapted equipment: (universal cuff, adaptive utensils, button hook, zipper pulls) Tenodesis splints Padded shower/commode chair Lightweight rigid or folding frame, with hand rim modifications Pressure-relieving wheelchair cushion Full electric hospital bed or full to king standard bed With or without transfer board Standing frame Modified vehicle with hand controls 2-4 hour attendant care

Based on Table 15-3, this patient has the potential to transfer across uneven surfaces with or without a transfer board. In order to begin transfer training, the environment should be set up so that the individual is transferring across a level surface or to a lower surface. This can be done with a transfer board in order to decrease the difficulty of the task. Prior to becoming independent with this task, she will need to improve her sitting balance abilities. However, as early as she can tolerate sitting

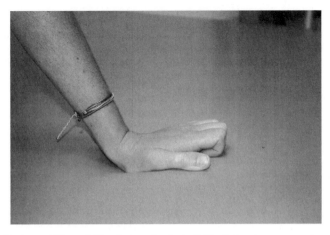

Figure 15-1. During mobility activities that require the individual's hand on a support surface, their fingers should be positioned in flexion to prevent overstretching of the long finger flexors, which protects an individual's tenodesis grip.

upright, she can begin learning how to transfer with the assistance of others. The most important aspect of teaching an individual with SCI to transfer is using the head/hips relationship. The individual must understand that wherever she wants to place her hips for the transfer, her head must go in the *opposite* direction. In the early stages of transfer training, the physical therapist guides the individual where to place her hands for the transfer, making sure that the patient maintains a flexed finger position to protect the tenodesis grasp (Fig. 15-1). The exact placement of the individual's hands varies depending on the surface being transferred to/from. The goal is to have a base that will allow the individual to bear weight on her hands while she uses momentum and the head/hips relationship to move her hips from one surface to another. This patient has innervation to the triceps and scapular depressors, which helps with elevation of her hips during the transfer. The physical therapist should stand in front of the patient while she is learning to transfer, but the therapist needs to allow the patient to use large movements of the head in order to gain required momentum for a successful transfer. The patient may need to perform two or more small scoots on a transfer board prior to gaining the skill to do the maneuver in one movement without a transfer board. As the patient continues to progress with her rehabilitation in the inpatient and outpatient settings, she can learn how to transfer to a variety of even and uneven surfaces without physical assistance, and also how to perform floor to wheelchair transfers.

To appropriately prescribe a wheelchair, the physical therapist must assess the individual's ability to propel a manual wheelchair or safely navigate a power wheelchair. The patient in this case has a complete SCI at the C7 neurologic level, so it is anticipated that she will be able to manually propel a wheelchair across level and sloping surfaces (Table 15-3). She is also young, strong, and active. At a C7 level, the patient has full bilateral innervation of her triceps, but is lacking innervation of the finger flexors. Once the patient is able to tolerate upright, she can begin learning to propel a manual wheelchair on level surfaces. Due to the lack of finger flexor innervation and inability to firmly grasp, she will not be able to grasp the hand rims fully and must be taught to press both of her palms into the hand rims and then push forward while pressing into the hand rims. Initially, the use of gloves and/or rubber tubing or hand rim adaptations can help increase friction to allow the patient to push more efficiently. There are a variety of hand rim modifications to increase the efficiency of propulsion for an individual without full hand innervation. The physical therapist may need to assist the patient with propulsion initially, transitioning to less assistance and fewer adaptations on the hand rim as the patient increases skill level. As the individual progresses, she will learn to perform advanced wheelchair skills including performing wheelies, negotiating ramps and curbs, and falling safely from the wheelchair.

An ultra-lightweight wheelchair would likely be the best choice for this patient to decrease the amount of weight she has to push. There are rigid frame and folding frame options, each with benefits and drawbacks. Rigid frame wheelchairs are more efficient and stable, but do not collapse easily for transportation in vehicles. However, the wheels are designed to pop off to facilitate getting the wheelchair into a vehicle. Folding frame wheelchairs collapse easily without having to remove parts, but they have more moveable parts which makes them less energy-efficient and less stable laterally.[7] There are many considerations when fitting an individual in a wheelchair including: seat depth, floor to seat height, back height, seat width, arm rests, type of foot plate or leg rests, and choice of cushions and back supports.[7] A customized seating system is required and should be performed by a physical therapist or a certified assistive technology professional with knowledge and experience in custom seating systems and the specific needs of the individual with SCI.

In addition to setting goals related to the level of the individual's SCI, inpatient rehabilitation focuses on discharge planning to the individual's home environment (if possible) with recommendations for modifications made to increase access to the environment. Barriers such as curbs, stairs, narrow doorways, small bathrooms, heights of kitchen counters and appliances must all be assessed with recommendations and referrals made for any necessary architectural modifications. This should be done early in the rehabilitation process to facilitate discharge and maximal independence within the individual's home.[6-8]

Sitting balance, stretching, bed mobility, wheelchair mobility, and transfer training are initiated in the inpatient rehabilitation setting. This training will likely continue at an outpatient rehabilitation facility due to continually shortened lengths of hospital stays. Physical therapy interventions for the current patient in the outpatient setting are discussed in Case 16.

Evidence-Based Clinical Recommendations

SORT: Strength of Recommendation Taxonomy

A: Consistent, good-quality patient-oriented evidence
B: Inconsistent or limited-quality patient-oriented evidence
C: Consensus, disease-oriented evidence, usual practice, expert opinion, or case series

1. Motor scoring on the Functional Independence Measure (FIM®) is valid for detecting changes in mobility in individuals with SCI. **Grade B**

2. The Spinal Cord Injury Independence Measure (SCIM III) is a reliable and valid functional mobility tool for use with individuals with SCI. **Grade B**

3. Guidelines from the Consortium for Spinal Cord Medicine can help the physical therapist with goal setting and expectations for functional outcome based on the individual's level of SCI. **Grade B**

COMPREHENSION QUESTIONS

15.1 What is an appropriate long-term goal for bed-to-wheelchair transfers for the patient in this case?

A. Modified independence with uneven transfers with or without a transfer board

B. Minimal assistance with uneven transfers with a transfer board

C. Modified independence with level transfers with or without a transfer board

D. Moderate assistance with level transfers with a transfer board

15.2 What is an appropriate long-term goal for bed mobility for the patient presented in this case?

A. Minimal assistance for rolling bilaterally

B. Modified independent for supine to sitting

C. Minimal assistance for lower extremity management

D. Moderate assistance for supine to sitting

ANSWERS

15.1 **A.** The patient in this case has a complete SCI at the level of C7. This indicates that the individual has innervation to the triceps, which increases the potential for increased independence with functional mobility. The patient in this case is young, athletic, and has a strong support system. A goal of modified independence with transfers from level and uneven surfaces is appropriate.

15.2 **B.** The first neurological level at which an individual with a complete SCI has the potential for modified independence with supine to sit is C6. The patient in this case (C7) has triceps innervation, which increases the individual's functional mobility potential.

REFERENCES

1. Medical Rehabilitation Program Descriptions. CARF, 2012. http://www.carf.org/WorkArea/DownloadAsset.aspx?id=23992. Accessed June 12, 2012.

2. *Guide for the Uniform Data Set for Medical Rehabilitation* (including the FIM® instrument), Version 5.0. Buffalo, NY: State University of New York; 1996.

3. Hall KM, Cohen ME, Wright J, Call M, Werner P. Characteristics of the functional independence measure in traumatic spinal cord injury. *Arch Phys Med Rehabil.* 1999;80:1471-1476.

4. Itzkovich M, Gelernter I, Biering-Sorensen F, et al. The Spinal Cord Independence Measure (SCIM) version III: reliability and validity in a multi-center international study. *Disabil Rehabil.* 2007;29:1926-1933.

5. Consortium for Spinal Cord Medicine, Paralyzed Veterans of America. *Outcomes Following Traumatic Spinal Cord Injury: Clinical Practice Guidelines for Health-Care Professionals.* Washington, DC: Consortium for Spinal Cord Medicine; 1999. www.pva.org. Accessed June 12, 2012.

6. Somers MF. *Spinal Cord Injury Functional Rehabilitation.* 3rd ed. New Jersey, NJ: Pearson; 2010.

7. O' Sullivan SB, Schmitz TJ. *Physical Rehabilitation.* Philadelphia, PA: FA Davis; 2007.

8. Umphred DA. *Neurological Rehabilitation.* 5th ed. St. Louis, MO: Mosby Elsevier; 2007.

Spinal Cord Injury—Outpatient Rehabilitation

Heather David

A 24-year-old female suffered a complete (AIS A) spinal cord injury at the neurological level of C7 as a result of a motor vehicle accident (MVA). She is an elementary school teacher and lives with her husband in a single story home. Prior to her injury, she enjoyed playing basketball, surfing, and playing with her dogs. She does not have children, but she and her husband planned on starting a family in a few years. The patient has just been discharged from an inpatient rehabilitation facility (Case 15). During her 6-week inpatient rehabilitation, she demonstrated the ability to tolerate upright sitting for over 5 hours and she no longer requires the use of an abdominal binder or lower extremity compression devices to prevent orthostatic hypotension. She had begun training in wheelchair propulsion, sitting balance, and transfers. She now presents to an outpatient physical therapy clinic and the physical therapist must help her develop appropriate goals for the next 6 months.

▶ What are possible complications interfering with physical therapy?
▶ Identify her functional limitations and assets.
▶ What is her rehabilitation prognosis?

Objectives

1. Identify the differences between compensatory and restorative approaches to rehabilitation.
2. List appropriate long-term (6-month) goals for the individual with a complete SCI at the neurological level of C7.
3. Describe appropriate physical therapy interventions in an outpatient setting for an individual with SCI.
4. Identify range of motion requirements for individuals with SCI and the need for selective stretching.
5. Describe methods of preventing upper extremity overuse injuries and pain for individuals with SCI.

Physical Therapy Considerations

PT considerations during management of the individual with loss of muscle activation, loss of sensation, decreased functional mobility, and multiple medical complications due to spinal cord injury:

▶ **General physical therapy plan of care/goals:** Improve functional mobility including bed mobility, sitting balance, transfers, and wheelchair propulsion

▶ **Physical therapy tests and measures:** Assessment of range of motion (ROM) and strength; reliable and valid tools for functional mobility, balance, gait, and participation restrictions

▶ **Precautions during physical therapy:** Orthostatic hypotension, autonomic dysreflexia, deep vein thrombosis, spinal instability, skin breakdown

▶ **Complications interfering with physical therapy:** Pain, spasticity, orthostatic hypotension, autonomic dysreflexia, spinal precautions, ROM restrictions, bowel and bladder management

Understanding the Health Condition

See Case 14 for understanding spinal cord injury.

Physical Therapy Patient/Client Management

Individuals with SCI are treated in a broad spectrum of facilities, including acute hospitals, inpatient rehabilitation centers, skilled nursing facilities, outpatient day programs, outpatient clinics, and within individuals' homes. Physical therapy management for an individual with SCI includes teaching functional mobility skills, self-care activities, and prevention of secondary complications. The physical therapist often works as part of a medical team including primary care physicians, neurologists, nurses, occupational therapists, speech therapists, mental health professionals, assistive technology professionals, and other allied health professionals. In addition, an individual with SCI will have many questions related to sexuality, sexual functioning, and fertility. The patient in this case has expressed a desire to have children someday and will need education on sexuality and fertility for individuals with SCI. The Consortium for Spinal Cord Medicine developed guidelines on a variety of topics related to individuals with SCI based on a 12-step process including choosing a panel of experts, reviewing literature, preparing evidence tables, grading and ranking the quality of evidence, and conducting statistical meta-analyses. The Consortium has published a clinical practice guideline related to sexuality and reproductive health; this guideline may be used as a foundation for answering patient's questions and making appropriate referrals related to sexuality and fertility education.[1]

Prior to her injury, this individual was very active and enjoyed playing basketball, surfing, and playing with her dogs. If available, the physical therapist can involve a recreational therapist in her treatment to work with her to explore opportunities for recreation based on her interests. Both therapists can help the patient locate community resources and programs that provide adaptive sporting and leisure opportunities.

Examination, Evaluation, and Diagnosis

A physical therapy examination is comprised of specific screening and testing procedures leading to a physical therapy diagnosis and referral to other members of the healthcare team when appropriate. The physical therapist has multiple tools to evaluate impairments and loss of functional mobility in an individual with SCI. Physical therapy evaluation of the individual with SCI should focus on examining vital signs, respiration function, skin integrity, sensation, ROM, strength, muscle tone, and functional mobility limitations. Detailed physical therapy examination of this patient was presented in Cases 14 and 15.

Plan of Care and Interventions

Rehabilitation approaches specific to the care of individuals with SCI typically include teaching the individual compensatory strategies by using substitution strategies and/or adaptive equipment to allow her to perform desired tasks in the absence of normal muscle innervation. Restorative strategies are typically used in the rehabilitation of patients with motor *incomplete* spinal cord injuries because the goal is recovery of normal movement with minimal compensations. It is common for therapists to utilize a blend of compensatory and restorative approaches. The extent to which each approach is used depends on the level and completeness of the SCI and the unique characteristics of the individual.[2] In general, the greater the amount of motor function an individual retains after SCI, the greater functional mobility independence he/she will have.[2] This individual with a complete SCI (AIS A) will likely rely on compensatory strategies (including the use of adaptive equipment) and substitution strategies more than an individual with a motor incomplete injury

(AIS C or D).[2] Goal setting is an important aspect of creating a physical therapy plan of care. Appropriate functional goals for the patient with a complete SCI at the neurological level of C7 include: (1) sitting at the edge of bed without upper extremity support and without loss of balance for 5 minutes to allow for upper body dressing; (2) transfer from bed to/from wheelchair with modified independence from level and uneven heights; (3) transfer from supine to long sitting with modified independence to allow for lower body dressing; (4) transfer from supine to sitting at the edge of bed with modified independence to prepare for transfers; (5) propel an ultra-lightweight wheelchair 1500 ft with modified independence over level surfaces to access long community distances; and (6) propel an ultra-lightweight wheelchair over inclines and declines and ascend/descend 4-inch curbs with modified independence.

The **level and completeness of the individual's injury determine the choice and emphasis of physical therapy interventions.** A 2007 study of 600 patients with SCI from six inpatient rehabilitation centers around the United States found that for individuals with high tetraplegia (C1-C4, AIS A, B, or C), the three most common individual therapeutic activities performed during physical therapy sessions were ROM/stretching, strengthening, and transfers, in that order.[3] For individuals with low tetraplegia (C5-C8, AIS A, B, or C), the three most common activities were ROM/stretching, transfers, and then strengthening. For individuals with paraplegia (AIS A, B, or C), the most common activities were transfers, ROM/stretching, and strengthening. Individuals with motor incomplete injuries at the AIS D level (see Case 14 for a review of American Spinal Injury Association classifications), the most common activities were gait training, strengthening, and balance exercises. In all injury categories, the most common group therapy activity was strengthening.[3]

Rehabilitation interventions related to ROM, skin protection, positioning, and selective stretching that began in the acute care setting are continued in the outpatient setting. The physical therapist must be aware of specific ROM requirements that allow individuals with tetraplegia to utilize various compensatory strategies required for functional mobility. Table 16-1 presents the ROM requirements for the current patient with motor complete tetraplegia.

Physical therapists need to incorporate stretching of specific muscle groups to prepare for the compensatory movement strategies the patient will need to perform functional activities. The patient needs adequate hamstring length (110° of straight leg raise) to prevent overstretching of tissues in the low back during long sitting activities.[2] Until adequate hamstring length is attained by stretching, long sitting activities may need to be modified to prevent overstretching of the low back.[2] Selective stretching of the hand and wrist musculature is also required. Due to her level of injury, the patient does not have innervation to the long finger flexors and she requires the use of a tenodesis grasp in order to perform many activities of daily living. A tenodesis grasp is accomplished by extending the wrist, which results in passive tension in the finger flexors. This causes the fingers to flex and the thumb to form a lateral pinch with the index finger.[2,6] Preservation of tightness in the finger flexors is *critical* for individuals with C5 to C7 tetraplegia to allow the individual to grasp and manipulate objects using the preserved active wrist extension. Although individuals with tetraplegia at C5 and above do not have active wrist extension, the finger flexors in these patients should still be allowed to tighten to allow use of the hand as a

Table 16-1   RANGE OF MOTION REQUIREMENTS FOR AN INDIVIDUAL WITH MOTOR COMPLETE TETRAPLEGIA[2,4,5]

	Range of Motion Goal	Function
Neck	Normal	Mat/bed mobility, sitting balance, transfers, upper body dressing
Low back	Mild tightness	Mat/bed mobility, sitting balance, transfers
Shoulders	Normal in all motions; greater than normal shoulder extension	Mat/bed mobility, transfers, upper body dressing, wheelchair mobility, floor to wheelchair transfers
	In the absence of triceps innervation, greater than normal combined extension with external rotation with elbow extension is required	*Mat/bed mobility, sitting balance*
Elbows and forearms	Normal in all motions, full extension is essential	Mat/bed mobility, transfers, wheelchair mobility, floor to wheelchair transfers
	In the absence of triceps innervation, combined full elbow extension with full forearm supination is required	*To "lock" elbows for extension in the absence of active triceps*
Wrists	Normal flexion and extension	Tenodesis grasp for performance of ADLs in the absence of active finger flexors
	In the absence of innervation to triceps, normal to greater than normal wrist extension is required	*Locking elbows for extension in the absence of active triceps*
Fingers	In the absence of innervation to finger flexors: • Normal metacarpophalangeal and interphalangeal motion • Mild tightness in extrinsic finger and thumb flexors	Tenodesis grasp for performance of ADLs
Hips	At least neutral extension Full flexion and full external rotation	Mat/bed mobility, lower body dressing, floor to wheelchair transfers
Hamstrings	110°-120° of passive straight leg raise	Long sitting, dressing, mat/bed mobility, floor to wheelchair transfers
Ankles	At least neutral dorsiflexion	Transfers, prevention of skin breakdown while seated in a wheelchair

Note: Italicized ROM requirements do not pertain to this patient case.

hook and because of the possibility for the return of voluntary motor function caudal to the neurological level of injury in the months and years following injury. Selective stretching must occur to promote *shortening* in the long finger flexors (Figs. 16-1A and B). Dynamic hand splints can be used to promote the use of a tenodesis grasp and resting hand splints can be used to promote the required muscle shortening that is needed to effectively use this type of grasp. The physical therapist must reinforce that when the patient is performing other functional mobility activities, the hand in contact with the support surface must have the fingers remained flexed to prevent overstretching of the long finger flexors during mobility training (Fig. 16-1C).

In addition to selective stretching, selective strengthening is appropriate for the patient with tetraplegia. In the first few weeks of rehabilitation, resistance exercises may be contraindicated due to the risk of spinal instability. Once the patient is allowed to perform resistance exercises, the use of *bilateral* upper extremity strengthening should be emphasized to avoid rotational and asymmetrical forces on the spine.[5] Strengthening can be performed with active assisted, active, or resisted motions depending on the strength of the muscle group being strengthened. Progressive resisted exercises can be performed bilaterally with manual resistance in straight planes, in diagonal patterns using proprioceptive neuromuscular facilitation (PNF), and/or with cuff weights. Strengthening for a patient with C7

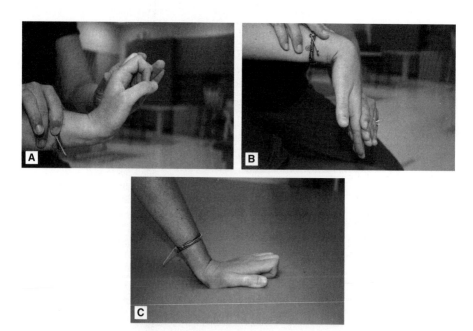

Figure 16-1. Protecting an individual's tenodesis grip. **A.** To stretch the wrist flexors, the therapist ensures the individual's fingers are in a flexed position while stretching the wrist into extension.
B. To stretch the short finger flexors, the therapist ensures that the individual's wrist is in a flexed position prior to stretching the fingers to a neutral position. **C.** During mobility activities that require the individual's hand on a support surface, his/her fingers should be positioned in flexion to prevent overstretching of the long finger flexors.

tetraplegia should focus on bilateral strengthening of scapular stabilizers, depressors, and protractors; shoulder flexors, extensors, and horizontal adductors; elbow flexors and extensors; and wrist extensors.[2,5]

Since this patient has already developed tolerance to sitting upright, she can begin working on increasing her sitting balance. This skill will be developed in short sitting and long sitting. It is easier to perform sitting balance tasks in long sitting as long as the patient has the requisite hamstring length. Sitting balance in short and long sitting can begin with the use of bilateral upper extremities and progress to unilateral upper extremity support, then sitting without upper extremity support. The patient must learn to use arm and head motions to maintain sitting balance.[2] These sitting skills assist the patient in performance of transfers and dressing.

Mobility training to allow the patient to meet her goals related to bed mobility includes rolling bilaterally, moving from supine to/from long sitting, moving from supine to/from prone, moving from supine to/from short sitting on the edge of the bed. These mobility skills require a blend of skill and strength.

In order to accomplish rolling from supine to sidelying or prone, the individual needs to use a movement strategy that uses momentum to produce the rolling motion. To initiate the roll, the individual throws her arms side-to-side and moves her head and neck in the same direction as her arms to gain enough momentum to roll herself onto her side (Fig. 16-2). To teach this activity, the physical therapist

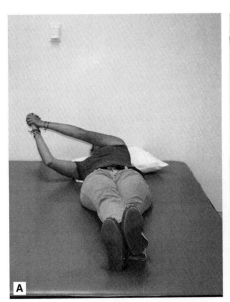 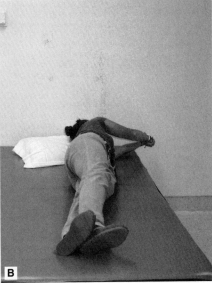

Figure 16-2. Rolling from supine to left sidelying in an individual with a complete (AIS A) SCI at the neurological level of C7. **A.** The individual starts the rolling motion by raising her arms and positioning them in the opposite direction of the roll in order to use momentum to complete the roll. **B.** To complete the roll, the individual continues the momentum from the right to the left and ends on her left side. To decrease the difficulty of the task, this individual is performing the roll with her legs crossed in the direction of the roll. In the early learning stages, the therapist will likely need to assist the patient with this lower extremity positioning.

can decrease the initial task difficulty by starting the individual in a half-sidelying position, propping her on wedges, and/or positioning the opposite leg crossed over the leg in the direction of the roll. As the individual develops competency in this task, the difficulty can be incrementally increased until she is able to perform a full roll from supine to sidelying and supine to prone without physical assistance or adaptive equipment. If the individual is not able to perform this task without physical assistance, the use of bed ladders or leg loops can be used to assist the individual with the performance of the task.

The individual needs to learn to move from supine to long sitting and short sitting. This patient has triceps innervation, which makes this task much easier to perform than for individuals with SCI at the C5 or C6 neurological levels. The ability to attain the long sitting position allows her to learn upper and lower body dressing in a more stable balance position than short sitting. The ability to attain short sitting allows the individual to prepare for transfers in a wheelchair. Depending on the choice of assistive devices and bowel and bladder management, it is important to teach the individual to transfer to and from a toilet or commode-shower chair. A commode-shower chair is a wheelchair that is waterproof and has a cut-out in the seat to serve as a commode (Fig. 16-3). This allows individuals to shower after

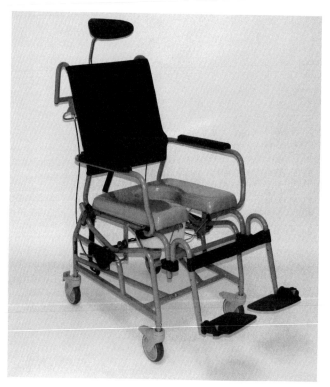

Figure 16-3. A waterproof commode-shower chair is a wheelchair that has a cut-out in the seat to serve as a commode to allow individuals to shower after performing a bowel program without having to transfer to another surface. (Reproduced with permission from Activeaid, Inc. Redwood Falls, MN. Activeaid Model 285/18.)

performing a bowel program without having to transfer to another surface.[7] The individual and caregivers must be trained in transferring to and from this type of chair in addition to the individual's regular wheelchair.

Individuals using a wheelchair for locomotion should be assessed for the ability to propel a manual wheelchair (if appropriate) or to safely navigate a power wheelchair. For individuals propelling manual wheelchairs, the physical therapist should assess a patient's ability to propel and perform advanced wheelchair skills such as wheelies (*i.e.*, lifting the front caster wheels up) and ascending/descending curbs, ramps, and stairs—skills that are important to increase mobility independence. The individual with a complete SCI at the C7 level has the potential to ascend and descend 2- to 4-inch curbs, although it is very challenging due to the lack of innervation to the finger flexors to allow griping of the rims of the wheelchair. Without active finger flexion, the individual must increase friction by pushing in on the wheelchair rims to control the acceleration and deceleration as needed. The **Wheelchair Skills Test** is an outcome measure designed to measure performance on a variety of wheelchair skills for a manual wheelchair; this assessment takes an average of 27 minutes to complete and requires an environment with a variety of incline heights, doorways, and stairs.[8] A recent study of manual wheelchair users with SCI found that those who had a higher total score on the Wheelchair Skills Test had increased community participation and higher life satisfaction as measured by the Hospital Anxiety and Depression Scale-Anxiety subscale, Satisfaction with Life Scale, Short Form Health Survey (SF-36), and Craig Handicap Assessment and Reporting Technique (CHART).[9] This study found that the single skill that was predictive of higher quality of life and higher community participation was the ability to descend a 15-cm curb.[9] There is also a version of the Wheelchair Skills Test to assess wheelchair mobility in a power wheelchair.[2]

To prevent overuse injuries to the shoulder due to poor pushing mechanics, the physical therapist needs to teach individuals who will be propelling a manual wheelchair the optimal mechanics. The Consortium for Spinal Cord Medicine has put forth **recommendations for upper extremity protection from overuse injuries and pain.**[10] These recommendations include emphasizing the importance of educating healthcare providers and persons with SCI about the risk and prevention of upper extremity injury and pain. The individual should be educated to minimize the frequency and force utilized during repetitive upper extremity tasks. The individual's equipment and ergonomics should also be routinely evaluated to ensure proper fit, use, and mechanics. The Consortium recommends that manual wheelchair users minimize the risk for injury by using long, smooth strokes to propel the wheelchair. Individuals should be positioned in the wheelchair to allow for 100° to 120° of elbow flexion when the individual's hand is at the top center of the pushrim. In addition, manual wheelchairs should be fully customized and made of the lightest possible material. The individual may also consider a power wheelchair system or power-assist wheels that can decrease the risk of upper extremity injury and pain by minimizing shoulder overuse. Depending on the level of injury, even individuals who are able to perform transfers without assistance may benefit from the use of adaptive transfer equipment and/or limiting the number of transfers they perform each day to promote upper extremity preservation. The patient in this case should be educated about the risk of overuse injuries and encouraged to use proper pushing mechanics for manual wheelchair propulsion, minimize the number of transfers performed per day, and she should be fitted for a fully customizable ultra-lightweight manual wheelchair. Individuals with C5 or C6 tetraplegia who use a manual chair for mobility should also consider the use of a power wheelchair or power-assist wheels for long distance wheelchair propulsion to assist with upper extremity preservation.

Evidence-Based Clinical Recommendations

SORT: Strength of Recommendation Taxonomy
A: Consistent, good-quality patient-oriented evidence
B: Inconsistent or limited-quality patient-oriented evidence
C: Consensus, disease-oriented evidence, usual practice, expert opinion, or case series

1. For individuals with low tetraplegia (C5-C8, AIS A, B, or C), the three most common physical therapy activities in inpatient rehabilitation facilities are range of motion/stretching, transfers, and then strengthening. **Grade B**

2. The Wheelchair Skills Test measures performance on a variety of manual wheelchair skills and the results may predict quality of life and community participation. **Grade B**

3. Education about manual wheelchair positioning and proper propulsion mechanics provided to individuals with SCI may help prevent upper extremity overuse injuries. **Grade B**

COMPREHENSION QUESTIONS

16.1 Which of the following statements is true regarding compensatory and restorative approaches to rehabilitation?

A. A compensatory approach focuses on regaining strength and resuming the performance of functional abilities.

B. A restorative strategy focuses on restoring the individual's ability to perform a task with the use of adaptive equipment using different movement strategies than the individual used before his/her injury.

C. A restorative approach is always the most appropriate approach.

D. A compensatory approach uses a variety of substitution movement strategies and/or adaptive equipment to accomplish desired tasks.

16.2 How much straight leg raise passive ROM is required for an individual with motor complete tetraplegia in order to perform bed mobility and lower body dressing activities?

A. 80° to 90°

B. 90°

C. 90° to 100°

D. 110° to 120°

16.3 Why would an individual with SCI use a tenodesis grasp?

A. A tenodesis grasp includes using active finger extension and flexion to manipulate small objects with precise fine motor skills.

B. A tenodesis grasp is used by individuals with T4 paraplegia to grasp and manipulate objects.

C. A tenodesis grasp is used in the absence of innervation to the long finger flexors.

D. A tenodesis grasp is used in the absence of innervation to the finger extensors.

ANSWERS

16.1 **D.** Rehabilitation approaches specific to the care of individuals with SCI typically include teaching compensatory strategies to allow them to perform tasks in the absence of normal muscle innervation using substitution strategies and/or adaptive equipment to accomplish desired tasks. A restorative approach to rehabilitation is typically used in rehabilitation of patients with motor incomplete spinal cord injuries with the goal of recovery of normal movement and minimal compensations.

16.2 **D.** 110° to 120° of straight leg raise is needed for individuals with tetraplegia to perform bed mobility skills including long sitting, transitioning from supine to long sitting, and dressing. An individual with SCI benefits from mild tightness of low back tissues for sitting posture and for improving the ability to move the lower body using movements generated by the upper body. Until 110° of straight leg raise is attained, long sitting activities may need to be modified to prevent overstretching tissues in the lower back.

16.3 **C.** A tenodesis grasp is accomplished by extending the wrist (using extensor carpi radialis longus and brevis), which results in passive tension in the finger flexors (flexor digitorum profundus, flexor digitorum superficialis, flexor pollicis longus). This causes the fingers to flex and the thumb to form a lateral pinch with the index finger.[2,6] Preservation of tightness in the finger flexors is critical for individuals with C5 to C7 tetraplegia to allow the individual to grasp and manipulate objects using preserved active wrist extension.

REFERENCES

1. Consortium for Spinal Cord Medicine. Sexuality and reproductive health in adults with spinal cord injury: a clinical practice guideline for health-care providers. *J Spinal Cord Med.* 2010;33:281-336.

2. Somers MF. *Spinal Cord Injury Functional Rehabilitation.* 3rd ed. New Jersey, NJ: Pearson; 2010.

3. Taylor-Schroeder S, LaBarbera J, McDowell S, et al. The SCIRehab project: treatment time spent in SCI rehabilitation. Physical therapy treatment time during inpatient spinal cord injury rehabilitation. *J Spinal Cord Med.* 2011;34:149-161.

4. Umphred DA. *Neurological Rehabilitation.* 5th ed. St. Louis, MO: Mosby Elsevier; 2007.

5. O' Sullivan SB, Schmitz TJ. *Physical Rehabilitation.* Philadelphia, PA: FA Davis; 2007.

6. Harvey L. Principles of conservative management for a non-orthotic tenodesis grip in tetraplegics. *J Hand Ther.* 1996;9:238-242.

7. Malassigne P, Nelson AL, Cors MW, Amerson TL. Design of the advanced commode-shower chair for spinal cord-injured individuals. *J Rehabil Res Dev.* 2000;37:373-382.

8. Kirby RL, Swuste J, Dupuis DJ, MacLeod DA, Monroe R. The Wheelchair Skills Test: a pilot study of a new outcome measure. *Arch Phys Med Rehabil.* 2002;83:10-18.

9. Hosseini SM, Oyster ML, Kirby RL, Harrington AL, Boninger ML. Manual wheelchair skills capacity predicts quality of life and community integration in persons with spinal cord injury. *Arch Phys Med Rehabil.* 2012;93:2237-2243.

10. Consortium for Spinal Cord Medicine, Paralyzed Veterans of America. Preservation of upper limb function following spinal cord injury. *A Clinical Practice Guideline for Health-Care Professionals.* Washington, DC: Consortium for Spinal Cord Medicine; 2005. www.pva.org. Accessed June 12, 2012.

Lumbar Spinal Stenosis

Annie Burke-Doe

CASE 17

A 67-year-old male with coronary artery disease and chronic low back pain went to the neurologist complaining of 4 months of disabling leg pain when walking. The pain was located in the buttocks and posterior thighs in a symmetric distribution, and began after 10 minutes of walking on a level surface. The pain would ease after sitting for several minutes, and then he was able to continue walking. He reported being able to climb stairs to his home and to ride his bicycle without pain. The neurologist ruled out vascular claudication with Doppler ultrasound (*i.e.*, no evidence of vascular insufficiency in his legs). Neurologic examination showed limited mobility of the lumbar spine, but no local tenderness or deformity. Right straight leg raise to 55° elicited pain in the back and right buttock. Muscle bulk, tone, and strength in the lower limbs were normal. Tendon reflexes were symmetrical at the knees and depressed at the right ankle. Proprioception and vibration sensation were slightly diminished at the toes. Magnetic resonance imaging of the lumbosacral spine showed widespread degenerative spine disease, central disc bulges at L3-L4 and L4-L5, and a focal, right-sided, posterolateral disc protrusion at L5-S1. Deformation of the thecal sac at the lower lumbar levels and multilevel neuroforaminal narrowing were also present. Needle electromyography (EMG) revealed mild chronic partial denervation with reinnervation in the medial head of the right gastrocnemius muscle. A diagnosis of neurogenic claudication secondary to lumbar spinal stenosis (LSS) associated with a mild right-sided S1 radiculopathy was made. The neurologist referred the patient to the physical therapist for evaluation and treatment.

- ▶ What examination signs may be associated with this diagnosis?
- ▶ What are the most appropriate examination tests?
- ▶ What is his rehabilitation prognosis?
- ▶ What are the most appropriate physical therapy outcome measures for pain and functional change?
- ▶ What are possible complications interfering with physical therapy?

KEY DEFINITIONS

CAUDA EQUINA SYNDROME: Loss of function of the lumbar plexus neurologic elements (nerve roots) of the spinal canal below the conus medullaris of the spinal cord

NEUROGENIC CLAUDICATION: Pain or discomfort in the low back, buttocks, and legs that is initiated or intensified with walking and is relieved by sitting

RADICULOPATHY: Neurologic condition characterized by dysfunction of a spinal nerve, its roots, or both; usually presents with unilateral pain, paresthesia, weakness, and/or reflex changes in the affected nerve root distribution

SPINAL STENOSIS: Narrowing of the spinal canal with encroachment on the neural structures by surrounding bone and soft tissue

Objectives

1. Describe lumbar spinal stenosis (LSS).
2. Identify the classic signs and symptoms of neurogenic claudication.
3. Discuss appropriate components of the examination.
4. Identify key components in the treatment of LSS.

Physical Therapy Considerations

PT considerations during management of the individual with chronic progressive low back pain, lower extremity pain, weakness, and neurogenic claudication due to LSS:

▶ **General physical therapy plan of care/goals:** Assess patient's need for understanding diagnosis; reduce pain and elucidate its relationship to posture and activity; improve range of motion (ROM), strength, and flexibility; improve functional activities; increase fitness level

▶ **Physical therapy interventions:** Mobilization and manipulation; muscle energy techniques; therapeutic exercise; joint protection; modalities for pain reduction; treadmill and/or bicycle training

▶ **Precautions during physical therapy:** Report signs/symptoms suggesting cauda equina syndrome, vascular, nonmechanical, or visceral sources to the physician; provocation testing prior to other tests may alter post-provocation test findings

▶ **Complications interfering with physical therapy:** Psychosocial factors, comorbidities, adverse drug reactions (ADRs) of nonsteroidal anti-inflammatories (NSAIDs)

Understanding the Health Condition

Spinal stenosis is defined as a narrowing of the spinal canal with encroachment on the neural structures by the surrounding bone and soft tissue.[1-3] Compression of nerve roots in the lumbar spine causes symptomatic LSS, which can be categorized into several distinct entities defined by the underlying reasons for the spinal nerve root compression.[4] Anatomically, narrowing may occur in the central spinal canal, in the area under the facet joints (subarticular stenosis), or more laterally, in the neural foramina.[4] Spinal stenosis is not always symptomatic and degenerative changes may not correlate with symptoms. In addition, abnormal anatomical findings can occur in the asymptomatic population.[4]

Arnoldi et al.[2] have classified LSS as either developmental (primary) or degenerative (secondary). The primary type is caused by developmental spinal anomalies[3] such as congenital shortening of the pedicles. Primary LSS typically presents in the third, fourth, and fifth decades of life when mild degenerative changes that would typically be tolerated result in narrowing sufficient to cause symptoms.[4,5] Secondary or acquired degenerative LSS is the most frequently observed type of spinal stenosis.[3-5] It typically occurs in those older than 60 years[3,6] and is associated with degeneration of the lumbar discs and facet joints.[4] It most frequently results from enlarging osteophytes at the facet joints, hypertrophy of the ligamentum flavum, and protrusion or bulging of intervertebral discs.[3,7] Other causes of acquired LSS include Paget's disease,[8] postsurgical changes, trauma, acromegaly,[9] ankylosing spondylitis,[5] and spondylolisthesis.[4]

Spinal stenosis is a prevalent and disabling condition with approximately 250,000 to 500,000 residents of the United States having symptoms.[10,11] This represents about 1 per 1000 persons and the number is estimated to grow as the population ages.[10] LSS remains the leading preoperative diagnosis for adults older than 65 years who undergo spinal surgery. It often results in considerable physical burden and is associated with significant healthcare costs.[12-14] Most persons older than 60 years have spinal stenosis to some degree. Because most patients with mild spinal stenosis are asymptomatic, the absolute frequency can only be estimated.[11]

Positive findings on plain radiographs of individuals with LSS include degenerative disc disease, osteoarthritis of the facets, spondylolisthesis, and narrowing of the interpedicular distance.[11] Although myelography was commonly used in the past to evaluate spinal cord or nerve root compression, it is an invasive procedure with possible adverse effects and is no longer routinely used.[13,15] Computed tomography (CT) is commonly used to evaluate the spinal elements; CT allows for accurate measurement of the canal dimensions when combined with contrast enhancement.[4,15] A dural sac with an anteroposterior diameter of less than 10 to 13 mm correlates with clinical findings of stenosis.[15,16] Magnetic resonance imaging (MRI) is comparable to contrast-enhanced CT in its ability to demonstrate spinal stenosis and is now the imaging modality of choice to assess the spinal canal and neural structures.[3,13,15]

Clinical manifestations of LSS range from asymptomatic to disabling. Symptomatic presentation is commonly associated with multilevel degenerative spine disease.[14] The etiology is typically due to mechanical compression on the neural elements or their blood supply.[14] Symptomatic spinal stenosis often presents with low back pain, signs and symptoms of focal nerve root injury, or neurogenic claudication.[14] Neurogenic claudication is classically described as poorly localized discomfort and aching pain in the lower back, buttocks, and legs that is precipitated by walking and relieved by sitting.[4,5,13,17,18] Some describe neuroclaudication symptoms as developing "spaghetti legs" or "walking like a drunken sailor."[9] Because the lumbar spinal canal volume increases with spinal flexion and decreases with extension,[19] some patients observe that they have fewer symptoms walking uphill,[9] resting, lying, sitting, or flexing the spine.[11,13,14] Neurologic changes are reported in 20% to 50% of patients[6,20] and cauda equina syndrome is considered rare.[2,21] Many patients are more troubled by poor balance, unsteady gait, or leg weakness that develops as they walk.[9]

Onset of symptoms with standing, location of maximal discomfort in the thighs, and preservation of pedal pulses help distinguish the "pseudoclaudication" of LSS from true claudication due to vascular insufficiency.[9] It can also be challenging to distinguish LSS from lumbar disc herniation since both conditions can produce pain radiating down the back of the thigh. Other features that lean toward a diagnosis of spinal stenosis include the *gradual* onset of symptoms, marked exacerbation with walking on level surfaces, and amelioration of symptoms with sitting or lumbar flexion.[9] In a study of 93 adults with back pain, Katz et al.[22] found that pain radiating into the buttocks or more distally had a sensitivity of 88% for the diagnosis of LSS, but a specificity of only 35%. In the same study, a history of back pain while standing, but no pain at all when sitting had a sensitivity of 46% and a specificity of LSS of 93%.[23] Thus, in those patients who present with pain radiating to the buttocks or further (high sensitivity) *and* have no pain when sitting (high specificity), it is more likely the diagnosis is LSS. In patients with LSS, Hall and colleagues[24] described symptoms involving the whole lower limb in 78% of cases, with 15% of the cases above the knee, and 6% of cases below the knee.

Restricted mobility, local lumbar spine tenderness, and evidence of root compression related to lumbar spinal degenerative disease are commonly associated with the diagnosis of LSS.[5] At rest, the neurologic examination is typically normal. Patients examined immediately after symptom-provoking treadmill stress tests may have minor motor, sensory, and reflex deficits that rapidly normalize with rest.[5] In a study by Fritz et al.[25], the authors suggested a **two-stage treadmill test (TSTT) as a diagnostic tool to determine the presence of LSS**. The TSTT is conducted by comparing a patient's walking tolerance on a level surface compared to a 15% incline at a self-selected pace. An earlier onset of symptoms with level walking, increased total walking time on an inclined treadmill, and prolonged recovery time after level walking were significantly associated with LSS. These findings are consistent with the fact that walking on a level surface places the spine in more extension (compression of spinal canal volume) than walking on an uphill incline, which increases spinal flexion (and lumbar spinal canal volume). Amundsen et al.[26] reported diminished or absent ankle reflexes in up to 50% of patients with LSS and weakness in 23% to 51% of that population. Tenhula et al.[27] have used the treadmill-bicycle test for differential diagnosis of LSS. In this study, 32 patients with LSS were evaluated pre- and post-spinal surgery. Patients had a significant increase in their symptoms from the start to the end of the treadmill test (lumbar spine in extension), but fewer patients had significant symptoms on bicycle testing (lumbar spine in flexion). Two years after lumbar spinal decompression surgery, the patients had an improvement in walking ability on treadmill testing, but showed no improvement in their ability to cycle. The authors believed the treadmill-bicycle test may be a useful tool for the differential diagnosis of neurogenic claudication.[27]

Conservative medical management for LSS frequently includes a combination of interventions such as bedrest, oral medications, epidural glucocorticoid injections, acupuncture, physical agents, postural and ergonomic advice, lumbar corsets, and flexion-based exercise programs.[24] When signs and symptoms persist despite conservative therapy, physicians typically offer the option of surgical intervention. The primary goal of surgery is to decompress the spinal canal and the neural foramina to eliminate pressure on the spinal nerve roots.[4] The traditional approach is a laminectomy or partial facetectomy.[16]

The natural history of LSS is not well understood.[10] A slow progression appears in all affected individuals. Even with significant narrowing, some patients show symptomatic and functional improvement or remain unchanged over time.[28] Sengupta and Herkowitz[29] summarized that in patients who have been followed for 5 to 10 years after LSS diagnosis, 45% stayed the same, 15% improved, and 30% reported progressive worsening of symptoms.

Physical Therapy Patient/Client Management

The efficacy of nonoperative treatment for spinal stenosis may depend greatly on the nature and severity of the patient's symptomatic and radiographic presentation.[23] There are few randomized controlled trials of nonoperative approaches to the management of spinal stenosis.[30] Nonoperative treatment is typically recommended for mild to moderate symptoms and is guided by clinical judgment, observational literature, and analogy to other spinal conditions.[4] Since spinal disorders are usually not caused by a single etiology and have similar signs and symptoms, classification systems have been developed to assist the clinician with making decisions, determining prognosis, evaluating the quality of care, conducting research, and selecting interventions.[21] Such classification systems categorize these disorders into syndromes based on a combination of pathology, clustering of signs and symptoms, and the duration of the symptoms.[20] A few classification systems for spinal disorders include the McKenzie Diagnostic Classification System, Delitto Treatment-Based Diagnostic Classification, and the Movement System Impairment-Based Classification.[20] The primary goals of physical therapy are to decrease symptoms and improve function. The physical therapist can suggest ways of modifying activities to avoid lumbar extension and teach the patient exercises to strengthen weak musculature.

Examination, Evaluation, and Diagnosis

Prior to the hands-on examination of this patient, the physical therapist needs to acquire information using a combination of open- and closed-ended questions. A patient with LSS should be asked questions related to medical history (comorbidities), social history (living situation), results of any diagnostic testing performed (imaging, EMG), medications (oral analgesics, epidural injections), prior level of function, and current complaints. Examples of questions include: "What are your symptoms?", "How long have you had low back pain or lower extremity symptoms?", "What increases your symptoms?", What relieves your symptoms?", "Have you fallen or stumbled recently?", "Do you live alone?", "What is your current level of activity?", "What activities have you modified in order to limit your symptoms?", and "What are your goals?" The therapist must screen the patient for any indicators of serious medical pathology or red flags (unexplained weight loss, constant pain that does not change with position, widespread neurologic signs) that increase the likelihood that the patient's problem is not of musculoskeletal origin. If red flags are present, the patient should be referred (back) to a physician.[20]

Physical therapists can use self-report outcome measures to help quantify progress in patients with LSS. The SF-36 Health Survey can assist with determination of general health and well being.[31] Condition-specific questionnaires such as the Oswestry Low Back Pain Disability Questionnaire[32] and the Roland-Morris Questionnaire[33] may be useful to determine improvement with treatment. Pain can be assessed with a visual analog scale (VAS) at rest and with activity (sitting, standing, and walking). When assessing pain related to activity level, it is important to closely monitor symptom changes and the time it takes before symptoms increase or improve.

The physical therapy examination begins with a systems review. It involves brief or limited examination of the status of the cardiovascular/pulmonary, integumentary, musculoskeletal, and neuromuscular systems as well as the communication ability, affect, cognition, language, and learning style of the patient.[34] The systems review helps the therapist determine areas that need further review and the overall psychological and emotional state of the patient.

The examination includes assessment of posture, ROM, flexibility, muscle performance, reflexes, neurodynamics, sensory changes, circulation, gait, and balance. The therapist should perform flexibility testing of the hip flexors and iliotibial band (Thomas test, Ober test), hamstrings, quadriceps, and gastrocnemius on a patient with suspected LSS because these structures are frequently shortened. Integrity of hip structures should also be assessed (e.g., by the scour test) to rule out other causes of buttock and thigh pain. Since almost all patients report that their lower extremity pain is altered by changes in position,[22] neurologic findings are often more pronounced after provocation testing (quadrant testing, joint mobility, neurodynamic testing). Therefore, it is critical to note whether any positive findings occur prior to or after provocation testing. Straight leg raise and reflexes at the ankle and knee may or may not be positive. Sensory testing should include the dermatomal distribution and level. Documentation of changes in severity of symptoms should be associated with a defined level of activity.

Patients with LSS who also have comorbidities of cardiovascular insufficiency, peripheral vascular disease, and/or polyneuropathy may describe signs and symptoms with walking—which may be difficult to differentiate from neurogenic claudication. The therapist should palpate pre- and post-activity bilateral distal peripheral pulses of the lower extremities and observe and record any skin changes (color, temperature). Neurogenic claudication can be clinically distinguished from vascular claudication by using graded treadmill testing.[27,35,36] The therapist records the time to the development of claudication pain and what the patient requires for symptoms to be relieved (flexion, sitting, or stopping activity). The graded treadmill testing protocol can assist the therapist with determination of the presence of neurogenic claudication and functional impact of spinal stenosis.[37] Neurogenic claudication improves with spinal flexion and increases with increasing lumbar lordosis even without activity.[3] In contrast, vascular claudication improves with rest in *any* position and is aggravated by lower extremity activity in any position, including cycling in a lumbar flexed position.[7] Functional ability (transfers, double and single leg balance, stair climbing) can also be assessed. When assessing gait, the therapist should particularly note stride, cadence, distance, any loss of balance, and potential need for assistive devices. Patients with LSS generally walk with a forward-stooped posture with lumbar flexion.[38] Special tests such as the Timed Up and Go[39] may be useful to determine baseline performance in patients with transfer and gait dysfunction. If balance impairment is noted or the patient has a history of falling, the Berg Balance Test[40] or Tinetti Assessment Tool of Gait and Balance[41] may be more appropriate.

Plan of Care and Interventions

Identified impairments and dysfunctions in this population may include deficits in knowledge related to the LSS diagnosis, pain, impaired muscle performance, impaired function, and decreased ROM. Goals based on findings and the patient's needs generally include independence in a home exercise program and pain management, improvement in functional abilities, improved muscle performance and flexibility, and improvement in aerobic fitness. **Treatments commonly used for patients with LSS** include therapeutic exercises (flexion bias,[21,42-44] stretching tight muscles,[45] strengthening,[45] lumbar stabilization,[21,28,43,44] postural awareness,[28] conditioning activities[20,21]), transfer and gait training (cadence, distance tolerated, use of assistive devices), manual therapy[17] (soft tissue and joint mobilization), lumbar traction (for hypomobility), education on diagnosis and avoiding symptom provocation[21] (extension/axial loading), postural awareness and body mechanics,[21] and pain-relieving modalities.[46,47] **The most appropriate conditioning activities** to maintain or improve aerobic fitness include inclined treadmill walking,[25] partial body-weight-support treadmill training,[48] bicycling[5,20] (which maintains spinal flexion bias to decrease spinal compression), and aquatic therapy[20] (which reduces spinal compression forces).

The physical therapist may refer the patient to other providers if he presents with lost or decreased ability to perform activities of daily living, needs assistance with a weight reduction program, may benefit from a lumbar orthosis, has increased emotional or psychiatric involvement, and/or is unable to manage his pain. If patients do not improve with conservative management, the therapist may also refer the patient for a surgical consultation.

Evidence-Based Clinical Recommendations

SORT: Strength of Recommendation Taxonomy

A: Consistent, good-quality patient-oriented evidence
B: Inconsistent or limited-quality patient-oriented evidence
C: Consensus, disease-oriented evidence, usual practice, expert opinion, or case series

1. Onset of symptoms with standing, location of maximal discomfort in the thighs, and preservation of pedal pulses distinguishes the "pseudoclaudication" due to lumbar spinal stenosis from true claudication due to vascular insufficiency. **Grade C**

2. Physical therapists can use a two-stage treadmill test (TSTT) as a diagnostic tool for lumbar spinal stenosis. **Grade B**

3. Therapeutic exercise for individuals with LSS should encourage flexion and unloading of the axial spine. **Grade B**

4. To promote spinal flexion bias, inclined treadmill walking, partial body-weight-support treadmill walking, and bicycling are recommended for general conditioning in individuals with LSS. **Grade C**

COMPREHENSION QUESTIONS

17.1 Which of the following statements is true regarding neurogenic claudication?

   A. Neurogenic claudication is characterized by vascular insufficiency after prolonged walking.

   B. Neurogenic claudication is characterized by lower extremity pain or cramping with reduction in pedal pulses.

   C. Neurogenic claudication is characterized by lower extremity pain or cramping with standing erect or walking; symptoms are relieved by sitting down.

   D. Neurogenic claudication is characterized by increased lower extremity pain with spinal extension due to an increase in spinal canal diameter.

17.2 In a patient with the diagnosis of lumbar spinal stenosis, what is the *most* likely gait deviation a physical therapist may observe?

   A. Narrow base of support

   B. Increased walking tolerance

   C. Trendelenburg sign

   D. Buttock and thigh pain

ANSWERS

17.1 **C.** In patients with lumbar spinal stenosis, symptoms of neurogenic claudication usually worsen with spinal extension and prolonged walking. Symptoms of neurogenic claudication are increased with spinal extension due to *decreased* spinal canal diameter (option D). Patients often assume a flexed spinal posture to reduce symptoms because this increases the spinal canal diameter and relieves pressure on the spinal cord.

17.2 **D.** Most patients with lumbar spinal stenosis demonstrate a wide-based gait and complain of buttock and thigh pain that increases with walking.

REFERENCES

1. Weinstein JN, Tosteson TD, Lurie JD, Tosteson AN, Blood E. Surgical versus nonsurgical therapy for lumbar spinal stenosis. *N Engl J Med*. 2008;358:794-810.

2. Arnoldi CC, Brodsky AE, Cauchoix J, et al. Lumbar spinal stenosis and nerve root entrapment syndromes. Definition and classification. *Clin Orthop Relat Res*. 1976;115:4-5.

3. Hellman DB, Imboden JJB. Musculoskeletal & immunologic disorders. In: McPhee SJ, Papadakis MA, Rabow MW, eds. *Current Medical Diagnosis & Treatment*. New York, NY: McGraw Hill; 2011.

4. Katz JN, Harris MB. Clinical practice. Lumbar spinal stenosis. *N Engl J Med*. 2008;358:818-825.

5. Medlink Neurology. Lumbar spinal stenosis. 2010. www.medlink.com. Accessed December 19, 2011.

6. Turner JA, Ersek M, Herron L, Deyo R. Surgery for lumbar spinal stenosis. Attempted meta-analysis of the literature. *Spine*. 1992;17:1-8.

7. Arbit E, Pannullo S. Lumbar stenosis: a clinical review. *Clin Orthop Relat Res*. 2001;384:137-143.

8. Weisz GM. Lumbar spinal canal stenosis in Paget's disease. *Spine*. 1983;8:192-198.

9. Epstein N, Whelan M, Benjamin V. Acromegaly and spinal stenosis. Case report. *J Neurosurg*. 1982;56:145-147.

10. Hsiang JK, Furnam MB, Nadalo LA, Pannullo RP. Spinal stenosis. In: Medscape. http://emedicine.medscape.com/article/1913265-overview. Accessed May 10, 2013.

11. Kalichman L, Cole R, Kim DH, et al. Spinal stenosis prevalence and association with symptoms: the Framingham Study. *Spine J*. 2009;9:545-550.

12. Elam K, Taylor V, Ciol MA, Franklin GM, Deyo RA. Impact of a worker's compensation practice guideline on lumbar spine fusion in Washington State. *Med Care*. 1997;35:417-424.

13. Ciol MA, Deyo RA, Howell E, Kreif S. An assessment of surgery for spinal stenosis: time trends, geographic variations, complications, and reoperations. *J Am Geriatr Soc*. 1996;44:285-290.

14. Fanuele JC, Birkmeyer NJ, Abdu WA, Tosteson TD, Weinstein JN. The impact of spinal problems on the health status of patients: have we underestimated the effect? *Spine*. 2000;25:1509-1514.

15. Hu SS, Tribus CB, Tay BK, Bhatia NN. Disorders disease and injury of the spine. In: Skinner HB, ed. *Current Diagnosis & Treatment in Orthopedics*. 4th ed. New York, NY: McGraw Hill; 2011.

16. Rao R. Neck pain, cervical radiculopathy, and cervical myelopathy: pathophysiology, natural history, and clinical evaluation. *Instr Course Lect*. 2003;52:479-488.

17. Whitman JM, Flynn TW, Fritz JM. Nonsurgical management of patients with lumbar spinal stenosis: a literature review and a case series of three patients managed with physical therapy. *Phys Med Rehabil Clin N Am*. 2003;14:77-101, vi-vii.

18. Bridwell KH. Lumbar spinal stenosis. Diagnosis, management, and treatment. *Clin Geriatr Med*. 1994;10:677-701.

19. Panjabi MM, Takata K, Goel VK. Kinematics of lumbar intervertebral foramen. *Spine*. 1983;8: 348-357.

20. Chiarello C. Spinal disorders. In: Cameron MH, Monroe LG, eds. *Physical Rehabilitation: Evidence-based Examination, Evaluation, and Intervention.* St. Louis, MO: Saunders Elsevier; 2007:140-193.

21. Fritz JM. Use of a classification approach to the treatment of 3 patients with low back syndrome. *Phys Ther.* 1998;78:766-777.

22. Katz JN, Dalgas M, Stucki G, et al. Degenerative lumbar spinal stenosis. Diagnostic value of the history and physical examination. *Arthritis Rheum.* 1995;38:1236-1241.

23. Simotas AC. Nonoperative treatment for lumbar spinal stenosis. *Clin Orthop Relat Res.* 2001;384: 153-161.

24. Hall S, Bartleson JD, Onofrio BM, Baker HL, Jr., Okazaki H, O'Duffy JD. Lumbar spinal stenosis. Clinical features, diagnostic procedures, and results of surgical treatment in 68 patients. *Ann Intern Med.* 1985;103:271-275.

25. Fritz JM, Erhard RE, Delitto A, Welch WC, Nowakowski PE. Preliminary results of the use of a two-stage treadmill test as a clinical diagnostic tool in the differential diagnosis of lumbar spinal stenosis. *J Spinal Disord.* 1997;10:410-416.

26. Amundsen T, Weber H, Lilleas F, Nordal HJ, Abdelnoor M, Magnaes B. Lumbar spinal stenosis. Clinical and radiologic features. *Spine*. 1995;20:1178-1186.

27. Tenhula J, Lenke LG, Bridwell KH, Gupta P, Riew D. Prospective functional evaluation of the surgical treatment of neurogenic claudication in patients with lumbar spinal stenosis. *J Spinal Disord.* 2000;13:276-282.

28. Fritz JM, Delitto A, Welch WC, Erhard RE. Lumbar spinal stenosis: a review of current concepts in evaluation, management, and outcome measurements. *Arch Phys Med Rehabil.* 1998;79:700-708.

29. Sengupta DK, Herkowitz HN. Lumbar spinal stenosis. Treatment strategies and indications for surgery. *Orthop Clin N Am.* 2003;34:281-295.

30. ECRI Health Technology Assessment Group. Treatment of degenerative lumbar spinal stenosis. *Evid Rep Technol Assess (Summ).* 2001;32:1-5.

31. Ware JE, Jr. SF-36 health survey update. *Spine*. 2000;25:3130-3139.

32. Fairbank JC, Couper J, Davies JB, O'Brien JP. The Oswestry low back pain disability questionnaire. *Physiotherapy.* 1980;66:271-273.

33. Roland M, Morris R. A study of the natural history of back pain. Part I: development of a reliable and sensitive measure of disability in low-back pain. *Spine*. 1983;8:141-144.

34. APTA. *American Physical Therapy Association: Guide to Physical Therapist Practice.* 3rd ed. Alexandria, VA: American Physical Therapy Association; 2003.

35. Yukawa Y, Lenke LG, Tenhula J, Bridwell KH, Riew KD, Blanke K. A comprehensive study of patients with surgically treated lumbar spinal stenosis with neurogenic claudication. *J Bone Joint Surg Am.* 2002;84-A:1954-1959.

36. Bal S, Celiker R, Palaoglu S, Cila A. F wave studies of neurogenic intermittent claudication in lumbar spinal stenosis. *Am J Phys Med Rehabil.* 2006;85:135-140.

37. Snowden ML, Haselkorn JK, Kraft GH, et al. Dermatomal somatosensory evoked potentials in the diagnosis of lumbosacral spinal stenosis: comparison with imaging studies. *Muscle Nerve.* 1992;15:1036-1044.

38. Thomas SA. Spinal stenosis: history and physical examination. *Phys Med Rehabil Clin N Am.* 2003;14:29-39.

39. Podsiadlo D, Richardson S. The timed "Up & Go": a test of basic functional mobility for frail elderly persons. *J Am Geriatr Soc.* 1991;39:142-148.

40. Bogle Thorbahn LD, Newton RA. Use of the Berg Balance Test to predict falls in elderly persons. *Phys Ther.* 1996;76:576-583; discussion 84-85.

41. Tinetti ME. Performance-oriented assessment of mobility problems in elderly patients. *J Am Geriatr Soc.* 1986;34:119-126.

42. Rademeyer I. Manual therapy for lumbar spinal stenosis: a comprehensive physical therapy approach. *Phys Med Rehabil Clin N Am.* 2003;14:103-110, vii.

43. Hilibrand AS, Rand N. Degenerative lumbar stenosis: diagnosis and management. *J Am Acad Orthop Surg.* 1999;7:239-249.

44. Rittenberg JD, Ross AE. Functional rehabilitation for degenerative lumbar spinal stenosis. *Phys Med Rehabil Clin N Am.* 2003;14:111-120.

45. Bodack MP, Monteiro M. Therapeutic exercise in the treatment of patients with lumbar spinal stenosis. *Clin Orthop Relat Res.* 2001:384:144-152.

46. DuPriest CM. Nonoperative management of lumbar spinal stenosis. *J Manipulative Physiol Ther.* 1993;16:411-414.

47. Onel D, Sari H, Donmez C. Lumbar spinal stenosis: clinical/radiologic therapeutic evaluation in 145 patients. Conservative treatment or surgical intervention? *Spine.* 1993;18:291-298.

48. Fritz JM, Erhard RE, Vignovic M. A nonsurgical treatment approach for patients with lumbar spinal stenosis. *Phys Ther.* 1997;77:962-973.

Nontraumatic Spinal Cord Injury

Timothy Harvey
Sharon L. Gorman

A 50-year-old male presented to the emergency department (ED) after worsening back pain and progressively decreasing strength in his legs. The patient had presented 6 months prior to an overseas ED and had a brief hospitalization after complaining of back pain and right leg radiculopathy. Imaging conducted during that admission found "nine bulging discs," but aside from this brief hospitalization, no interventions were undertaken for his back pain. The patient's prior medical history consists of chronic back pain that the patient attributes to his work in the military. Additional medical history includes hypertension, obesity (body mass index = 32.4 kg/m^2), left ventricular hypertrophy, and recurrent kidney stones. He has had a long military career and he was working in security prior to his current presentation at the ED. He has an active lifestyle with regular motorcycle riding, swimming, skydiving, and other activities that give him an "adrenaline rush." The patient was urgently admitted to the hospital and he received an emergency decompression laminectomy from T11 to L4 with hardware placement. Immediately postoperatively, the patient was unable to move his lower extremities. The postoperative computed tomography (CT) scan showed large disc herniations from T6 to T10, so a second surgery for transpedicular decompression from T9 to T10 was conducted. Two days after admission, the patient had his third and final surgery to place pedicular screws from T6 to L4. The patient spent 3 weeks in the acute hospital with minimal mobility or physical therapy interventions. He has just been admitted to an inpatient rehabilitation facility (IRF) for physical and occupational therapy.

▶ Based on his health condition, what do you anticipate will be the contributors to activity limitations and impairments?
▶ What are the examination priorities?
▶ What are the most appropriate physical therapy interventions?
▶ What is the prognosis for independent ambulation for this patient?

KEY DEFINITIONS

AMERICAN SPINAL INJURY ASSOCIATION (ASIA) CLASSIFICATION OF SPINAL CORD INJURY: Systematic assessment of sensation, motor, and reflex activity designed for consistent description of persons after spinal cord injury; classification includes determination of a spinal level of injury (*e.g.*, T4) and assignment of an impairment category (*i.e.*, A through E)

COMPUTED TOMOGRAPHY (CT) SCAN: Series of radiographic images taken from many different angles that uses computer processing to create cross-sectional images

OVERGROUND AMBULATION TRAINING: Locomotor retraining conducted on the ground without the use of body-weight support and/or treadmills; requires higher equilibrium demand from the patient and is more task-oriented than locomotor training with body-weight unloading

Objectives

1. Examine an individual with spinal cord injury to determine his/her American Spinal Injury Association Impairment Scale (AIS) classification.

2. Identify standardized outcome measures that can detect improvements related to gait and balance for persons with spinal cord injury.

3. Describe factors that inform prognosis for improvements in gait in persons with spinal cord injury.

4. Prescribe interventions that increase weightbearing and encourage upright posture to enhance function for persons with spinal cord injury.

Physical Therapy Considerations

PT considerations during management of the individual with nontraumatic spinal cord injury:

▶ **General physical therapy plan of care/goals:** Increase activity and participation; increase strength; prevent or minimize loss of range of motion (ROM), strength, and aerobic functional capacity; improve quality of life

▶ **Physical therapy interventions:** Neuromuscular re-education; functional training; pre-gait and gait training, including body-weight-supported treadmill training (BWSTT); patient/family education and training on positioning and ROM exercises; coordination of care with interprofessional team; prescription of supportive devices

▶ **Precautions during physical therapy:** Monitor vital signs; coordination with medical team for pain management; progressive weightbearing during gait training; protection of joints and protection of skin in insensate areas

► **Complications interfering with physical therapy:** Postsurgical movement restrictions; patient safety; nonsurgical spinal stabilization methods; integument damage due to immobility; deep vein thrombosis, pulmonary embolism

Understanding the Health Condition

Spinal cord injury (SCI) can occur from many different injuries or diseases. Spinal cord injuries are classified as either traumatic or nontraumatic. A traumatic SCI occurs due to a definable or nonrandom event causing damage to the spinal cord. A nontraumatic SCI (NTSCI) occurs due to etiologies such as spinal stenosis, tumorous compression, vascular ischemia, infection, or congenital disorders.[1] These etiologies cannot be traced back to specific events and often occur over a period of time. As a result, increased age is associated with an increased risk of developing NTSCI.[2] Regardless of the cause, spinal cord injuries are further classified into one of two categories: complete or incomplete. A person with a complete SCI is described as having "no preservation of sensory function and/or motor function more than three segments below the neurological level of injury."[3] A person with an incomplete SCI has *some* sensory and/or motor function more than three segments below the neurological level of injury. Based on the limb involvement, the terms "paraplegia" or "tetraplegia" may be used. Paraplegia is impairment or loss of motor and/or sensory function of the lower body with involvement of both legs, whereas tetraplegia involves all four limbs and the trunk. In the United States, 12,000 new spinal cord injuries occur yearly and in 2010 it was estimated that 265,000 people were living with some sort of SCI.[4] In 1979, the average age of a person with SCI was 28.7 years. By 2005, the average age had increased to 40 years.[4] Approximately 81% of spinal cord injuries occur in males. Of all the individuals newly diagnosed with SCI, half have an incomplete SCI.[5]

A common cause of NTSCI is compression of the spinal cord. The vertebral disc is often the cause of the compression. The vertebral canal is a small opening for the spinal cord to travel through. When a bulging or herniated disc invades the vertebral canal, it can compress the spinal cord (Fig. 18-1). If not treated in a timely manner, permanent damage to the spinal cord can occur. This patient's first surgery—a decompression laminectomy with hardware from T11 to L4—involved removal of the spinous processes through incisions in the laminae to allow the spinal cord more space by opening the vertebral canal posteriorly. The patient's second surgery, a transpedicular decompression at T9-T10, involved increasing the size of the vertebral canal via incisions at the pedicles. The patient's third and final surgery stabilized the spine from T6 to L4 using screws from pedicle to pedicle. A CT scan of this patient's spine after his surgeries shows multiple pedicle screws (Fig. 18-2).

The strongest predictor of neurologic recovery after SCI is the degree of completeness of the injury. This can be categorized using the **American Spinal Injury Association (ASIA) Impairment Scale, or AIS.** Persons with complete SCI have a decreased chance of neurologic motor recovery. A study by Geisler et al.[6] examined 760 patients with SCI over a 6-year period to determine prognostic factors and found that patients with complete SCI demonstrated less return of motor function

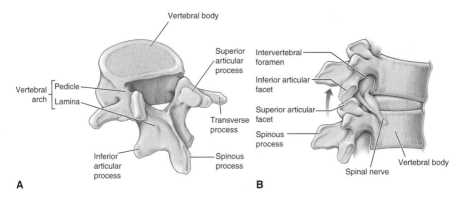

Figure 18-1. A. Single vertebra showing the narrow vertebral canal between the vertebral body and arch. **B.** Sagittal view of two vertebrae with vertebral disc between them and spinal cord running through vertebral canal. (Reproduced with permission from Morton DA, Foreman KB, Albertine KH, eds. *The Big Picture: Gross Anatomy.* New York: McGraw-Hill; 2011. Figures 1-4B and D.)

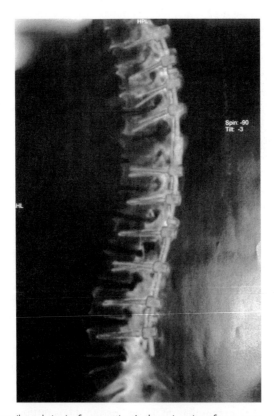

Figure 18-2. CT scan (lateral view) of case patient's thoracic spine after surgery.

compared to those with incomplete SCI. A recent systematic review of 10 articles assessing prognostic factors for functional recovery concluded that patients with complete SCI had less functional recovery and an increased mortality rate compared to those with incomplete SCI.[7]

Other good prognostic indicators include preservation of motor and sensory function, early neurologic return, younger age at time of SCI, and certain patterns of SCI. In two separate studies by Waters et al.,[8,9] patients with paraplegia and tetraplegia were assessed. Both studies concluded that preserved motor function after SCI was critical for the best functional prognosis. Less than 1% of patients with SCI experience complete neurologic recovery while in the hospital. Most patients plateau in functional gains approximately 6 months post-SCI and a few individuals continued to improve up to 1 year after SCI. Individuals who do not lose pinprick sensation also have a greater chance of motor recovery. In 59 patients with SCI, Poynton et al.[10] discovered that 85% of the motor segments graded 0/5 that *still* had preserved pinprick sensation in the corresponding dermatomes returned to functional strength of at least 3/5. In a small study of 21 patients with cervical SCI, 75% of those with preserved pinprick sensation regained the ability to walk at follow-up (average of 49.6 months after initial pinprick examination).[11] *Early* neurologic return is a positive prognostic indicator for functional recovery after SCI. Ishida et al.[12] examined 22 patients with acute central cervical SCI over a 2-year period and concluded that more improvement in the first 6 weeks after the injury predicted increased motor and sensory recovery. Neurologic recovery is also directly related to age; the younger the person is at the time of the SCI, the greater the probability of functional return.[13,14] In a review on age-related outcomes, McKinley et al.[14] concluded that "functional independence was negatively affected by age in both paraplegic and tetraplegic individuals." Last, the *pattern* of neurological injury also influences prognosis. In a retrospective review of 412 patients with traumatic, incomplete cervical SCI, those with Brown-Sequard or central cord syndrome had the greatest chance of motor recovery.[13] Factors that had no influence on motor recovery were early anterior decompressions, sex, race, type of fracture, or mechanism of injury.[13]

Neuroplasticity is the concept that the brain "remaps" itself after injury, allowing other areas of the brain to compensate and adapt where information is processed and executed. There are two types of plasticity that should be considered with SCI recovery. Spontaneous plasticity describes the structural changes occurring in the nervous system after SCI. This includes sprouting that occurs in the axons of spared intersegmental interneurons to form new synapses.[15,16] Activity-dependent plasticity includes the adaptive neuronal changes that occur as a result of sensory input and repetitive limb movement. These neuronal changes are task-specific; if the activity is halted, the changes will disappear.[15-18] Physical therapy interventions can be directed toward enhancing activity-dependent plasticity for persons with SCI. **Body-weight-supported treadmill training (BWSTT)** is hypothesized to work in this fashion. BWSTT allows patients to ambulate and eventually make structural changes in the brain and spinal cord with practice. This is crucial because without the use of BWSTT, the patient could not make the necessary structural changes in the brain due to the inability to ambulate without the assistance provided by BWSTT. During BWSTT, the patient uses a harness that supports a predetermined percentage of his weight and prevents him from falling when he attempts to walk on a treadmill. This system allows the physical therapist to assist the patient during each phase of gait in order to improve his gait pattern. BWSTT has been shown to be effective in improving ambulatory status in patients with SCI.[19-21] In a pilot study, four out of five patients who utilized a wheelchair for locomotion improved to over-ground ambulation after 36 hours of BWSTT over a 3-month period.[19] In three participants with incomplete SCI, BWSTT increased walking speed and distance and decreased oxygen consumption per meter by 65%.[20] BWSTT has also been shown to partially reverse muscle atrophy after SCI.[21]

Many individuals with SCI have doubts and fears about what their life will be like once they return home. A common question many patients ask is, "Will I ever be able to walk again?" This can be challenging for physical therapists to answer. Therapists must use reliable research and clinical experience to answer this question appropriately. While there is published evidence to support BWSTT as a beneficial intervention, there is no evidence confirming that it is the *best* technique to improve ambulation in persons with SCI. In a study by Alexeeva et al.[22] with patients with incomplete SCI, traditional physical therapy interventions were compared to body-weight-support on a fixed track and to BWSTT. The authors concluded that all three groups experienced significant improvements in walking speed, muscle strength, and well-being. However, the BWSTT group did not make improvements in balance compared to the body-weight-support on fixed track and the traditional physical therapy groups. Nooijen et al.[23] randomized 51 subjects with SCI into one of four groups: BWSTT with manual assistance, BWSTT with electrical stimulation of the peroneal nerve, overground ambulation with electrical stimulation of the peroneal nerve, and treadmill training with a locomotor robot. These authors concluded that all of these approaches were beneficial, but that no single approach demonstrated superior improvements in gait quality and speed.

Physical Therapy Patient/Client Management

Assessments and interventions during inpatient rehabilitation for an individual with SCI should include muscle strength and sensation testing to determine the extent of neurologic injury with periodic reassessments to determine either improvement or progression. The physical therapist must examine functional mobility to identify compensatory techniques that will enable the patient to perform bed mobility and transfer skills. Locomotion should be assessed. This may consist of wheelchair mobility or gait. Both skills may be examined depending on the patient's level of injury, motor and sensory preservation, and the likelihood that the patient will transition from wheelchair to ambulation. In later stages, thorough examination informs the therapist and orthotist regarding appropriate orthotics and assistive devices necessary for gait. SCI can significantly change a person's ability to perform activities of daily living, so the therapist should monitor the patient for signs of depression or maladaptive responses to this large life change. Referral to a psychologist, counselor, or psychiatrist should be made when appropriate.

Examination, Evaluation, and Diagnosis

During the patient interview, the physical therapist determined that the patient was alert and oriented to person, place, time, and purpose. Prior to these surgeries, he was independent in all activities. He does not have access to medical equipment that he may need upon discharge. Following his inpatient rehabilitation stay, the patient is planning to live nearby with his sister and brother-in-law. Their home does not have any steps; however, there is a one-step threshold down to what will be the patient's bedroom. This area has carpeted floors, while the rest of the home has hardwood floors. The bathroom is "about 100 feet" from his room and up the one-step threshold. When the therapist collaborated with the patient regarding goals, he stated his desire to be independent with all mobility so that he is "not a burden" on his sister and family. He is motivated and cooperative, has good family support, and was previously very active. He states he "wants as much therapy as possible" and wants to work as hard as possible while in inpatient rehabilitation.

During the systems review, the physical therapist identified many systems needing further examination (Table 18-1).

Pain was assessed before any functional or movement assessment. The patient rated his pain (located in the thoracic region of his surgeries) as 2/10 on the numeric rating scale.[24] He also described an intermittent dull ache around the surgical incision site just inferior to the scapulae. Any movement made the pain worse and rest with medication decreased the pain. To minimize the interference of pain on the patient's performance, the therapist made sure that he received analgesic medications prior to continuing the physical examination.

Due to the nature of the patient's presenting complaint and status as documented in the medical record after his surgical procedures, the therapist performed an ASIA examination to determine the extent of the patient's SCI.[25] The physiatrist examined deep pressure appreciation upon admission to the IRF and the physical therapist used those results. The patient's ability to sense pinprick and light touch was normal in all dermatomes on both the left and the right. The patient was classified as L1 incomplete AIS D (Fig. 18-3). The neurological level was determined based

Table 18-1 RESULTS OF SYSTEMS REVIEW FOR CASE PATIENT	
Cardiovascular and pulmonary	BP: 118/75 mm Hg; HR: 86 bpm; RR: 13 breaths/min No further examination indicated
Musculoskeletal	Further examination indicated due to decreased functional mobility and inability to ambulate without assistive device
Neuromuscular	Further examination indicated due to patient's symptoms prior to surgery and surgical interventions received
Integumentary	Further examination indicated due to episode of *Staphylococcus* infection at incision site following surgery
Cognitive	Alert and oriented to person, place, time, and purpose; no signs of compromise during interview or documented in medical record No further examination indicated

Abbreviations: BP, blood pressure; bpm, beats per min; HR, heart rate; RR, respiratory rate.

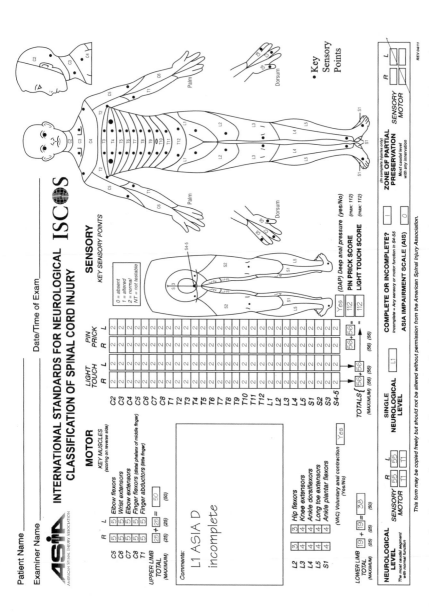

Figure 18-3. ASIA Neurological Classification of Spinal Cord Injury form for the current patient upon admission to the inpatient rehabilitation facility. (Reproduced with permission from American Spinal Injury Association: International Standards for Neurological Classification of Spinal Cord Injury, revised 2011; Atlanta, GA. Reprinted 2011.)

Table 18-2 LOWER EXTREMITY MANUAL MUSCLE TESTING RESULTS FOR CASE PATIENT		
Lower Extremity Movement	Left Lower Extremity	Right Lower Extremity
Hip flexion	3–/5	3–/5
Hip extension	3–/5	3–/5
Hip adduction	4/5	4/5
Hip abduction	3–/5	3/5
Knee flexion	4/5	4/5
Knee extension	4/5	4/5
Dorsiflexion	4/5	4/5
Plantarflexion	4–/5	4–/5

on his 3/5 motor score at L2, coupled with intact sensation throughout all dermatomes. According to ASIA classification, the neurological level of injury is the *lowest* level with intact motor and sensory function. The patient had intact deep pressure appreciation in all areas tested, classifying him as having an incomplete SCI. Because the strength in all muscles below the neurological level tested > 3/5, the patient was classified as AIS D. Since ASIA examination involves testing the strength of only a single muscle to represent each myotome, the therapist conducted additional lower extremity manual muscle testing (MMT). Although the goal was to assess the strength of the lower extremity muscles in the positions described by Reese,[24] the patient's inability and/or inefficiency of getting into the standardized positions was not practical. Lower extremity MMT was performed with the patient in a seated position due to lack of functional mobility, spinal precautions, and to be more efficient with examination time (Table 18-2). Of significant note were his weak hip flexors and extensors, which will impact transfers and gait. The MMT has been reported as having good inter-rater reliability (with therapists agreeing 82% of the time) and good validity.[26,27]

The ASIA examination considers proprioception an additional test. Altered proprioception may influence balance and gait abilities. Results of the patient's proprioception testing using the ASIA additional protocol are described in Table 18-3.

Table 18-3 ASIA PROPRIOCEPTION RESULTS FOR CASE PATIENT		
Joint	Right	Left
Wrist	Intact	Intact
Thumb	Intact	Intact
Little finger	Intact	Intact
Knee	Absent	Intact
Ankle	Absent	Intact
Great toe	Absent	Absent

During the ASIA examination, the patient complained that the plantar aspect of his right foot was numb. The therapist tested this region and found the patient had impaired sensation to light touch and pinprick stimuli. This region is not included in standardized dermatome testing for the ASIA examination, so it was not considered in his ASIA classification. However, these results are considered when developing his plan of care and during interventions.

Next, the therapist examined the patient's functional mobility. Movement restrictions due to the extensive spinal surgeries dictated that the patient "log roll" and avoid hip flexion >90°. The patient required minimal assistance for supine to sit and used bilateral upper extremities on the bedrails to complete the log roll prior to coming to a seated position. The sit-to-stand transfer required moderate assistance with the patient using bilateral upper extremities to push off the plinth. Sitting balance was independent for both static and dynamic balance with normal balance reactions in all directions. The patient was able to withstand mild resistance in all directions at the trunk. In sitting, the patient had a forward head posture and excessively rounded shoulders. In static standing without upper extremity support, the patient required minimal assistance due to trunk instability. He required moderate assistance for all reaching activities in standing. The patient was able to ambulate 50 ft with a front-wheeled walker (FWW) on a flat surface with moderate assistance, primarily for trunk and pelvic control during weight shifting. The patient also needed verbal cueing for proper right lower extremity foot placement, possibly due to absent proprioception on this side. During all phases of gait, the patient demonstrated decreased smoothness of contraction and mild ataxic movements in the right lower extremity. He required minimal assistance for safe wheelchair set-up and supervision for wheelchair propulsion over 100 ft on level surfaces. Although it is necessary to examine stair negotiation prior to discharge, this was deferred on initial examination due to the patient's decreased dynamic standing balance, trunk motor control during gait, right lower extremity proprioception, and his extensive recent surgical history.

At this point in the examination, the patient was becoming fatigued so the therapist decided to conduct additional less strenuous impairment level testing. Active cervical spine ROM in all directions and bilateral passive shoulder flexion, abduction, external rotation, and internal rotation were greater than corresponding normative values.[28] Trunk and pelvic movement were not tested due to the patient's postsurgical precautions: no bending, lifting, or twisting of the thoracic or lumbar spine. All lower extremity passive ROM was greater than normative values except hip flexion, which was tested only to 90° due to postsurgical precautions. The patient did not exhibit abnormal muscle tone in any muscles during passive ROM of extremities.

Over the next three physical therapy sessions, additional outcome measures were performed including the Functional Independence Measure (FIM®), the Timed Up and Go (TUG), and the Berg Balance Scale (BBS). Due to IRF regulations and facility accreditation requirements, it was necessary to complete the FIM® within the first 3 days of admission. The therapist selected the TUG and the BBS to gather more data specific to gait, balance, and fall risk.

The scores for the FIM® are recorded by the appropriate corresponding discipline (see Case 15). A systematic review investigated the psychometrics of the locomotor aspects of the FIM® in patients with SCI.[29] The Functional Independence Measure Locomotor (FIML) includes the FIM® scores for ambulation, wheelchair propulsion, and stairs. FIML has a standard error of measurement of 1.6 points and smallest real difference (smallest change that represents a change exceeding that of the error of the measurement) of 4.4 points. The FIML exhibits a ceiling effect; this means that once a patient reaches a score of complete independence, improvement cannot be detected. Table 18-4 shows the scoring descriptors for the FIML. At admission to the IRF, the patient scored "2" on ambulation using the FWW and ambulating 50 ft, "2" with wheelchair propulsion for < 50 ft, and "0" on stairs due to this task not being examined on admission due to safety concerns.

The Timed Up and Go (TUG) was administered to ascertain baseline gait characteristics and fall risk. The TUG has high intra- and inter-rater reliability (0.979 and 0.973, respectively) in patients with SCI.[31] In a systematic review by Lam et al.[29] on the psychometrics of the TUG in patients with SCI, the standard error of measurement was 3.9 seconds while the minimal clinically important difference (MCID) was described as 10.8 seconds. According to these authors, there was good concurrent validity with the 10-Meter Walk Test (10MWT), Six-Minute Walk Test (6MWT), and the Walking Index for Spinal Cord Injury (WISCI). On the patient's third day in the IRF, the therapist administered the TUG. The patient completed three trials of the TUG using the FWW (allowed during this test) with an average time of 37.31 seconds, classifying him as being at a high risk for falls.[32,33]

The physical therapist also selected to have the patient perform the Berg Balance Scale (BBS) for two reasons. First, there is a lack of standardized balance outcome measures in individuals with SCI. Second, the therapist wanted to select an outcome measure in which the patient was *not* allowed to use an assistive device. The patient scored 18/56 on the BBS, placing him at a high fall risk.[32] In a study comparing validity of the BBS with the WISCI, TUG, 10MWT, and Spinal Cord Index

Table 18-4 FUNCTIONAL INDEPENDENCE MEASURE LOCOMOTOR SCORING SCALE[30]	
Complete Independence (7)	Timely and safe without assistive device
Modified Independence (6)	Requires extra time, assistive device, or safety risk
Supervision (5)	Set up or requires cueing without physical contact
Minimal Assistance (4)	Patient performs > 75% of activity
Moderate Assistance (3)	Patient performs 50% to 74% of activity
Maximum Assistance (2)	Patient performs 25% to 49% of activity with locomotion; patient must travel > 150 ft and greater than one flight of stairs to score higher than a 2 with activity
Total Assistance (1)	Patient performs < 25% of activity or requires two helpers
Activity Did Not Occur (0)	Unsafe, patient's medical condition restricts, or patient refuses

for Functional Ambulation Inventory (SCI-FAI), the BBS had good concurrent validity for standing balance in patients with SCI who had an AIS D classification.[34]

This patient's physical therapy diagnosis was a 50-year-old male with T6-L4 vertebral fusion presenting with decreased trunk and lower extremity strength, impaired lower extremity proprioception, decreased endurance with ambulation, and decreased standing balance. These contributed to his inability to ambulate independently, transfer safely, ride his motorcycle, and continue working in the security field. This is consistent with the medical diagnosis of a nontraumatic L1 incomplete SCI (AIS D) followed by a decompressive spinal fusion surgery.

The physical therapist set the physical therapy goals in collaboration with the patient. The prognosis for achieving these goals in 3 weeks is good due to the patient's motivation, good family support, and independent prior level of function. In addition, the patient has good prognostic factors including an incomplete SCI, preserved motor function and pinprick sensation, and relatively young age. The physical therapy goals included: (1) standby assistance for all transfers with the FWW for bilateral upper extremity support to allow for family and friends to assist patient with daily activities; (2) modified independence with all bed mobility to decrease the likelihood of pressure ulcers; (3) ambulate 50 ft with the FWW on flat surfaces with minimal assistance to allow patient and nursing staff the option for patient to walk without physical therapy; (4) ascend and descend four stairs with bilateral upper extremity support and railings on both sides with minimal assistance to allow patient to increase endurance. The expected outcomes for discharge from the IRF were also set in collaboration with the patient. These included that the patient would be at Modified Independence level with bed mobility, transfers, sitting balance, standing balance, ambulation, wheelchair mobility, stairs and functional mobility around the house without any family member at home to assist patient. Frequency and duration of physical therapy sessions were set at 120 min/d, 6 d/wk while in the IRF for the anticipated 3-week length of stay determined by the interprofessional team.

Plan of Care and Interventions

Gait training, balance training, and targeted strengthening exercises for the lower extremities were the focus of most physical therapy interventions. The patient participated in 17 days of physical therapy prior to discharge. Overground ambulation, BWSTT, and strengthening using the recumbent cycle (with and without electrical stimulation) are described in detail.

Overground training was implemented in 12 of the 17 therapy sessions. The patient ambulated with the FWW on a flat surface for the first eight therapy sessions of overground training with distances varying from 50 to 150 ft, depending on the patient's reported fatigue. During the last four overground training sessions, the assistive device was advanced to bilateral quad canes and/or single point canes. This was done to give the patient less stability via the assistive device during ambulation and to emphasize hip extension during the stance phase of the gait cycle. During each therapy session, the physical therapist or physical therapist assistant determined requisite guarding and corrected identified gait deviations. The number of gait bouts per session was based on the patient's self-report or objective signs of fatigue (increased respiratory rate and/or degradation of gait pattern).

Five therapy sessions included BWSTT for 20 to 30 minutes with 30% to 60% of body weight supported. Each session started with the therapist assisting the patient with different sequences of advancement of his right lower extremity. Next, the patient ambulated independently on the treadmill to allow him the opportunity to make the necessary gait corrections *without* manual assistance. Last, the patient ambulated overground in an attempt to transfer the skills gained through BWSTT to actual ambulation. During each therapy session, the therapist determined speed of the treadmill and length of the session based on the patient's fatigue and/or increasing gait deviations. Modifications were added to BWSTT to improve endurance, balance, and proprioception. These included 3 sessions of walking at varying treadmill speeds and 2 sessions of walking over obstacles placed on the treadmill (*e.g.*, small wooden blocks, pencil, crumpled sheet of paper, small bean bag).

Over 17 days in the IRF, the patient received 120 minutes of physical therapy daily. Individual therapy sessions ranged from 30 to 90 minutes, depending on the schedule of the patient and physical therapist. This made treadmill training impractical during every session of therapy, so overground training was used more frequently. Periodically, a physical therapist assistant worked with the patient. During these sessions, BWSTT was not used because physical therapist assistants in this IRF could only treat patients for 30-minute sessions, which did not allow enough time for set-up and performance of BWSTT. Because the patient needed two to three people for safe set-up and performance, there were occasions when insufficient staffing prevented use of BWSTT.

There are no published reports of negative impacts resulting from BWSTT or overground training in patients with SCI. However, there is evidence suggesting that patients with certain AIS classifications benefit more than others from BWSTT and/or overground training.[17] Individuals with less motor function and lower AIS classifications have a lower probability that BWSTT or overground training will improve functional mobility.[35] People with incomplete SCI (either AIS C or D) typically benefit more from locomotor training than those with complete SCI (AIS B or A).[36] Given this patient's high AIS classification (AIS D), it was likely that he would benefit from BWSTT and overground training.

Overground training is also an effective intervention to improve ambulation in patients with SCI. Dobkin et al.[35,37] reported improvement with both BWSTT and overground training, but found neither intervention to be superior. A systematic review of 17 studies involving patients with incomplete SCI reported that overground training should be used in favor over BWSTT to achieve higher levels of independent ambulation.[38] In this patient's rehabilitation, both interventions were used with success. The overground training allowed him to ambulate at his own speed and he had to pay attention to foot placement to receive visual and sensory feedback with stepping. Overground training was also effective because it simulated real-life circumstances while allowing him to be challenged in a safe environment.

Lower extremity strength training was implemented using the NuStep recumbent bicycle with neuromuscular electrical stimulation. The patient received this intervention for 15 minutes on each of the 12 days he received overground ambulation training. Electrodes were placed on bilateral gluteus maximus muscles to facilitate hip extension during the hip and knee extension phase of cycling. The therapist used a remote control to turn the electrical signals on and off during the appropriate cycling phase. This was done to allow the patient to vary his cycling speed and to utilize interval training for lower extremity strengthening. While this intervention was intended to improve his lower extremity strength and proprioception using increased resistance, there is some evidence that this intervention may be effective for improving a patient's ambulation ability. A case series by Gregory et al.[39] concluded that lower extremity resistance and plyometric training can improve gait speed and decrease neuromuscular impairments in persons with incomplete SCI. In a case report of a patient with incomplete SCI, functional electrical stimulation during cycling was used.[40] This case report concluded that there was no increase in lower extremity strength, but the patient noted improvement in lower extremity function that included ambulation of short distances with a single crutch and an increased ability to pick items up from the floor.

From the results of the FIM®, BBS, and TUG, the patient demonstrated substantial improvements in functional mobility during the 17 days of acute rehabilitation. After 18 days in the IRF, the patient was able to reach all four of his anticipated goals. Per the policy of the IRF, all expected outcomes were based on FIM® scores.[30] The patient was expected to reach Modified Independence with all aspects for the FIML. Table 18-5 summarizes the patient's FIM® scores at admission and at discharge. He was able to reach Supervision with ambulation using the FWW, and was only able to ascend and descend four steps, putting him at a Maximum Assistance with FIM® scoring. The patient's FIML score increased by 9 points from admission to discharge (double the smallest real difference of 4.4 points).

It is impossible to determine which of the weightbearing interventions had the most impact on this patient's functional return. However, overground ambulation was the most utilized intervention during his treatment. Overground ambulation

Table 18-5   PATIENT'S FIM® SCORES AT ADMISSION AND DISCHARGE

FIM® Task	Admission	Discharge
Bed to Wheelchair Transfer	3 Moderate Assistance	6 Modified Independence
Ambulation	2 Patient ambulated 50 feet with front-wheeled walker	5 Patient ambulated greater than 300 feet with front-wheeled walker
Wheelchair Propulsion and Set Up	2 Patient was able to propel wheelchair 50 feet	6 Patient was able to propel wheelchair 150 feet
Stairs	0 Not Tested	2 Maximum Assistance

Copyright © 1997 Uniform Data System for Medical Rehabilitation, a division of UB Foundation Activities, Inc. Reprinted with permission.

was utilized outside of physical therapy sessions with the patient ambulating in his room with other healthcare providers. Other disciplines added to the patient's dose of overground training by having him ambulate as often as safely possible around the rehabilitation unit.

The patient's standing balance improved significantly on the BBS. Three days after admission, the patient scored 18/56. On the day of discharge 2 weeks later, he scored 37/56. This indicates that his fall risk decreased from high to moderate, and his discharge score was only 2 points away from classifying him as a low fall risk. On the BBS, the patient exceeded the 7-point MCID for stroke patients (there is no reported MCID for persons with SCI).[41]

The patient also improved his TUG scores. Three days following IRF admission, he averaged 37.31 seconds over three trials. At discharge, he averaged 20.26 seconds over three trials—an improvement of 17 seconds—which exceeds the MCID of 10.8 seconds for the TUG.[29] Using the patient's TUG score to determine fall risk is more complicated. A study by Shumway-Cook[42] suggested that patients who score over 14 seconds on the TUG should be classified as a high fall risk. However, Podsiadlo and Richardson[33] suggested that individuals whose TUG performance is under 30 seconds should no longer be considered at high fall risk. Thus, the patient decreased his fall risk according to one study but not according to another. During ambulation, the patient appeared as if he could easily fall. Combining evidence and clinical judgment, the therapist determined that he was at a higher risk for falls.

BWSTT is a very popular intervention for patients with SCI and there is growing evidence to support the efficacy of this intervention. In a retrospective study utilizing BWSTT with 35 patients with SCI, 25 were classified as wheelchair-bound at the start of the study.[43] Of those 25 wheelchair-bound participants, 20 were classified as independent walkers following BWSTT. Preliminary data also suggest that BWSTT is associated with improvement in overground walking speed.[44] In another retrospective study, Wernig et al.[45] reported that improvements in ambulation were sustained 6 months to 6.5 years following initial BWSTT for individuals with both chronic SCI ($n = 35$) and acute SCI ($n = 41$). Further follow-up would be necessary to see if this patient maintained his gains in ambulation.

The patient's ASIA examination was repeated prior to discharge. There was no change in proprioception, but strength in the hip flexors improved to 4/5 and knee extensors and left ankle dorsiflexors to 5/5. The patient was still classified as AIS D because improvement to an AIS E would mean that the patient had no residual sensory or motor deficits. In a study with patients following traumatic SCI, patients were assessed using the AIS multiple times from 2 weeks after SCI up to 12 months postinjury.[46] The authors concluded that 90% of patients classified as AIS D did not convert to either AIS C or AIS E. These data suggest that the current patient's likelihood of improving to AIS E is low. This patient may have benefited from the locomotor training because of his medical diagnosis of incomplete SCI and AIS D classification. BWSTT was utilized in an attempt to reconnect or retrain the patient's neural connections from the brain to the body. This fits in the current neuroplasticity research in patients with SCI.

Using the described weightbearing interventions to improve ambulation and functional mobility, the patient demonstrated significant improvements over the

17 days of physical therapy he received during his IRF stay—less than the majority of research that supports ambulation recovery. A systematic review assessing studies using BWSTT for patients with SCI described study lengths between 3 and 23 weeks.[5] Twelve-week BWSTT programs (with and without electrical stimulation supplementation) resulted in improvements in ambulation in patients with SCI.[35,47] A case report with a young adult with an incomplete SCI suggested that lower intensity and frequency of locomotor retraining over a longer period of time using both overground and BWSTT may also show improvement.[48] The current patient's case reflects that lower frequency (5 BWSTT sessions over 17 days of therapy) may have contributed to his functional and measurable gains. More research into frequency, duration, and dosage of interventions aimed at improving locomotion after SCI are needed.

The patient was discharged from the IRF to his sister's home. He was given a home exercise program (HEP) and prescribed follow-up with home health physical therapy. The facility's policy stated that home health follow-up needed to occur 48 to 72 hours following discharge. The patient's HEP included three simple exercises targeting the remaining deficits he exhibited. First, bridging for 10 to 20 repetitions for 3 to 5 sets while holding each bridge for 3 to 5 seconds. This exercise was given to address decreased bilateral hip extension strength and to improve upright posture during ambulation. Dose was set at the level where the patient began to demonstrate a breakdown in form. The patient was instructed to prioritize maintaining form over performing any particular number of repetitions or sets. Second, the patient was instructed to perform sit-to-stand transfers for 10 to 15 repetitions for three sets daily. This exercise was to improve hip extension strength for upright posture during ambulation. Last, he was instructed to draw the alphabet with his toe gently touching the ground while sitting. This exercise was selected to work on improving the patient's proprioception. Even though there had not been any improvement in proprioception during his IRF stay, this exercise was designed to improve his ability to place his lower extremities directly where he was aiming. Eventually, this may translate into improved gait mechanics by allowing him to have improved foot placement during gait and increased safety with daily activities.

Evidence-Based Clinical Recommendations

SORT: Strength of Recommendation Taxonomy

A: Consistent, good-quality patient-oriented evidence
B: Inconsistent or limited-quality patient-oriented evidence
C: Consensus, disease-oriented evidence, usual practice, expert opinion, or case series

1. The ASIA impairment scale (AIS) isolates factors related to the severity of a spinal cord injury and can guide physical therapists' determination of prognosis related to gait recovery. **Grade B**

2. Body-weight-supported treadmill training (BWSTT) and overground locomotor training improve ambulation in persons with spinal cord injury. **Grade A**

3. Strength training using a recumbent bicycle with electrical stimulation of selected muscles improves lower extremity strength and gait speed, and decreases neuromuscular impairments in persons with incomplete spinal cord injuries. **Grade C**

COMPREHENSION QUESTIONS

18.1 Which of the following interventions is *most* effective at improving gait for persons with SCI?

A. Body-weight-supported treadmill training (BWSTT)

B. Overground ambulation training

C. Strength training

D. A and B

18.2 Which of the following results indicate that the patient made a clinically significant improvement in balance *and* is at a low risk for falls?

A. FIML score increased by 12 points

B. BBS improvement of 18 points for a total of 41 out of 56

C. TUG time improved by 29 seconds to 32 seconds (average of three trials)

D. BBS increased by 8 points to 36 out of 56 in 2 weeks

ANSWERS

18.1 **D.** Current evidence shows that BWSTT and overground ambulation training improve ambulation in persons with SCI. Many studies have not found a significant difference between using BWSTT and overground training (options A and B). While strength training may be important for increasing strength in selected muscles used during gait and has been shown to improve function in some persons with SCI, it may be less effective in persons who are classified as AIS A, B, and C (option C).

18.2 **B.** The MCID for BBS is 6 points and the threshold for classification of low fall risk is ≥ 41 points out of 56. The smallest real change for FIML is 4.4 points, but there is no standard for the FIML related to fall risk prediction (option A). Approximately 11 seconds is the MCID for the TUG and scores under 13.5 seconds indicate low fall risk (option C).

REFERENCES

1. McKinley WO, Seel RT, Gadi RK, Tewksbury MA. Nontraumatic vs. traumatic spinal cord injury: a rehabilitation comparison. *Am J Phys Med Rehabil.* 2001;80:693-699.

2. Sturt RN, Holland AE, New PW. Walking ability at discharge from inpatient rehabilitation in a cohort of non-traumatic spinal cord injury patients. *Spinal Cord.* 2009;47:763-768.

3. Waters RL, Adkins RH, Yakura JS. Definition of complete spinal cord injury. *Paraplegia.* 1991;29:573-581.

4. Spinal Cord Facts and Figures at a Glance. National Spinal Cord Injury Statistical Center. Updated 2011. https://www.nscisc.uab.edu/PublicDocuments/nscisc_home/pdf/Facts%202011%20Feb%20Final.pdf. Accessed March 13, 2012.

5. Lam T, Eng JL, Wolfe DL, Hsieh JT, Whittaker M. A systematic review of the efficacy of gait rehabilitation strategies for spinal cord injury. *Top Spinal Cord Inj Rehabil.* 2007;13:32-57.

6. Geisler FH, Coleman WP, Grieco G, Poonian D, Sygen Study Group. Measurements and recovery patterns in a multicenter study of acute care spinal cord injury. *Spine.* 2001;26:S68-S86.

7. Al-Habib AF, Attabib N, Ball J, Bajammal S, Casha S, Hurlbert RJ. Clinical predictors of recovery after blunt spinal cord trauma: systematic review. *J Neurotrauma.* 2011;28:1431-1443.

8. Waters RL, Adkins RH, Yakura JS, Sie I. Motor and sensory recovery following complete tetraplegia. *Arch Phys Med Rehabil.* 1993;74:242-247.

9. Waters RL, Yakura JS, Adkins RH, Sie I. Recovery following complete paraplegia. *Arch Phys Med Rehabil.* 1992;73:784-789.

10. Poynton AR, O'Farrell DA, Shannon F, Murray P, McManus F, Walsh MG. Sparing of sensory to pin prick predicts recovery of a motor segment after injury to the spinal cord. *J Bone Joint Surg Br.* 1997;79:952-954.

11. Katoh S, El Masry WS. Motor recovery of patients presenting with motor paralysis and sensory sparing following cervical spinal cord injuries. *Paraplegia.* 1995;33:506-509.

12. Ishida Y, Tominaga T. Predictors of neurologic recovery in acute central cervical cord injury with only upper extremity impairment. *Spine.* 2002;27:1652-1658.

13. Pollard ME, Apple DF. Factors associated with improved neurologic outcomes in patients with incomplete tetraplegia. *Spine.* 2003;28:33-39.

14. McKinley W, Cifu D, Seel R, et al. Age-related outcomes in persons with spinal cord injury: a summary paper. *NeuroRehabilitation.* 2003;18:83-90.

15. Lynsky JV, Belanger A, Jung R. Activity-dependent plasticity in spinal cord injury. *J Rehabil Res Dev.* 2008;45:229-240.

16. Berhman AL, Bowden MG, Nair PM. Neuroplasticity after spinal cord injury and training: an emerging paradigm shift in rehabilitation and walking recovery. *Phys Ther.* 2006;86:1406-1425.

17. Somers MF. *Spinal Cord Injury Functional Rehabilitation.* 3rd ed. Upper Saddle River, NJ: Pearson Education Inc.; 2010:21-26.

18. Dunlop SA. Activity-dependent plasticity: implications for recovery after spinal cord injury. *Trends Neurosci.* 2008;31:410-418.

19. Nymark J, DeForge D, Barbeau H, et al. Body weight support treadmill gait training in the subacute recovery phase of incomplete spinal cord injury. *J Neuro Rehabil.* 1998;12:119-138.

20. Protas E, Holmes SA, Qureshy H, Johnson A, Lee D, Sherwood AM. Supported treadmill ambulation training after spinal cord injury: a pilot study. *Arch Phys Med Rehabil.* 2001;82:825-831.

21. Giangregorio LM, Hicks AL, Webber CE, et al. Body weight supported treadmill training in acute spinal cord injury: impact on muscle and bone. *Spinal Cord.* 2005;43:649-657.

22. Alexeeva N, Sames C, Jacobs PL, et al. Comparison of training methods to improve walking in persons with chronic spinal cord injury: a randomized clinical trial. *J Spinal Cord Med.* 2011;34:362-379.

23. Nooijen CF, Ter Hoeve N, Field-Fote EC. Gait quality improved by locomotor training in individuals with SCI regardless of training approach. *J Neuroeng Rehabil.* 2009;6:36.

24. Reese NB. *Muscle and Sensory Testing.* 2nd ed. St. Louis, MO: Elsevier Saunders; 2005.

25. ASIA Learning Center. American Spinal Injury Association. http://www.asialearningcenter.com. Accessed July 16, 2012.

26. Cuthbert SC, Goodheart GJ, Jr. On the reliability and validity of manual muscle testing: a literary review. *Chiropr Osteopat.* 2007;15:4.

27. Perry J, Weiss WB, Burnfield JM, Gronley JK. The supine hip extensor manual muscle test: a reliability and validity study. *Arch Phys Med Rehabil.* 2004;85:1345-1350.

28. Norkin CC, White DJ. *Measurement of Joint Motion: A Guide to Goniometry*. 4th ed. Philadelphia, PA: F.A. Davis Company; 2009:425-428.

29. Lam T, Noonan VK, Eng JJ. A systematic review of functional ambulation outcome measures in spinal cord injury. *Spinal Cord*. 2008;46:246-254.

30. Functional independence measure and functional assessment measure. Measurement Scales Used in Elderly Care. http://www.dementia-assessment.com.au/symptoms/FIM_manual.pdf. Accessed April 19, 2012

31. van Hedel HJ, Wirz M, Dietz V. Assessing walking ability in subjects with spinal cord injury: validity and reliability of 3 walking tests. *Arch Phys Med Rehabil*. 2005;86:190-196.

32. Shumway-Cook A, Brauer S, Woollacott M. Predicting the probability of falls in community-dwelling older adults using the Timed Up & Go Test. *Phys Ther*. 2000;80:896-903.

33. Podsiadlo D, Richardson S. The timed "Up & Go": a test of basic functional mobility for frail elderly people. *J Am Geriatr Soc*. 1991;39:142-148.

34. Lemay JF, Nadeau S. Standing balance assessment in ASIA D paraplegic and tetraplegic patients: concurrent validity of the Berg Balance Scale. *Spinal Cord*. 2010;48:245-250.

35. Dobkin B, Barbeau H, Deforge D, et al. The evolution of walking-related outcomes the first 12 weeks of rehabilitation for incomplete traumatic spinal cord injury: the multicenter randomized Spinal Cord Injury Locomotor Trial. *Neurorehabil Neural Repair*. 2007;21:25-35.

36. Fawcett JW, Curt A, Steeves JD, et al. Guidelines for the conduct of clinical trials for spinal cord injury as developed by ICCP Panel: spontaneous recovery after spinal cord injury and statistical power needed for therapeutic clinical trials. *Spinal Cord*. 2007;45:190-205.

37. Dobkin B, Apple D, Barbeau H, et al. Weight-supported treadmill training versus over-ground training for walking after acute incomplete SCI. *Neurology*. 2006;66:484-493.

38. Wessels M, Lucas C, Eriks I, de Groot S. Body weight-supported gait training for restoration of walking in people with an incomplete spinal cord injury: a systematic review. *J Rehabil Med*. 2010;42:513-519.

39. Gregory CM, Bowden MG, Jayaraman A, et al. Resistance training and locomotor recovery after incomplete spinal cord injury: a case series. *Spinal Cord*. 2007;45:522-553.

40. Donaldson N, Perkins TA, Fitzwater R, Wood DE, Middleton F. FES cycling may promote recovery of leg function after incomplete spinal cord injury. *Spinal Cord*. 2000;38:680-682.

41. Stevensen TJ. Detecting change in patients with stroke using the Berg Balance Scale. *Aust J Physiother*. 2001;47:29-38.

42. Shumway-Cook A, Baldwin M, Pollissar NL, Grubar W. Predicting the probability for falls in community-dwelling older adults. *Phys Ther*. 1997;77:812-819.

43. Wernig A, Nanassy A, Muller S. Laufband (treadmill) therapy in incomplete paraplegia and tetraplegia. *J Neurotrauma*. 1999;16:719-726.

44. Field-Fote EC. Spinal cord control of movement: implications for locomotor rehabilitation following spinal cord injury. *Phys Ther*. 2000;80:477-484.

45. Wernig A, Nanassy A, Muller S. Maintenance of locomotor abilities following Laufband (treadmill) therapy in para- and tetraplegic persons: follow-up studies. *Spinal Cord*. 1998;36:744-749.

46. Spiess MR, Muller RM, Rupp R, Schuld C, EM-SCI study group, van Hedel HJ. Conversion of ASIA impairment scale during the first year after traumatic spinal cord injury. *J Neurotrauma*. 2009;26:2027-2036.

47. Field-Fote EC, Tepavac D. Improved intralimb coordination in people with incomplete spinal cord injury following training with body weight support and electrical stimulation. *Phys Ther*. 2002;82:707-715.

48. Young DL, Wallman HW, Poole I, Threlkeld AJ. Body weight supported treadmill training at very low treatment frequency for a young adult with incomplete cervical spinal cord injury. *NeuroRehabilitation*. 2009;25:261-270.

Acute Transverse Myelitis

Rolando T. Lazaro
Helen Luong

CASE 19

The patient is a 57-year-old female who has had acute and progressive onset of numbness and tingling in the lower extremities, mild mid- to low back pain, and bowel and urinary incontinence over the past 10 days. She reports that the signs and symptoms have plateaued. She is currently unable to walk and was admitted to the hospital for a complete medical work-up. She has no significant prior medical history, but relevant family history includes a paternal grandmother with multiple sclerosis. Prior to this hospitalization, the patient was living in a single-level home with her spouse and was independent in all activities of daily living. She is unemployed, and does not currently exercise on a regular basis. She reports an inability to walk and numbness and tingling in her legs as if she has been out in the cold too long. She states that she has been unable to get around the house independently since the onset of her symptoms. Since admission to the hospital, she has not been out of bed. Magnetic resonance imaging of the thoracic and lumbar spine showed abnormal increased T2 signal and enhancement along the posterior half of the spinal cord from approximately T10 to T12. The neurologist diagnosed idiopathic acute transverse myelitis. The patient was started on high-dose intravenous glucocorticoid therapy, and was referred to physical therapy for evaluation and management.

▶ Based on her diagnosis, what do you anticipate will be the contributors to activity limitations?
▶ What are the examination priorities?
▶ What are the most appropriate physical therapy interventions?
▶ What precautions should be taken during physical therapy examination and interventions?
▶ What are the complications interfering with physical therapy?
▶ How would her contextual factors influence or change your patient/client management?

KEY DEFINITIONS

AUTONOMIC DYSFUNCTION: Malfunction of the autonomic nervous system; signs include urinary incontinence or retention, bowel incontinence or constipation, and sexual dysfunction

PAROXYSMAL TONIC SPASMS: Involuntary temporary dystonic contractions of limb or trunk muscles

T2-WEIGHTED MAGNETIC RESONANCE IMAGING (MRI): Type of MRI scan in which fluid appears bright in the image; in the case of acute transverse myelitis, bright areas (denoting increased signal) indicate inflammation

Objectives

1. Describe the typical signs and symptoms of acute transverse myelitis.

2. List pertinent physical therapy tests and measures for the individual with acute transverse myelitis.

3. Discuss appropriate physical therapy interventions for an individual with acute transverse myelitis.

Physical Therapy Considerations

PT considerations during management of the individual with acute transverse myelitis in the acute care setting:

▶ **General physical therapy plan of care/goals:** Improve functional mobility; prevent or minimize loss of range of motion (ROM) and aerobic functional capacity; identify and address secondary complications of immobility; maintain skin integrity

▶ **Physical therapy interventions:** Patient education regarding skin care and ROM; functional mobility training; task-specific training; trunk stability training with augmented (visual) feedback

▶ **Precautions during physical therapy interventions:** Close physical supervision to decrease risk of falls; skin breakdown; monitor vital signs

▶ **Complications interfering with physical therapy:** Development of pressure ulcers due to decreased mobility; decreased cardiopulmonary endurance secondary to inactivity and deconditioning

Understanding the Health Condition

Idiopathic acute transverse myelitis (ATM) is a disabling neurologic disorder in adults and children. While transverse myelitis can have various causes, the condition often occurs as an autoimmune phenomenon after infection or as a result of an underlying systemic autoimmune or demyelinating disease. ATM has been associated with bacterial or viral infections, multiple sclerosis, systemic lupus erythematosus, and Sjogren's syndrome.[1] Approximately 15% to 30% of cases are idiopathic in origin.[2] The abnormal activation of the immune system results in inflammation and injury to the spinal cord, resulting in demyelination.[3-5]

Diagnosis of ATM is rare—the condition affects between 1 and 8 individuals per million annually.[4,5] Generally, diagnosis is made by excluding other differential diagnoses.[6] It is often misdiagnosed as Guillain-Barré syndrome because both conditions frequently present with rapidly progressive sensory and motor loss in the lower extremities. Table 19-1 highlights clinical characteristics of these two conditions.[5]

Additional differential diagnoses that must be ruled out include demyelination (*e.g.*, multiple sclerosis, neuromyelitis optica), infection (*e.g.*, herpes simplex virus), and other inflammatory disorders (*e.g.*, systemic lupus erythematosus, neurosarcoidosis).[7]

ATM usually follows a monophasic course. As an immune-mediated disorder, it involves inflammation within the spinal cord that can damage myelin and axons. This inflammatory process results in motor, sensory, and autonomic dysfunction that progressively worsens over a period of 4 hours to 21 days and then plateaus.[5]

The clinical presentation of ATM includes pain and sensory, motor, and autonomic dysfunction.[2,5] Between 80% and 94% of people with ATM have sensory disturbances.[5] Sensory disturbances typically present at a well-defined truncal level below which the sensation of pain, light touch, and temperature is altered or lost.[5] Since the spinal cord carries motor nerve fibers to the limbs and trunk, inflammation within the spinal cord can cause weakness in the trunk and/or limbs corresponding to the areas of the spinal cord affected.[5] Due to motor impairments, 50% of affected individuals are unable to ambulate.[3] Because the mid-thoracic region is a common area affected in adults with ATM,[5] trunk muscles may be affected,[8]

Table 19-1   COMPARISON OF SIGNS AND SYMPTOMS OF ACUTE TRANSVERSE MYELITIS AND GUILLAIN-BARRÉ SYNDROME

Characteristics	Acute Transverse Myelitis	Guillain-Barré Syndrome
Motor findings	Weakness in all extremities, or lower extremities only	Ascending weakness: greater in lower extremities than upper extremities
Sensory findings	Sensory abnormalities below a specific spinal level	Ascending sensory loss: greater in lower extremities than upper extremities
Autonomic findings	Early impairment in bowel and bladder control	Cardiovascular system autonomic dysfunction may be present
Spinal MRI findings	Increased T2 signal within a focal area with or without gadolinium enhancement (indicative of spinal cord inflammation)	Normal

Reproduced with permission from Krishnan C, Kaplin AI, Deshpande DM, Pardo CA, Kerr DA. Transverse myelitis: pathogenesis, diagnosis, and treatment. Front Biosci. 2004;9:1483-99.

resulting in balance impairments. Paroxysmal tonic involuntary spasms of limb or trunk muscles have also been reported.[2] Autonomic dysfunction, including urinary incontinence or retention, bowel incontinence or constipation, and sexual dysfunction may also occur.[2]

Recovery begins when signs and symptoms reach a plateau.[3,5] Most of the recovery occurs over the course of the first 3 months after the initial onset of signs and symptoms, although patients can experience some improvements for up to 2 years.[5] Roughly 42% of individuals with ATM have good recovery, 38% have fair recovery, and 20% have poor recovery from the condition.[5] Patients with good recovery demonstrate normal gait, mild urinary symptoms, and minimal sensory and upper motor neuron signs. Those with fair recovery ambulate independently, but may demonstrate urinary urgency and/or constipation. Those with poor recovery are unable to walk or have severe sensory deficits and/or gait disturbances, and no sphincter control. During recovery, there can be additional complications related to immobility such as skin breakdown (pressure ulcers), contractures that lead to loss of ROM, deterioration of bone and muscle architecture, urinary tract infections, and deep vein thromboses.

Medical management of ATM includes glucocorticoid therapy, plasmapheresis, and/or immunotherapy to decrease the inflammatory process, heparin for prophylaxis against deep vein thrombosis, baclofen for spasticity, alpha adrenergic medications for genitourinary dysfunction, and additional medications for pain, mood, and anxiety.[2]

Physical Therapy Patient/Client Management

The majority of the current literature on physical therapy management of transverse myelitis is based on chronic long-term management and not acute management.[2,5] To address weakness, strengthening programs or splinting and orthotics, when necessary, have been recommended. Daily land-based and/or water-based therapy for 8 to 12 weeks, with daily weightbearing for 45 to 90 minutes and functional mobility training have also been recommended. Based on the similarities between the pathophysiology of idiopathic ATM and acute spinal cord injury (SCI), similar rehabilitation management strategies are used for these populations. The roles of the physical therapist are to prescribe interventions that improve functional skills such as bed mobility, transfers, and gait or wheelchair mobility and to institute preventative measures against secondary complications of immobility such as skin breakdown, decreased ROM, and contractures.[9,10] This process starts with identifying the factors that may affect the patient's current and future health as well as those that contribute to activity limitations and participation restrictions.

Examination, Evaluation, and Diagnosis

Prior to seeing this patient, the therapist should perform a thorough chart review to obtain information about the patient's course of hospitalization. Reviewing the patient's medical imaging, laboratory values, and consultation reports from other medical specialties assists in determining the physical therapy plan of care. Systems review of the cardiovascular and integumentary systems may reveal other problems that require physical therapy interventions.

The **Spinal Cord Independence Measure (SCIM)** is a comprehensive functional assessment tool designed specifically for individuals with SCI.[9] This tool is reliable, valid, and more sensitive to functional changes in individuals with SCI than the Functional Independence Measure (FIM®).[11,12] Based on its reported validity in individuals with SCI, this tool has face validity for use in those with ATM. The SCIM examines the patient's ability to perform 17 activities of daily living (ADLs). It is grouped into three functional subscales: (1) self-care, (2) respiration and sphincter management, and (3) mobility. There are different scoring scales based on each item. A lower score indicates that more assistance is required to perform the activity, or use of medical devices or interventions is required (*e.g.*, parenteral feeding, assisted ventilation, or indwelling catheter). In the respiration and sphincter management and mobility subscales, an individual can receive a score from 0 to 40 points. For the self-care subscale, the score ranges from 0 to 20 points. Scores in the three subscales can be added to generate a total score from 0 to 100 points, with lower scores indicating a lower level of independence.[13] The SCIM is available at www.rehab. research.va.gov/jour/07/44/1/pdf/catzappend.pdf.

The therapist may also perform sensory and motor examinations to determine the individual's neurological level of injury by using the American Spinal Injury Association (ASIA) Classification Scale.[9] This tool is a comprehensive system of tests of sensation and motor function that provide information on the extent and severity of the patient's spinal cord injury. (See Case 14 for details regarding the ASIA examination.) In the acute care setting, the SCIM can provide the physical therapist a way to quantify functional improvement due to physical rehabilitation interventions (and/or the natural course of the disease process), especially for the self-care and mobility subsections. However, the therapist may choose to perform the ASIA examination to identify specific sensory and motor impairments that may contribute to the individual's activity limitations.

Tests of proprioception[10] and kinesthesia should be performed to obtain information regarding the patient's ability to sense joint position and movement. There is high reliability for position sense testing (r = 0.90).[14] To determine the patient's upright postural control, tests of balance in sitting and standing[10] should be performed. Data obtained from these tests can provide important clues about the patient's current ability and potential for performance of functional tasks.

Plan of Care and Interventions

Specific physical therapy goals are set after the evaluation and must take into consideration the patient's optimal discharge plans. Goals related to preventing skin breakdown and decreasing fall risk must be incorporated. Physical therapy interventions include ROM and strengthening exercises, pulmonary interventions, seating and positioning, mobilization (bed mobility, transfers, gait/wheelchair mobility), and education to the patient, family, and caregivers on maintaining skin integrity and ROM. **Rehabilitation during the acute recovery stage of ATM** is important to prevent inactivity-related problems such as skin breakdown and soft tissue contractures that lead to loss of ROM and decreased functional mobility.

Since idiopathic ATM often affects the spinal cord at mid-thoracic level, patients frequently present with trunk weakness resulting in poor sitting balance. One aim of rehabilitation is to regain the trunk stability necessary to perform functional activities from a seated position and to tolerate upright body position.[15] Benefits of upright posture include fewer respiratory complications, reduced pressure on the sacrum, and skin protection.[16] To improve trunk strength with the current patient, the physical therapist could have her perform and practice functional mobility training, with an emphasis on supine or sidelying-to-sit performance and transfer training. Proprioceptive neuromuscular facilitation (PNF) techniques can also be incorporated. It is beneficial for the patient to have a schedule in which she is sitting up in a chair, with the length of time in sitting progressively increased to improve her sitting tolerance and trunk strength.

It is especially important to address sitting balance because a poor short-sitting position increases the fear of falling, fall risk, and mobility limitations, all of which create greater patient dependence in basic and instrumental ADLs. Poor sitting balance also affects self-confidence, potentially resulting in further decreased physical activity and quality of life.[16] Activities that challenge the patient to progressively move her center of gravity while maintaining the base of support can improve trunk stability. This may start with the patient sitting on a firm (noncompliant) surface with upper extremity support (e.g., patient holding onto the edge of the bed) and physical assistance from the therapist, as necessary, to maintain this position. The therapist can start by having the patient perform weight-shifting activities in sitting. For example, the therapist can ask the patient to lean her trunk forward, backward, and then return to upright midline. The therapist should progressively increase the balance challenge by increasing the excursions of the weight shifts and removing the upper extremity support and physical assistance. As the patient's sitting balance improves, additional challenge may be provided by having the patient sit on a foam (compliant) surface while performing dynamic weight shifts and excursions out of her base of support. PNF activities such as rhythmic stabilization can be incorporated, which may facilitate activation and co-contraction of the trunk muscles.

Decreased or lost proprioception in the trunk and lower extremities that can occur in ATM also contribute to problems with sitting balance. Training the patient to use other intact sensory systems to augment feedback can improve balance. The use of **visual feedback** has been shown to improve trunk stability and functional mobility.[17] Visual feedback can be used to match or recalibrate proprioceptive sensory input that may be impaired.[18] This can easily be done in the acute care setting by placing a long-length rolling mirror in front of the patient while she performs static and dynamic activities in sitting. As the patient improves, the mirror can be used progressively less.

Evidence-Based Clinical Recommendations

SORT: Strength of Recommendation Taxonomy

A: Consistent, good-quality patient-oriented evidence
B: Inconsistent or limited-quality patient-oriented evidence
C: Consensus, disease-oriented evidence, usual practice, expert opinion, or case series

1. The Spinal Cord Independence Measure (SCIM) is a comprehensive functional assessment tool that is reliable, valid, and sensitive to functional change in individuals with spinal cord injury, including those with acute transverse myelitis. **Grade B**

2. Physical therapy interventions during the acute recovery stage of ATM improve functional mobility and help prevent secondary complications such as pressure ulcers and contractures. **Grade C**

3. Use of visual feedback during trunk stability training improves balance and functional performance in individuals with spinal cord injury. **Grade B**

COMPREHENSION QUESTIONS

19.1 A patient with acute transverse myelitis was referred to physical therapy. Examination reveals that the patient has poor sitting balance. Which of the following interventions may be beneficial?

    A. Lower extremity strengthening 2 days after the initial onset of signs and symptoms

    B. Direct current electrical stimulation to the trunk musculature for 30 minutes twice daily to improve trunk strength and mobility

    C. Use of visual feedback during sitting balance training to improve balance and upright trunk stability

    D. All of the above

19.2 A patient with acute transverse myelitis was referred to physical therapy. Which of the following physical therapy tests and measures may be appropriate to use for this patient?

    A. Tests of joint position and movement sense

    B. Spinal Cord Independence Measure (SCIM)

    C. American Spinal Injury Association (ASIA) examination

    D. All of the above

ANSWERS

19.1 **C.** Visual feedback may be used to improve trunk stability. This feedback can be used to match and recalibrate proprioceptive input that may be impaired in individuals with acute transverse myelitis.

19.2 **D.** All of these tests and measures provide appropriate information regarding possible motor and sensory impairments and activity limitations of individuals with acute transverse myelitis.

REFERENCES

1. Lynn J. Transverse myelitis: symptoms, causes and diagnosis. http://www.myelitis.org/tm.htm. Accessed February 1, 2012.

2. Frohman EM, Wingerchuk DM. Clinical practice. Transverse myelitis. *N Engl J Med.* 2010;363:564-572.

3. Kerr DA, Ayetey H. Immunopathogenesis of acute transverse myelitis. *Curr Opin Neurol.* 2002;15:339-347.

4. Bruna J, Martinez-Yelamos S, Martinez-Yelamos A, Rubio F, Arbizu T. Idiopathic acute transverse myelitis: a clinical study and prognostic markers in 45 cases. *Mult Scler.* 2006;12:169-173.

5. Krishnan C, Kaplin AI, Deshpande DM, Pardo CA, Kerr DA. Transverse myelitis: pathogenesis, diagnosis and treatment. *Front Biosci.* 2004;9:1483-1499.

6. Persaud D, Leedom CL. Spinal cord impairment: acute transverse myelitis. *SCI Nurs.* 1999;16: 122-125.

7. Jacob A, Weinshenker BG. An approach to the diagnosis of acute transverse myelitis. *Semin Neurol.* 2008;28:105-120.

8. Neumann DA. *Kinesiology of the Musculoskeletal System: Foundations for Physical Rehabilitation.* St. Louis, MO: Mosby Inc.; 2002.

9. Somers MF. *Spinal Cord Injury: Functional Rehabilitation.* 3rd ed. Upper Saddle River, NJ: Pearson Education Inc.; 2010.

10. O'Sullivan SB, Schmitz TJ. *Physical Rehabilitation.* 5th ed. Philadelphia, PA: FA Davis; 2007.

11. Catz A, Itzkovic M. Spinal cord independence measure: comprehensive ability rating scale for the spinal cord lesion patients. *J Rehabil Res Dev.* 2007;44:65-68.

12. Itzkovich M, Gelerneter I, Biering-Sorensen F, et al. The spinal cord independence measure version III: reliability and validity in a multi-center international study. *Disabil Rehabil.* 2007;29:1926-1933.

13. Catz A, Itzkovich M, Tesio L, Biering-Sorensen F, Weeks C, et al. A multicenter international study on the Spinal Cord Independence Measure, version III: Rasch psychometric validation. *Spinal Cord.* 2007;45:275-291.

14. Kent BE. Sensory-motor testing: the upper limb of adult patients with hemiplegia. *Phys Ther.* 1965:45:550-561.

15. Chen CL, Yeung KT, Bih LI, Wang CH, Chen MI, Chien JC. The relationship between sitting stability and functional performance in patients with paraplegia. *Arch Phys Med Rehabil.* 2003;84:1276-1281.

16. Consortium for Spinal Cord Medicine. Early acute management in adults with spinal cord injury: a clinical practice guideline for health-care professionals. *J Spinal Cord Med.* 2008;31:403-479.

17. Sayenko DG, Alekhina MI, Masani K, et al. Positive effect of balance training with visual feedback on standing balance abilities in people with incomplete spinal cord injury. *Spinal Cord.* 2010;48:886-893.

18. Betker AL, Desai A, Nett C, Kapadia N, Szturm T. Game-based exercise for dynamic short-sitting balance rehabilitation of people with chronic spinal cord and traumatic brain injuries. *Phys Ther.* 2007;87:1389-1398.

Guillain-Barré Syndrome

Kristen Barta

A 78-year-old male was admitted to a rehabilitation facility with the diagnosis of Guillain-Barré syndrome. He initially developed numbness and tingling in bilateral feet and lower legs that progressed to his hands and arms over a 3-day period. Upon visiting his primary care physician, he was transferred directly to the hospital for further monitoring. He underwent a spinal tap and nerve conduction velocity test, ultimately leading to a diagnosis of Guillain-Barré syndrome. While in the hospital for 3 weeks, he developed complete bilateral lower extremity paralysis with decreased sensation. He developed some upper extremity weakness, but maintained at least a grade of 3/5 for all upper extremity muscles. His pulmonary and respiratory function remained adequate and he did not require mechanical ventilation. After the third week, his signs and symptoms began to plateau and he started to regain minimal motor function. The patient was then transferred to an inpatient rehabilitation facility (IRF). At admission to the IRF, the physical therapist is asked to evaluate and treat the patient to improve functional mobility and independence to enable a discharge home with his wife to a one-story home with level-entry access.

▶ What are the most appropriate physical therapy goals?
▶ What are the most appropriate physical therapy interventions?
▶ What precautions should be taken during the physical therapy examination and interventions?
▶ What are possible complications interfering with physical therapy?

KEY DEFINITIONS

GUILLAIN-BARRE SYNDROME (GBS): Disorder in which the body's immune system attacks the peripheral nervous system, resulting in progressive weakness of the limbs, trunk, and possibly respiratory muscles

NERVE CONDUCTION VELOCITY: Diagnostic test to measure how nerves and muscles respond to electrical stimuli; aids in diagnosis of GBS

SPINAL TAP: Procedure in which a small amount of cerebrospinal fluid is removed from the spinal canal for examination; high levels of protein aid in diagnosis of GBS

Objectives

1. Describe the pathophysiology of GBS.
2. List lab values that should be checked frequently during the patient's disease course.
3. Describe overwork weakness and its negative impact on recovery.
4. Discuss an appropriate progression of treatment strategies to improve function and independence in the patient with GBS.

Physical Therapy Considerations

PT considerations for management of the patient recovering from an episode of GBS:

▶ **General physical therapy goals:** Improve bilateral lower extremity strength and functional activity tolerance; improve ankle and hip strategies for balance reactions; normalize gait pattern; improve functional mobility and independence

▶ **Physical therapy interventions:** Patient education regarding energy conservation techniques and GBS-related fatigue; muscle strengthening, balance activities, gait training, functional training

▶ **Precautions during physical therapy:** GBS-related fatigue; physical supervision to decrease fall risk; frequent skin assessments to decrease risk of skin breakdown (due to sensory impairments); frequent monitoring of lab values to decrease risk of overwork weakness resulting from denervated muscles

▶ **Complications interfering with physical therapy:** Deep vein thrombosis (due to immobility), compromised sensation, contractures

Understanding the Health Condition

A person who is diagnosed with GBS or acute inflammatory polyradiculoneuropathy has undergone a process of demyelination of the peripheral nerves. While the etiology of GBS is unknown, a few events are more prevalent in individuals diagnosed.

Typically, GBS is preceded by Epstein-Barr virus, respiratory infection, cytomegalo-virus, mononucleosis, swine flu inoculation, or *Campylobacter jejuni* enteritis.[1,2] The annual incidence in the United States is 1.3 cases per 100,000, with men affected more frequently than women. The overall mortality rate is 10%, and 20% of individuals with GBS have lasting severe disability.[3]

GBS is an autoimmune disorder that results from the immune system's organized attack against Schwann cells that form the myelin sheath wrapping around motor and sensory axons within the peripheral nervous system. The myelin sheath's primary function is to increase the *speed* of action potentials traveling along axons. In GBS, antibodies trigger macrophages and lymphocytes to migrate to the nodes of Ranvier and attack the Schwann cells. Antibodies against peripheral nervous system tissue have been identified in patients with GBS.[3] As the immune system attacks the myelin sheath, demyelination occurs and the individual develops weakness of the extremities and trunk. In severe cases, the respiratory muscles are also affected. The progressive weakness takes place over a period of days to weeks, averaging about 4 weeks.[3]

GBS is diagnosed by subjective examination and clinical presentation along with a spinal tap and nerve function studies. In the early stages, the clinical presentation of muscular weakness and diminished reflexes may be similar to other neurological diseases. However, the accelerated rate of progressive weakness points toward a diagnosis of GBS. A person must present with extremity weakness at the onset to lead to a diagnosis of GBS. Presence of only pulmonary dysfunction and respiratory involvement without muscular weakness of the limbs and diminished reflexes would not indicate GBS.[4] In patients with GBS, a spinal tap often reveals cerebrospinal fluid containing elevated levels of protein without an elevated cell count.[5] Nerve function tests demonstrate delayed conduction velocities that are a result of the demyelination.

Upon diagnosis, the individual is often monitored in the intensive care unit of the hospital. This is because of the risk of respiratory muscle weakness and the potential urgent need for mechanical ventilation. Taly et al.[6] found that individuals with GBS who presented with impairments of joint position and vibration sense of the extremities tended to have a greater need for ventilator support.

Initial medical intervention in the hospital includes plasmapheresis and administration of immunoglobulin. These medical interventions are given during the progressive phase to slow the disease process and maintain the integrity of the peripheral nervous system. By slowing the disease process, more muscular strength and sensory function can remain intact. Plasmapheresis removes the patient's whole blood, extracting the plasma (containing antibodies) from the blood, and then transfuses the blood with the red and white cells back into the person. Plasmapheresis is a common treatment for some autoimmune diseases because it removes the circulating antibodies that are thought to be involved in the disease process. Plasmapheresis often occurs daily for a number of days to inhibit or stop the progression of the demyelination.[7] In patients with GBS, this treatment can reduce the duration of skeletal muscle paralysis and decrease the need for mechanical ventilation by 50%.[8] Immunoglobulin therapy is the intravenous administration of high doses of antibodies that are collected through donors. These transfused antibodies can overpower the patient's own destructive antibodies, decreasing the rate at which they harm the peripheral nervous system. A patient usually receives this treatment over a 12-hour period for 5 consecutive days.[9]

Physical Therapy Patient/Client Management

GBS causes a quick and progressive decline in muscular strength and sensory function. This rapid progression can occur within a few days to several weeks and can present with a variety of impairments based on the severity of demyelination. An individual could have involvement of only the lower extremities or the upper extremities, all extremities, trunk musculature, and possibly respiratory muscles. A general presentation of GBS is symmetrical weakness that begins distally and progresses proximally.[4] About 10% to 30% of patients have respiratory complications and an estimated 14% to 25% require mechanical ventilation support due to demyelination of the nerves innervating the diaphragm.[10,11] As progression of the condition ceases, the person enters a plateau phase (of unpredictable duration) in which there is neither a decline nor an improvement in symptoms. This is a temporary phase followed by a recovery phase. During the recovery phase, remyelination occurs and the individual begins to regain sensory and motor function. If the individual has been placed on mechanical ventilator support, this is weaned as the diaphragm strengthens and he recovers from any other pulmonary complications. Intensive therapy or exercise should be *avoided* prior to the recovery phase to decrease the risk of any potential complications during the demyelination process.[10]

A patient recovering from an episode of GBS can present with a wide range of dysfunction depending on the severity of demyelination, length of progression time, and presence of respiratory involvement. The physical therapist's role during the demyelination phase is to educate the patient, family, and nursing staff regarding physical changes resulting from the disease process, proper positioning techniques to maintain skin and joint integrity, an appropriate stretching program, and the signs and symptoms of overwork fatigue. The physical therapist becomes more involved in the patient's physical recovery after completion of the plateau phase and entry into the recovery phase.

Examination, Evaluation, and Diagnosis

Because this patient did not require ventilator support and he regained minimal strength in bilateral upper extremities, the prognosis for rehabilitation and recovery of function is positive. In 3 weeks, he reached the plateau phase in which he began to medically stabilize, did not develop additional weakness, and started to regain muscular strength and function. Patients typically reach this phase in 2 to 3 weeks after initiation of the progressive phase.[9] The physical therapy examination should include appropriate strength and sensory testing, balance assessment, functional mobility assessment, gait observation, and overall functional activity tolerance.

This information provides a baseline of function and safety and allows the therapist to establish goals necessary to achieve a discharge home.

In the inpatient rehabilitation setting, the **Functional Independence Measure (FIM®)** is an appropriate tool to measure functional mobility and progress during the course of the patient's rehabilitation. Using the FIM®, the physical therapist measures a person's bed mobility and transfer status, gait dysfunction, and ability to manage stairs. The FIM® is a reliable tool to assess the severity of a person's disability and level of caregiver burden and it has been validated on individuals with a variety of neurological disorders.[12,13]

Sensory testing provides valuable information regarding the patient's ability to recognize pressure points and any deficits in proprioception that lead to joint position awareness limitations. A body chart can be used to help identify patterns of sensory changes and location of pain, which can indicate areas of the body at risk of injury. To reduce the risk of skin breakdown due to immobility and decreased sensation, the therapist should educate the patient, family, and nursing staff on proper positioning of the patient when he is in the bed or sitting in a chair. Orthotics or splints to prevent joint contractures and promote function may be used, but with caution. These devices should be removed frequently for regular skin checks to assess for pressure points. Adjustments should be made accordingly if any areas of skin show signs of increased pressure. As the patient becomes more mobile, deficits in proprioception decrease awareness of his body position in space, which leads to an increased fall risk. Appropriate assistive devices and training are imperative to improve his safety.

Muscular weakness and a decline in functional activity tolerance are often the most disabling problems a patient encounters on the road to recovery. A decline in strength tends to be the first sign a person notices during the initial stages of the disease. This decline progresses to a certain level, stabilizes, and then begins to improve. This patient had progressed to complete paralysis of bilateral lower extremities, which indicates that during his plateau phase he was not able to move his legs voluntarily. Thus far in his recovery phase, he has shown improvement in muscular strength and has become medically stable enough to transfer to an inpatient rehabilitation facility for intensive rehabilitation therapy to address his decline in functional status. Functional limitations, balance deficits, and gait dysfunction are expected as a result of his muscular weakness. In addition to the FIM® for functional assessment, the **Tinetti Performance Oriented Mobility Assessment** has been shown to predict fall risk in the elderly population.[14] While the Tinetti assessment has not been validated specifically for use on patients with GBS, it would be an appropriate assessment tool to use with this patient. The Tinetti assesses sitting and standing balance and gait. The maximum score between the balance and gait subsets is 28. A lower score indicates a *higher* risk of falling; patients are considered a high fall risk if they score < 19.[14]

A patient recovering from GBS is at risk of experiencing overwork weakness, or fatigue-related relapse. Overwork weakness is defined as "a prolonged weakness in the absolute strength and endurance of a muscle due to excessive activity."[15] The patient is at risk of overwork weakness because as the nerves are remyelinating during the recovery phase, repair of the motor units is not consistent. When the patient is actively contracting a muscle during a functional or strengthening activity, the same motor units may be repeatedly firing due to the limited number of motor units available. This leads to a risk of these motor units being overworked. Signs and symptoms of overwork weakness are an increase in serum creatine kinase (CK) levels along with onset of muscle soreness that persists for 1 to 5 days after activity.[15] The patient may also state that he feels weaker and less stable in subsequent therapy sessions (typically the next day). The physical therapist must continuously assess for overwork weakness during the course of rehabilitation. This includes checking routine blood lab values prior to therapy, evaluating for weakness, using caution with eccentric contractions, and strengthening muscles in gravity-eliminated positions until the muscle is able to withstand resistance without signs or symptoms of overwork weakness.

Plan of Care and Interventions

Physical therapy begins with education for the patient and family regarding how to facilitate a safe and effective recovery of functional mobility. Educating the patient and family about the risk of **fatigue-related relapse** and its signs and symptoms decreases the risk of the patient working too hard and damaging nerves and muscles that are healing. It is crucial to remember to educate patients that nerve regeneration does *not* occur at a faster rate with an increase in exercise intensity.[16] While it is beneficial for a patient to begin a therapeutic exercise program, caution must be used to not overwork muscles. Persistent fatigue lasting longer than a day or abnormal sensations of numbness or tingling are typical symptoms of overwork. Patients and family must immediately report any signs or symptoms to the therapist and physician. Exercise and therapy will be held until symptoms have resolved and the patient is medically cleared to participate.

Strengthening should begin in the recovery phase starting at a low intensity and slowly progressing. A typical therapy session may begin with the patient on a sitting schedule to develop upright posture tolerance (*e.g.*, building up to sitting in a chair for 60 minutes, 4 times per day). Despite the patient's high level and transition to the recovery phase upon entering the IRF, he is still at risk of overwork weakness of the axial musculature. Posting a sitting schedule in the patient's room facilitates compliance by the patient, family, and the entire medical team. The patient's upper extremities did not weaken to the degree that he was not able to move them against gravity. He can be started on a program of gentle active range of motion against gravity or resistance with low loads. Since his lower extremities weakened to the level of paralysis, extra precaution should be used when initiating a strengthening program in order to avoid overstressing denervated muscles. The physical therapist should begin with isometric and concentric contractions in gravity-eliminated positions and progress to gravity-resisted positions only when he is able to maintain a grade of 2+/5 in this position. Overwork injury typically occurs more with eccentric than with concentric contractions, but this does not mean that interventions should avoid all eccentric muscle-strengthening activities.[17] For the patient to be safe and prepared for home discharge, functional eccentric contractions are necessary for transitions from standing to sitting, squatting, and walking down ramps. Due to the increased work required by muscle fibers during eccentric contractions, it is recommended that a patient demonstrate adequate concentric contraction to lift the weight of the limb or trunk against gravity (*e.g.*, during bed mobility) before progressing to eccentric muscle strengthening. Depending on the patient's rate of reinnervation and recovery, this training may not be initiated until later in the therapy program. Initially, the exercise program should include a low number of repetitions (*e.g.*, 10) with a high number of sets, but spread throughout the course of the day (*e.g.*, 5-6 sets per day).[18]

Due to the patient's lower extremity and trunk weakness, he needs to be trained to perform safe, functional transfers. The therapist can teach the patient how to use a leg lifter to manage his lower extremities in bed, giving him more independence during supine to sitting transitions. During transfers into and out of bed, he needs to use a sliding board because his lower extremities do not have adequate strength to complete a stand pivot transfer. Using a sliding board can decrease risk of fatigue-related relapse because he can use his legs for positioning and support but this strategy will likely not overwork the recovering motor units. A stand pivot transfer requires the use of concentric contractions of the quadriceps and gluteal muscles for the lift-off portion and eccentric contractions of these muscles for lowering into the sitting position. His rate of strength return will determine how quickly he can progress to a squat pivot transfer with physical assistance and then with an appropriate assistive device.

As the patient's functional mobility and strength improve through therapy interventions and reinnervation of motor units, gait training can be initiated. Once he has progressed to standing with an assistive device with minimal assistance, pre-gait interventions can be introduced. Basic weight shifting and stepping strategies allow a slow progression to the single limb stance required for ambulation. Body-weight-supported training through use of a mechanical lift system can allow the patient to be upright and begin a stepping sequence without having full weightbearing on the lower extremities. This training can allow the patient to advance each lower extremity in the swing phase while decreasing the risk of overwork weakness by supporting his partial or full weight in the stance phase. Progress over several training sessions can be demonstrated by gradually increasing the amount of the patient's body weight he has to support. In a case report, Tuckey and Greenwood[19] described the use of a body-weight-supported system to train a nonambulatory patient recovering from GBS to effectively and safely progress from static standing with two-person assistance to ambulation overground. Without body-weight support, the patient was able to ambulate < 3 m with a rollator and two-person assistance; after 3 m, the patient's legs unpredictably buckled—an obvious safety issue. With partial body weight support, the patient ambulated 110 m on the treadmill. This treatment strategy allowed the patient to complete longer training sessions in a task-specific and safe manner. Within 3 weeks of the partial-body-weight-supported gait training, the patient progressed from ambulating 3 m to ambulating 100 m without body weight support. In the pre-gait phases of the rehabilitation program for the patient recovering from GBS, a body-weight-supported system can allow the patient to practice and train for tasks too difficult or too unsafe to complete, thereby facilitating his coordination and muscular strength required for ambulation.

The main focus of physical therapy interventions for patients recovering from GBS is to complete exercises and functional mobility at low-intensity loads, few repetitions, with multiple sets to be performed throughout the day. Caution must be taken to not work the same muscle group day after day and to allow rest breaks during the training program for muscle recovery. The physical therapist provides extensive and consistent education to the patient and family regarding signs and symptoms of fatigue-related relapse and strategies to decrease this risk. Treatment strategies including strengthening, functional mobility, and gait training that have been used for a variety of diagnoses such as multiple sclerosis, amyotrophic lateral sclerosis, and post-polio syndrome can be modified for the patient recovering from GBS.[20]

Evidence-Based Clinical Recommendations

SORT: Strength of Recommendation Taxonomy

A: Consistent, good-quality patient-oriented evidence
B: Inconsistent or limited-quality patient-oriented evidence
C: Consensus, disease-oriented evidence, usual practice, expert opinion, or case series

1. Physical therapists can use the Functional Independence Measure (FIM®) to measure functional limitations and caregiver burden for individuals with Guillain-Barré syndrome in the inpatient rehabilitation setting. **Grade B**

2. Physical therapists can use the Tinetti Performance Oriented Mobility Assessment to determine dysfunctions in ambulation and balance and determine fall risk in individuals with GBS. **Grade B**

3. Individuals with GBS may exercise to muscle fatigue, but must avoid exercise that leads to abnormal sensory sensations or weakness, or fatigue that persists longer than a day because this could increase risk of fatigue-related relapse. **Grade C**

COMPREHENSION QUESTIONS

20.1 A physical therapist is asked to evaluate a patient in an acute care hospital. The patient was diagnosed with Guillain-Barré Syndrome 3 days ago and is currently experiencing a gradual loss of strength and sensation. What is the *most* appropriate treatment plan for this patient?

A. Initiate an exercise program of supine therapeutic exercise including straight leg raises, gluteal squeezes, hip abduction, and ankle pumps to improve strength.

B. Do not perform the evaluation and educate the patient not to move while in the bed.

C. Educate patient and family on proper positioning in bed and gentle passive range of motion for ankles, knees, and hips to decrease risk of skin breakdown and development of joint contractures.

D. Gradually progress the patient daily from sitting at the edge of the bed to eventually ambulating with appropriate assistive device to decrease his potential for losing functional mobility.

20.2 A physical therapist is treating a patient with Guillain-Barré Syndrome in an outpatient clinic 3 d/wk. Upon arrival for his second treatment session, the patient reports that yesterday and today he has felt weaker and less stable when ambulating. What is the *most* appropriate course of action for his scheduled treatment session?

A. Hold his therapy session for the day and recommend that he visit his physician for an assessment and blood work.

B. Perform fewer repetitions and lower intensity of the already established exercises.

C. Tell the patient that this is a normal part of muscle strengthening and continue current treatment plan.

D. Eliminate any eccentric exercises and train muscles only concentrically for remainder of rehabilitation.

ANSWERS

20.1 **C.** The patient has recently been diagnosed and is currently in a phase of decline in which he is experiencing progressive muscular weakness and sensation loss. Aggressive exercise and mobilization (options A and D) should not occur until after he has gone through the plateau phase and has begun the recovery phase. Due to the high risk of skin breakdown and joint contractures associated with prolonged bed rest, the patient should not be told to avoid all movement (option B). It is important to educate the patient and family on proper techniques of positioning and gentle range of motion to decrease these risks. This will reduce additional complications in his functional recovery once he is cleared for mobilization.

20.2 **A.** The patient may be experiencing overwork weakness, which is a serious contraindication to therapy. The patient needs to be evaluated by his physician and have lab work done to check for increased serum levels of creatine kinase. He must be cleared by his physician to resume exercise.

REFERENCES

1. Hund EF, Borel CO, Cornblath DR, Hanley DF, McKhann GM. Intensive management and treatment of severe Guillain-Barre syndrome. *Crit Care Med.* 1993;21:433-446.

2. Ropper AH. Critical care of Guillain-Barre syndrome. In: Ropper AH, ed. *Neurological and Neurosurgical Intensive Care.* 3rd ed. New York, NY: Raven Press; 1993.

3. Kuwabara S. Guillain-Barré syndrome: epidemiology, pathophysiology and management. *Drugs.* 2004;64:597-610.

4. van Doorn PA, Ruts L, Jacobs BC. Clinical features, pathogenesis, and treatment of Guillain-Barre syndrome. *Lancet Neurol.* 2008;7:939-950.

5. National Institute of Neurological Disorders and Stroke. www.ninds.nih.gov. Accessed August 25, 2012.

6. Taly AB, Veerendrakumar M, Das KB, et al. Sensory dysfunction in GB syndrome: a clinical and electrophysiological study of 100 patients. *Electromyogr Clin Neurophysiol.* 1997;37:49-54.

7. van der Meche FF, Schmitz PI. A randomized trial comparing intravenous immune globulin and plasma exchange in Guillain-Barre syndrome. Dutch Guillain-Barre Study Group. *N Engl J Med.* 1992;326:1123-1129.

8. Melillo EM, Sethi JM, Mohsenin V. Guillain-Barre syndrome: rehabilitation outcome and recent developments. *Yale J Biol Med.* 1998;71:383-389.

9. All About Guillain-Barre Syndrome. www.jsmarcussen.com. Accessed October 31, 2011.

10. Teitelbaum JS, Borel CO. Respiratory dysfunction in Guillain-Barre Syndrome. *Clin Chest Med.* 1994;15:705-714.

11. Hughes RA, Rees JH. Guillain-Barre syndrome. *Curr Opin Neurol.* 1994;7:368-392.

12. Hamilton BB, Laughlin JA, Fiedler RC, Granger CV. Interrater reliability of the 7-level functional independence measure (FIM). *Scand J Rehabil Med.* 1994;26:115-119.

13. The Inpatient Rehabilitation Facility Patient Assessment Instrument (IRF-PAI) Training Manual. UB Foundations Activities, Inc. (UBFA, Inc.). 2004. http://www.cms.gov/Medicare/Medicare-Fee-for-Service-Payment/InpatientRehabFacPPS/Downloads/IRFPAI-manual-2012.pdf. Accessed February 14, 2013.

14. Tinetti ME, Williams TF, Mayewski R. Fall risk index for elderly patients based on number of chronic disabilities. *Am J Med.* 1986;80:429-434.

15. Curtis CL, Weir JP. Overview of exercise responses in healthy and impaired states. *Neurol Rep.* 1996;20:13-19.

16. Steinberg JS. *Guillain-Barre Syndrome (Acute Idiopathic Polyneuritis): An Overview for the Layperson.* Wynnewood, PA: The Guillain-Barre Syndrome Support Group International; 1987.

17. Newham DJ, Mills KR, Quigley BM, Edwards RH. Pain and fatigue after concentric and eccentric muscle contractions. *Clin Sci (Lond).* 1983;64:55-62.

18. Stillwell GK. Rehabilitative procedures. In: Dyck PJ, et al. eds. *Peripheral Neuropathy.* 2nd ed. Philadelphia, PA: WB Saunders; 1984.

19. Tuckey J, Greenwood R. Rehabilitation after severe Guillain-Barre Syndrome: the use of partial body weight support. *Physiother Res Int.* 2004;9:96-103.

20. Umphred DA. *Neurological Rehabilitation.* 4th ed. Philadelphia, PA: Mosby; 2001.

Post-polio Syndrome

Rolando T. Lazaro
Sharon L. Gorman

CASE 21

The patient is a 53-year-old, right-hand dominant, obese male (BMI 34.2 kg/m^2) who was referred to outpatient physical therapy. During the initial physical therapy interview, he reports that he is "getting weaker" in his legs and trunk. He also states that he gets tired easily, especially at the end of the day, and more than usual. He reports having several falls in the past few months. He recounts that his most recent fall happened in a grocery store 2 weeks ago; he had no injuries except for some bruising. He states that it was the end of the day and he was very tired but had forced himself to go. While inside the store, he reported that he tripped and fell, landing on his right shoulder. The patient reports that he was diagnosed with poliomyelitis at 30 months of age. As a child, he ambulated with bilateral hip-knee-ankle-foot orthoses (HKAFOs) and forearm crutches. During his teens, he abandoned the use of bilateral HKAFOs because "they took a long time to put on," and he "didn't really need them and walked fine without them." Instead, he used an ankle-foot orthosis (AFO) on the right foot and forearm crutches, and has used these devices since then. The patient lives with his wife and teenage son. He retired from a sales job 11 years ago. His hobbies include gardening, attending baseball games, and going to the movies with his family. He describes himself as outgoing and a high achiever with a "type A personality" because he is very determined and "never gives up on anything." He states that he is frustrated that he does not have the energy and strength to do activities that he has done in the past, like going on long walks or gardening. The patient recently had a complete medical work-up including laboratory work and diagnostic imaging of the brain and spinal cord that revealed no active pathological conditions.

▶ Based on his health condition, what do you anticipate will be the contributors to activity limitations?

▶ What are the examination priorities?

▶ What are the most appropriate physical therapy outcome measures for gait and balance?

▶ What are possible complications interfering with physical therapy?

KEY DEFINITIONS

ANKLE-FOOT ORTHOSIS (AFO): Externally applied orthosis (usually plastic) that surrounds the ankle and at least part of the foot to control position and motion of the ankle, compensate for weakness, or correct deformities; commonly used in the treatment of disorders affecting muscle function such as stroke, spinal cord injury, muscular dystrophy, cerebral palsy, polio, multiple sclerosis, and peripheral neuropathy

HIP-KNEE-ANKLE-FOOT ORTHOSIS (HKAFO): Device used for patients requiring more stability of the hip, knee, and lower torso due to paralysis and/or weakness (secondary to paraplegia, spina bifida, recurrent hip dislocation, other neurological impairments); provides pelvic stability in several planes (rotation, side-to-side, front-to-back motions), reduces unwanted motion, increases steps per minute, and reduces energy expenditure

NON-FATIGUING EXERCISE: Patient uses submaximal effort or maximal contraction with limited repetitions[1]

Objectives

1. Describe the typical signs and symptoms of post-polio syndrome.
2. List pertinent tests and measures used in a physical therapy examination for an individual with post-polio syndrome.
3. Discuss appropriate physical therapy interventions for a person with post-polio syndrome.

Physical Therapy Considerations

PT considerations during management of the individual with gait instability, weakness, pain, and balance dysfunction due to post-polio syndrome:

▶ **General physical therapy plan of care/goals:** Assessment of muscle strength to identify specific strength deficits and to establish baseline; assessment of impairments affecting cardiopulmonary endurance; examination of functional mobility, transfers, and locomotion; assess need for orthotic devices to maximize function and joint protection; decrease pain

▶ **Physical therapy interventions:** Patient education on energy conservation, joint protection, and weight loss; functional mobility training; gait training using appropriate assistive devices and orthotics

▶ **Precautions during physical therapy:** Appropriate guarding during physical therapy interventions to minimize risk of falls; appropriate exercise grading to manage fatigue and overexertion; appropriate exercise dosage to maintain or improve strength and prevent further muscular overuse

▶ **Complications interfering with physical therapy:** Overexertion in regaining muscle strength; decreased ability to exercise at levels required for aerobic conditioning; development of biomechanical damage to joints lacking sufficient muscular stabilization

Understanding the Health Condition

To understand post-polio syndrome, it is important to first discuss acute paralytic poliomyelitis. Acute paralytic poliomyelitis ("polio") is caused by a virus that damages or kills the anterior horn cells of the spinal cord, causing asymmetrical, flaccid, muscular paralysis.[2] The paralysis typically involves the lower extremities, although muscles of respiration and upper extremities may also be affected. Individuals who have recovered from this initial bout of polio have varying degrees of activity limitation and participation restriction, based on the severity of the initial attack and the physical rehabilitation following the initial onset.[3] While the condition remains relatively stable in subsequent years, some individuals complain of pain, new muscle weakness, generalized whole-body and muscular fatigue, and muscle atrophy many years after the initial infection. This condition is termed post-polio syndrome (PPS). There is no evidence to suggest that these new symptoms are due to reactivation of the poliovirus.[4]

The presence of new or increased muscle weakness in individuals who have recovered from acute polio is the most important clinical presentation that indicates PPS.[5] Although there are no definitive diagnostic tests for PPS, experts have developed criteria to assist in diagnosing PPS,[3,6] with the following being common: (1) diagnosed previous episode of acute poliomyelitis resulting in loss of motor neurons; (2) period of neurological and functional recovery at least 15 years or more following the initial episode of acute poliomyelitis; (3) slow onset of new muscle weakness, generalized whole-body and muscular fatigue, and muscle atrophy, and (4) symptoms that cannot be explained by other medical conditions. In this patient case, review of the prior medical history and patient interview revealed that the patient satisfied all of these criteria for a diagnosis of PPS.

PPS is a very slowly progressing condition marked by long periods of stability. Severity depends on the degree of residual weakness and limitations an individual has after the original polio infection. People who had only minimal symptoms from the original attack and subsequently develop PPS will most likely experience only mild PPS symptoms. People originally hit hard by the poliovirus and left with severe residual weakness may develop a more severe case of PPS with a greater loss of muscle function, difficulty in swallowing, and more periods of fatigue.[7] Nollet and colleagues[5] found that individuals with PPS are more prone to fatigue and have more physical mobility restrictions than those who have recovered from acute polio but do not have PPS.

Several medical interventions have been investigated for their effectiveness in alleviating signs and symptoms of PPS. Preliminary studies indicate that **intravenous immunoglobulin therapy** may reduce pain, increase quality of life, and modestly improve strength.[8,9] Preliminary results also indicate that lamotrigine (an antiseizure drug) may reduce pain, fatigue, and muscle cramps and may increase quality of life in people with PPS.[10] Pain from joint deterioration and increasing skeletal deformities such as scoliosis are common. Medical management includes analgesic and anti-inflammatory medications. Surgical procedures may be indicated to provide more joint stability and thereby decrease pain. Some individuals with PPS experience only minor symptoms, while others develop more visible muscle weakness and atrophy. While PPS is rarely life-threatening, symptoms can interfere significantly with an individual's capacity to function independently.[7]

Physical Therapy Patient/Client Management

Physical therapy management for patients/clients who have PPS must focus on optimizing activity and participation, while protecting the remaining motor units from further degeneration. Because PPS affects older individuals, age-related changes in the neuromusculoskeletal system must also be considered as potential contributing factors that may affect recovery. A thorough assessment of muscular strength and endurance allows for an individualized strengthening and endurance program that will optimize function. Cardiopulmonary assessment and interventions must also be included in the management priorities. Interventions may include energy conservation and modification of the environment to facilitate functional performance. Reassessment of the patient's orthotic and supportive devices and ambulatory aids is necessary as part of the goal of conserving energy. Falls are a major consideration, and therefore patient education to decrease this risk should also be incorporated.

Examination, Evaluation, and Diagnosis

A thorough patient interview is important to obtain information regarding the current complaints and how recent symptoms affect activity and participation. Specific questions that allude to changes in muscular performance must be investigated. For example, the therapist may ask: "Can you think of activities that you recently find difficult to perform?" Typically, individuals with PPS will state that they are experiencing difficulties in doing certain things that they have otherwise done easily in the past. This patient stated that he had more trouble completing everyday tasks such as shopping; he noted an overall increase in his general fatigue and had been experiencing more falls than usual. Obtaining information about the patient's ability to perform activities of daily living (ADLs) may also allow the therapist to make appropriate recommendations to other healthcare providers such as occupational therapists or speech-language pathologists. Given this patient's problems with shopping and general endurance, an occupation therapy referral was discussed with the patient. Moreover, specific questions pertaining to pain and fatigue (both in specific muscle groups and generalized whole-body fatigue) must be investigated. Since PPS may affect the muscles of respiration, it is important to pose screening questions pertaining to the cardiovascular and pulmonary systems (*e.g.*, "Do you notice any shortness of breath or difficulty breathing?"). In this case, the patient only complained of general fatigue and muscular fatigue, with no indications of difficulty breathing or shortness of breath. Use of any orthotic or assistive devices in the past must also be clarified, including an investigation on the frequency of their use and any changes in the devices through the years.

Patients who recovered from an acute bout of polio typically were prescribed orthotic devices to facilitate function as well as to support or protect the joints in affected regions. These devices frequently take a long time to don and doff, so many individuals tend not to use them. As a result, they overuse the muscles that the orthotic devices were intended to protect and submit the joints to excessive biomechanical stresses. In this case, the patient had self-selected to use a right AFO and forego his bilateral HKAFOs years ago, but continued to use his forearm crutches. With his new diagnosis of PPS, the therapist obtained a referral for an orthotist to coordinate replacement of his old and worn right AFO and for consideration of additional bracing. Given the patient's active lifestyle, the therapist also initiated a discussion with the patient regarding obtaining a wheelchair for community-level mobility to address his fatigue.

The prevalence of pain in individuals with PPS ranges from 75% to 91%.[11,12] Pain in the lower extremities is more commonly reported than in the upper extremities and trunk, and pain during movement or physical activity (ambulation) is more common than at rest. The visual analog scale (VAS), pain questionnaire, and pain drawing are appropriate tools to quantify pain in patients with PPS. The patient reported a pain rating of 7-8 out of 10 in the right shoulder, both thighs, and low back. He reported using over-the-counter analgesics for most of this pain; after taking medications, he rates the pain as 3/10. The patient also specified that his pain was worse on days when he walked a lot and when he let himself get fatigued.

It is important to perform a detailed strength assessment to determine the strength of each muscle group. This must be done for both the muscles affected and unaffected by the initial bout of polio because PPS can cause changes in muscles that seemingly recovered fully from the initial bout of polio.[5] Manual muscle testing (MMT) is frequently used to assess strength and monitor progress in persons with PPS. Because many individuals with PPS have significant weakness, MMT can accurately measure strength better than other assessment methods that detect strength changes in stronger muscles, such as hand-held dynomometry.[13] Table 21-1 lists the MMT results for key muscles for this patient. Note the significant weakness in muscles around the right shoulder and both lower extremities. The MMT grades serve as a baseline and guide for selecting appropriate interventions to optimize activity and participation.

Muscular fatigue plays a pivotal role in PPS. Many patients do not have the endurance in a specific muscle for repeated contractions due to the decreased number of active motor units in the areas affected by the initial polio attack. This can have significant effects on activities that require repeated motor pattern activation, such as walking. For example, as the muscular endurance of the quadriceps deteriorates after multiple contractions, this can significantly limit walking distance and gait endurance.

Balance is another impairment that requires thorough examination. The therapist must select a measure sensitive enough to detect changes in the patient's abilities. Balance measures that can be used in individuals with PPS include Romberg, Sharpened Romberg, single-leg stance (with eyes open and eyes closed), and the Berg Balance Scale (BBS). The BBS may not be an appropriate assessment tool for this patient due to his use of assistive devices and/or orthotics for stability in standing, which is not allowed with the BBS. Other balance measures capture more dynamic standing abilities and include significant test items related to gait. Because this patient has the ability to stand and walk, other higher level balance measures

Table 21-1 MANUAL MUSCLE TEST RESULTS FOR CASE PATIENT		
Upper Extremities	Right	Left
Scapular adduction and downward rotation	3+	4
Scapular abduction and upward rotation	3+	4
Shoulder depression	0	3+
Shoulder flexion	0	3+
Shoulder extension	0	4
Shoulder abduction	0	4
Shoulder internal rotation	1	4
Shoulder external rotation	2	3+
Elbow flexion	3+	5
Elbow extension	0	5
Wrist flexion	2	4
Wrist extension	3	4
Grip[a]	20 kg	36 kg
Lower Extremities		
Hip flexion	1	2
Hip extension	1	1
Knee flexion	2−	2
Knee extension	2	2
Ankle dorsiflexion	0	0
Ankle plantarflexion	1	2

[a]Mean grip strength norms for this patient's age and sex are: 50.6 kg (right); 45.2 kg (left).[14]

may be indicated such as the Dynamic Gait Index (DGI), Functional Gait Assessment, or Timed Up and Go (TUG)—including the modified TUG, manual TUG, and/or the cognitive TUG. The TUG is a reliable measure of gait in PPS.[15] For this patient, the physical therapist selected the TUG and the DGI. He completed the TUG with his forearm crutches and right AFO in 16.25 seconds. While normative values are not available for the TUG in persons with PPS, a TUG score of ≥ 13.5 seconds has been associated with an increased risk for falls in community-dwelling elderly.[16] On the DGI, he scored 17/24. Research has shown that in community-dwelling elderly, a score < 19 on the DGI indicates an increased fall risk.[17] During the DGI, the patient had difficulties changing gait speed, stepping over and around obstacles, and negotiating stairs. This information can indicate difficulty with muscular power or endurance and problems with stability when in single limb stance. This information can help the therapist choose interventions to address specific balance deficits.

Activity level assessments need to examine functional mobility skills and gait. Other activities may be examined based on patient complaints or other information gained during the patient interview. The patient was able to perform supine-to-sit and sit-to-stand transfers independently. He ambulated independently with right AFO and bilateral forearm crutches for 20 ft, limited by right shoulder pain (7/10 pain rating) and shortness of breath. The therapist may want to see the patient perform ADLs both with and without his usual orthotics to assess the improvements in biomechanical stability, support, and performance when using the orthotics. Many patients with PPS have a long history of orthotic use, but there may be technological advances in the orthotics they require. The therapist should consult an orthotist to determine whether a lighter-weight version, more modern design, or more/less stability can be obtained with a new orthotic. The patient has been using the same right AFO for mobility and ambulation for about 7 years and it is visibly worn. Due to MMT results in the left ankle region (0-2/5), he may also benefit from a left AFO.

Because PPS increases fatigue and decreases endurance, the therapist must examine the cardiovascular and pulmonary systems. Outcome measures such as the **Piper Fatigue Scale,**[18] **Fatigue Impact Scale,**[19] **and Fatigue Severity Scale**[20] have demonstrated reliability and validity for measuring post-polio fatigue. The therapist chose the Fatigue Severity Scale for this patient. This measure consists of nine items that describe the severity of fatigue and how this symptom affects selected activities and functions. The patient is asked to rate his agreement with each statement on a 1 to 7 scale, with the higher number indicating strong agreement. Responses to each item are added; scores > 36 indicate that the patient is suffering from fatigue. This patient received a score of 52/63, consistent with his complaints of fatigue.

The Six-Minute Walk Test (6MWT) may allow adequate assessment of endurance and aerobic capacity and it has been noted to be reliable in individuals with PPS.[15] In considering whether to have a patient perform this test, the therapist needs to be cognizant of whole-body fatigue and its effect on each patient. Given the 20-ft ambulation distance limitation for this patient, he was not appropriate for the 6MWT. In addition, because of the onset of dyspnea on exertion (DOE) and fatigue occurring with this limited ambulation distance, the therapist deferred further testing and carefully recorded information about his fatigue level and DOE in order to assess endurance in future visits.

The therapist documented the patient's physical therapy diagnosis upon completion of the examination. The patient presented with activity limitations in ambulation, causing participation restrictions in leisure activities such as long walks, instrumental ADLs, and gardening, which also put him at a high risk for falls. Impairments in body structure and function include pain, fatigue, significant weakness, decreased balance, and limited endurance.

Plan of Care and Interventions

Patient education and training play an important role in the plan of care for patients with PPS. Part of the conversation and collaboration with the patient may include a discussion on pacing or grading activities. Patient education on possible lifestyle modifications and energy conservation techniques may help decrease general fatigue. Suggestions include taking more frequent breaks, and especially taking breaks when (or before) feeling tired. Tasks can be broken up into smaller components to decrease fatigue and/or pain. Work modifications must also be explored to investigate whether there are more efficient ways of performing these duties. Adherence to the prescribed home program, which includes physical exercises and the use of orthotics and assistive devices during ambulation, is very important in the achievement of these goals. With this patient, the therapist spent "rest time" during treatment sessions on education regarding energy conservation, adherence, and lifestyle modifications. The biggest change for this patient was obtaining a motorized wheelchair for community-level mobility. The motorized wheelchair's purpose was to allow the patient to conserve his energy and increase participation by limiting fatigue. By limiting his ambulation with forearm crutches, a secondary goal was to decrease his right shoulder pain, since he relied heavily on this arm when ambulating. In terms of ambulation, it was appropriate to advise him to ambulate only short distances, and possibly use his motorized wheelchair when covering longer distances. For example, he was advised to bring his wheelchair to baseball games to minimize overuse and fatigue; for short trips to the grocery store, his AFOs and forearm crutches could suffice.

It is important to discuss the role of exercise to improve weakness and optimize the function of persons with PPS. There is some concern that high-intensity strengthening exercises may cause overuse and further deterioration of the remaining motor units. Some authors report that strengthening can be safely performed with muscles that have a strength grade of fair plus $(3+/5)$ or higher with **non-fatiguing exercises** and rest periods between sets.[1] There have been several suggestions on how to implement a regimen of non-fatiguing strengthening exercises in persons with PPS. One suggestion from a Canadian post-polio clinic is for the physical therapist to determine the patient's 5-repetition maximum (5RM), which is the maximum amount of weight with which a patient can do only 5 repetitions without signs of fatigue (e.g., decrease in form or quality of movement). The patient is then asked to start the subsequent exercise session using 50% of the 5RM weight and to perform up to 30 repetitions using that weight, but stop at the first sign of fatigue. When the patient is able to perform 30 repetitions during two successive sessions, the weight is increased to 75% of 5RM.[21] In terms of exercising to increase aerobic endurance, the 20% rule has been suggested.[22] In this method, after the patient's maximum exercise capability has been determined, the patient is instructed to perform the exercise during the subsequent sessions at 20% of this level, 3 to 4 times per week for 1 month, and then increase this exercise intensity by 10%. For example, if it was determined that the patient could ride an exercise bicycle maximally for an hour 4 times per week, the patient is instructed to perform this exercise for 12 minutes (which is 20%) 3 to 4 times per week and then increase it by 6 minutes (10%) for a total of 18 minutes after a month of training.

Strengthening exercises for the upper extremities may be beneficial to ensure better support of the patient's body, especially when ambulating using the forearm crutches. This patient was prescribed non-fatiguing exercises for the right upper extremity. Balance exercises included weight shifting in standing on non-compliant and compliant surfaces. Physical therapy interventions to manage muscular pain may include the use of physical agent modalities and electrotherapy as appropriate.[1]

A consultation with an orthotist was obtained to investigate replacing the patient's worn right AFO and potentially obtaining a new left AFO due to new left ankle weakness. Based on the patient's weakness and fatigue, the orthotist and therapist recommended that the patient obtain bilateral HKAFOs. However, the patient was clear that he did not want braces that were that restrictive. Given his prior history with HKAFOs, consensus was reached on replacing the right AFO and obtaining a left AFO, both made with lighter-weight plastic to decrease the energy demand during gait as much as possible. The therapist ensured the delivery of the AFOs would occur with at least two therapy treatment sessions remaining to allow the patient to work on gait training with the new AFOs with the therapist.

At discharge from physical therapy, patients should be given education, resources, and referrals to assist them in long-term management of PPS. Stressing the need for non-fatiguing exercises to avoid overuse and fatigue is one example. For this patient, referral to a pool exercise class was a good way of accomplishing a follow-up exercise plan. Aquatic exercise provides the opportunity to safely exercise within appropriate submaximal limits while at the same time protecting vulnerable joints from overuse. The pool program also included exercises aimed at improving cardiopulmonary and aerobic endurance. Last, education on weight reduction is appropriate to assist in decreasing the stress and load to the joints and muscles that occur with increased body mass.

Evidence-Based Clinical Recommendations

SORT: Strength of Recommendation Taxonomy

A: Consistent, good-quality patient-oriented evidence
B: Inconsistent or limited-quality patient-oriented evidence
C: Consensus, disease-oriented evidence, usual practice, expert opinion, or case series

1. Intravenous immunoglobulin therapy may reduce pain, increase quality of life, and improve strength modestly in persons with post-polio syndrome. **Grade B**

2. The Piper Fatigue Scale, Fatigue Impact Scale, and Fatigue Severity Scale are reliable and valid for measuring post-polio fatigue. **Grade B**

3. Non-fatiguing exercise protocols can prevent overuse and progressively strengthen muscles weakened by PPS. **Grade C**

COMPREHENSION QUESTIONS

21.1 Each of the following is an appropriate criterion to diagnose post-polio syndrome *except*:

A. A previously diagnosed episode of acute poliomyelitis resulting in loss of motor neurons

B. Period of neurological and functional recovery lasting ≥15 years following the initial episode of acute poliomyelitis

C. Laboratory tests that indicate the presence of poliovirus in the cerebrospinal fluid

D. Slow onset of new muscle weakness, generalized whole-body and muscular fatigue, and muscle atrophy

21.2 The following are appropriate physical therapy management strategies in patients with post-polio syndrome *except*:

A. Patient education on weight loss, energy conservation, and environmental modifications

B. Use of physical agent and electrotherapeutic modalities to decrease pain

C. Non-fatiguing exercises with submaximal contractions or maximal contractions with rest periods in between sets

D. All of the above are correct.

ANSWERS

21.1 **C.** There are currently no laboratory tests or medical imaging studies that can confirm PPS. Moreover, there is no evidence that PPS results from the reactivation of the poliovirus.

21.2 **D.** All of the above interventions are appropriate in the physical therapy management of persons with PPS. Non-fatiguing exercises have been noted to be beneficial in improving strength in people with PPS in the muscles graded fair plus (3+) or higher.

REFERENCES

1. Eskew RA, Quiben MU, Hallum A. Aging with dignity and chronic impairments. In: Umphred DA, ed. *Neurological Rehabilitation*. 5th ed. St. Louis, MO: Mosby Elsevier; 2007, 952.

2. Latham J, Foley G, Nolan R, et al. *Post Polio Syndrome Management and Treatment in Primary Care*. Dublin, Ireland: Post Polio Support Group; 2007. http://www.ppsg.ie/dloads/PostPolioBooklet.pdf. Accessed April 25, 2012.

3. Jubelt B. Post-polio syndrome. *Curr Treat Options Neurol*. 2004;6:87-93.

4. Kilmer DD. Response to resistive strengthening exercise training in humans with neuromuscular disease. *Am J Phys Med Rehabil*. 2002;81(suppl):S121-S126.

5. Nollet F, Beelen A, Prins MH, et al. Disability and functional assessment in former polio patients with and without postpolio syndrome. *Arch Phys Med Rehabil*. 1999;80:136-143.

6. Farbu E, Gilhus NE, Barnes MP, et al. EFNS guidelines on diagnosis and management of post polio syndrome. Report of an EFNS task force. *Eur J Neurol.* 2006;13:795-801.

7. National Institute of Neurological Disorders and Stroke (NINDS). NINDS post-polio syndrome information page. http://www.ninds.nih.gov/disorders/post_polio/post_polio.htm. Accessed March 21, 2012.

8. Gonzalez H, Sunnerhagen KS, Sjöberg I, Kaponides G, Olsson T, Borg K. Intravenous immunoglobulin for post polio syndrome: a randomized controlled trial. *Lancet Neurol.* 2006;5:493-500.

9. Farbu E, Rekand T, Vik-Mo E, Lygren H, Gilhus NE, Aarli JA. Post-polio syndrome patients treated with intravenous immunoglobulin: a double-blinded randomized controlled pilot study. *Eur J Neurol.* 2007;14:60-65.

10. On AY, Oncu J, Uludag B, Ertekin C. Effect of lamotrigine on the symptoms and life qualities of patients with post polio syndrome: a randomized controlled study. *NeuroRehabilitation.* 2005;20:245-251.

11. Willen C, Grimby G. Pain, physical activity, and disability in individuals with late effects of polio. *Arch Phys Med Rehabil.* 1998;79:915-919.

12. Halstead LS, Rossi CD. Post-polio syndrome: clinical experience with 132 consecutive outpatients. In: Halstead LS, Wiechers DO, eds. *Research and Clinical Aspects of the Late Effects of Poliomyelitis.* Vol 23. New York, NY: March of Dimes Birth Defects Foundation; 1987.

13. Bohannon RW. Manual muscle testing: does it meet the standards of an adequate screening test? *Clin Rehabil.* 2005;19:662-667.

14. Bohannon RW, Peolsson A, Massy-Westropp N, Desrosiers J, Bear-Lehman J. Reference values for adult grip strength measured with a Jamar dynamometer: a descriptive meta-analysis. *Physiotherapy.* 2006;92:11-15.

15. Flansbjer U, Lexell J. Reliability of gait performance tests in individuals with late effects of polio. *Phys Med Rehabil.* 2010;2:125-131.

16. Shumway-Cook A, Brauer S, Woollacott M. Predicting the probability for falls in community-dwelling older adults using the Timed Up & Go Test. *Phys Ther.* 2000;80:896-903.

17. Shumway-Cook A, Baldwin M, Polissar NL, Gruber W. Predicting the probability for falls in community-dwelling older adults. *Phys Ther.* 1997;77:812-819.

18. Strohschein FJ, Kelly CG, Clarke AG, Westbury CF, Shuaib A, Chan KM. Applicability, validity and reliability of the Piper Fatigue Scale in postpolio patients. *Am J Phys Med Rehabil.* 2003;82:122-129.

19. Frith J, Newton J. Fatigue Impact Scale. *Occup Med.* 2010;60:159.

20. Oncu J, Durmaz B, Karapolat H. Short-term effects of aerobic exercise on functional capacity, fatigue, and quality of life in patients with post-polio syndrome. *Clin Rehabil.* 2009;23:155-163.

21. Saskatchewan Awareness of Post Polio Society Inc. The benefit of exercise in PPS. http://poliosask.org/exercise.html. Accessed February 14, 2013.

22. Yarnell SK. Non-fatiguing general conditioning program (the 20% rule). *Post Polio Health.* Summer 1991;7(3). http://www.post-polio.org/edu/pphnews/pph7-3a.html. Accessed April 21, 2012.

Carpal Tunnel Syndrome

Jennifer Junkin

CASE 22

A 22-year-old college athlete had his cast removed 2 days ago. Eight weeks ago, he sustained a Colles' fracture of his dominant right wrist when he fell on an outstretched hand during a basketball game. He presents to an outpatient physical therapy clinic today for his initial evaluation. He reports some pain in his forearm and hand with numbness and tingling in his thumb, index, middle, and half of his ring finger. His right grip strength is 50% weaker than the left. There is observable atrophy in the right thenar eminence, and he describes a "pressure" sensation at his wrist. He notices that his right hand falls asleep sometimes when doing homework on the computer. Motion at end-range wrist flexion and extension increases his pain and neurologic symptoms. The patient has a positive Phalen's test and a positive Tinel's sign at the wrist. His signs and symptoms are consistent with carpal tunnel syndrome.

▶ What examination signs may be associated with this suspected diagnosis?

▶ What are the most appropriate physical therapy interventions?

▶ Describe a physical therapy plan of care based on each stage of this health condition.

KEY DEFINITIONS

DOUBLE CRUSH SYNDROME: Type of peripheral nerve compression syndrome in which there is a central compression that impacts a nerve bundle (*e.g.*, at the thoracic or pelvic outlet) and a second more peripheral compression (*e.g.*, at the carpal or tarsal tunnel)

GANGLION CYST: Noncancerous fluid-filled lumps that most commonly develop along the tendons or joints in the hands or feet

RAYNAUD'S PHENOMENON: Intermittent ischemia of the fingers or toes usually caused by exposure to cold or due to emotional stimuli

Objectives

1. Identify the contents and borders of the carpal tunnel.
2. Discuss key steps of the examination that would lead the physical therapist toward a diagnosis of carpal tunnel syndrome.
3. Describe lifestyle and environmental factors that could contribute to developing carpal tunnel syndrome.
4. Discuss evidence-based treatment strategies and precautions for each stage of the condition (acute, subacute, chronic).

Physical Therapy Considerations

PT considerations during management of the individual with progressive weakness and atrophy of the thenar muscles and first two lumbricals, sensory disturbances in the median nerve distribution, pain in the wrist and hand with repetitive use, and functional loss due to carpal tunnel syndrome:

▶ **General physical therapy plan of care/goals:** Assess muscle strength and sensation in the median nerve distribution distal to the carpal tunnel; ergonomic work space assessment; patient education on positioning and possible benefits of bracing or night splint; maximize function with repetitive work activities such as typing and gripping

▶ **Physical therapy interventions:** Increase space and mobility of the carpal tunnel by stretching and manual therapy techniques; strengthen thenar muscles and first two lumbricals; stretches to increase flexibility of forearm flexor muscles; patient education on positioning and bracing; functional task training; home exercise program

▶ **Precautions during physical therapy:** Increasing pressure in the carpal tunnel when performing exercises in end-range flexion or extension; sensory disturbances in the median nerve distribution; double crush syndrome

▶ **Complications interfering with physical therapy:** Double crush syndrome; ganglion cyst; Raynaud's phenomenon

Understanding the Health Condition

The carpal tunnel is a confined space in the wrist. When viewing the anterior surface of the wrist, the carpal bones are the floor and walls of the tunnel, and the flexor retinaculum makes up the roof.[1] The forearm flexor tendons travel through the carpal tunnel along with the median and ulnar nerves. Any space-occupying lesion or dysfunction in this area will produce signs and symptoms that are collectively defined as carpal tunnel syndrome (CTS). Common causes of CTS include thickening of the tendons (tendinitis), scarring down of the tendons (tendinosis), swelling, inflammation, fractures or dislocations, malunion fractures, sustained abnormal postures, and any other etiologic factor that decreases the space in the carpal tunnel and compresses the median nerve.[2] CTS is frequently classified as an overuse syndrome or as a cumulative trauma. Office workers with poor ergonomic design of their workstations and whose job responsibilities include keyboarding are frequently affected by CTS. Sustained wrist flexion or extension can increase compressive forces at the wrist that may result in median nerve sensory and motor disturbances. A study in 1981 by Gelbermen et al.[3] revealed that intercarpal pressure increased fourfold in wrist extension and threefold in wrist flexion compared to the pressure in the neutrally positioned wrist.

CTS is a very common disorder. The incidence in the general population is estimated at 4.4 cases per 10,000 individuals and it accounts for 2% of all workers' compensation claims.[4] The carpal tunnel release is the most commonly performed operation of the hand.[5] While the syndrome more commonly affects the dominant hand, this is largely based on environmental factors and history of the individual.[5] CTS affects females 2.5 times more often than males.[6]

Typically, the onset of CTS is gradual and initial symptoms vary from case to case. The syndrome can also occur after a traumatic incident such as a fracture or dislocation of the wrist or distal radius.[6] CTS affects the median nerve distribution in the hand and therefore causes sensory changes in the palmar side of the thumb as well as the index, middle, and half of the ring finger (Fig. 22-1). Discomfort and pain in the wrist and fingers typically starts gradually and can present as a change in sensation within the median nerve distribution. Pain at night is a common complaint[7] since many people sleep with flexed wrists. A person with CTS may wake up feeling the need to "shake out" the affected hand or wrist. Decreased grip strength may make it difficult to form a fist, grasp small objects, or perform other manual tasks, causing limitations in activities at home and work.[7] Long-term effects include progressive weakness or atrophy of the thenar muscle compartment in the affected hand.[1]

The prognosis for individuals diagnosed with CTS is good. Cases can be treated conservatively or surgically. The main goals of conservative nonsurgical treatment include relieving pressure in the carpal tunnel, increasing hand strength in the thenar muscles and lumbricals, patient education regarding avoidance of awkward postures and positions, and ergonomic assessment and modifications of workplace or home workstations. A resting hand splint for nighttime management is frequently recommended because a splint can keep the wrist in the neutral position that is associated with the least amount of compression to the structures in the carpal tunnel.[6] Manual therapy techniques such as nerve gliding, tendon gliding, and soft tissue mobilization are components of conservative management that have been shown to provide short-term symptom relief.[6]

Median Nerve

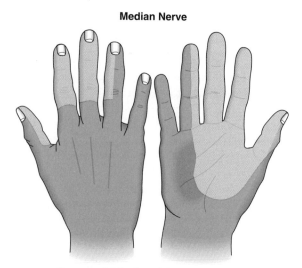

Sensory distribution of the median nerve

Figure 22-1. Lighter shaded areas show the sensory distribution of the median nerve. On the dorsal surface of the hand, the nerve supplies the index and middle fingers, and half of the fourth finger. On the palmar surface, the median nerve supplies the lateral two-thirds of the palm, the thumb, second and third fingers, and the lateral half of the fourth finger. (Reproduced with permission from Simon RP, Greenberg DA, Aminoff MJ. *Clinical Neurology.* 7th ed. New York, NY: McGraw-Hill; 2009. Figure C-2A.)

In persistent cases in which conservative management has failed, surgical intervention may be undertaken to relieve increased pressure within the carpal tunnel. Research into the effectiveness of conservative versus surgical management of CTS has shown conflicting data. In an older study, **conservative management through physical therapy** interventions was reported to relieve symptoms of mild CTS effectively enough to spare individuals from having to go through a surgical carpal tunnel release.[8] However, in a 2008 Cochrane Review, surgical intervention was found to be superior to conservative treatment in relieving symptoms.[9] Authors of the most recent systematic review[10] that included 20 randomized controlled trials concluded that nonsurgical interventions (*i.e.*, physical therapy, oral and injected medications, splinting, ergonomic modifications, etc.) were effective for short-term management of CTS symptoms (ranging from 2 to 7 weeks). The authors concluded that more research should be done to evaluate the long-term effectiveness of conservative interventions.[10]

Physical Therapy Patient/Client Management

Patients with CTS generally present with some sort of wrist and hand pain, sensory disturbances in the median nerve distribution, weakness and/or atrophy in the thenar muscle compartment of the hand, and loss of grip strength. Each patient can have a slightly different presentation—with some or all of these signs and symptoms. During the initial examination, the physical therapist's goal is to identify impairments related to sensation changes, range of motion (ROM), strength, decreased joint mobility, soft tissue mobility, and flexibility that contribute to or cause the patient's complaints. The plan of care is developed based on the impairments found for each individual. A team approach should be used when managing patients with CTS and continued care by a general practitioner during physical therapy treatment is helpful. The general practitioner can recommend or prescribe nonsteroidal anti-inflammatory drugs (NSAIDs) that may help reduce swelling in the carpal tunnel and provide some pain relief. Physician-administered injections of glucocorticoids (*e.g.*, hydrocortisone) directly into the carpal tunnel may be an additional option for some patients. In one study, a single glucocorticoid injection that was given proximal to the carpal tunnel improved symptoms in 77% of the patients at 1 month after the injection. In half of those patients, the symptoms were still relieved 1 year after injection.[11] In 2007, the authors of a systematic review evaluated the effectiveness of glucocorticoid injections in treating CTS. The authors concluded that a single injection caused symptom relief when compared to a placebo at 1-month postinjection; at 6 months postinjection, there was no significant difference in symptoms between the patients that received a glucocorticoid injection and those that received splinting and NSAIDs.[12] These options are often considered before surgical decompression.

Examination, Evaluation, and Diagnosis

The examination of a patient—subjective history, systems review, and administration of tests and measures—must be performed before the clinician performs any interventions. It is important to ask questions regarding the patient's current symptoms. From the initial history, the physical therapist obtains information such as length of time since the symptoms began, symptom provocation and relief, degree and location of pain, mechanism of injury (if a specific incident can be recalled), previous episodes of a similar problem, job status and function, medications, and the results of any imaging performed. Questions specific to CTS should include questions about median nerve sensory disturbances, night pain, problems with handling and/or dropping items, perceived loss of grip strength, job demands, and ergonomic design of workstation. Past and current medical history questions must be asked as well. Screening questions that may suggest a systemic problem (*e.g.*, recent unintended weight loss or weight gain, general fatigue, fever, dizziness, etc.) should be asked and any significant past medical problems should be addressed for how these may affect implementation of physical therapy interventions.

Table 22-1 outlines tests and measures that should be performed on the individual presenting with suspected CTS. Findings suggestive of CTS include sensory disturbances and strength loss in the median nerve distribution, decreased grip strength, decreased length of the forearm flexors, decreased ROM of the wrist and fingers, decreased mobility of the carpal bones, increased wrist girth due to edema, positive special tests, and tenderness to palpation in the affected wrist, hand, and forearm.

Although there are numerous special clinical tests for CTS, there is no clinical "gold standard" diagnostic test for CTS. Therefore, a combination of positive clinical findings is important when considering the diagnosis. Phalen's test is a common provocative test in which the patient sits comfortably with his wrist fully flexed for approximately 60 seconds. The test is considered positive if wrist flexion reproduces the patient's symptoms of numbness or tingling in the median nerve distribution.[13] The diagnostic accuracy of Phalen's test is only minimally to

Table 22-1   TESTS AND MEASURES FOR THE INDIVIDUAL WITH SUSPECTED CTS
Sensory testing in the median nerve distribution (Fig. 22-1)
Strength testing of muscles supplied by the median nerve: pronator teres, flexor carpi radialis, palmaris longus, flexor digitorum superficialis, lateral half of flexor digitorum profundus, flexor pollicis longus, pronator quadratus, first and second lumbricals, opponens pollicis, abductor pollicis brevis, flexor pollicis brevis
Grip strength
Flexibility of forearm and hand muscles
Range of motion of the wrist and hand
Passive joint mobility testing of the forearm, wrist, and fingers
Girth measurements around the wrist
Special clinical tests (Carpal Compression Test, Phalen's, Tinel's, reverse Phalen's)
Palpation for tenderness around the wrist, hand, and forearm

moderately acceptable since the sensitivity has been reported to range from 34% to 88% and specificity from 40% to 100%.[13] To perform Tinel's test, the therapist gently taps the anterior surface of the wrist where the median nerve crosses the carpal tunnel. A positive Tinel's sign is if the tapping reproduces sensation changes in the median nerve distribution in the hand.[14] The diagnostic accuracy of Tinel's test also has wide reported ranges: sensitivity ranges from 23% to 74% and specificity from 56% to 100%. Reverse Phalen's test is similar to Phalen's test, except that the wrist is held in end-range extension rather than flexion. A positive test is when sensory changes occur in the median nerve distribution after holding the position for 60 seconds.[13] Although the reverse Phalen's test has high reported specificity (82%), it has near coin-toss probability for sensitivity (55%).[15] Thus, while a positive reverse Phalen's test is more likely to lead the physical therapist toward a diagnosis of CTS, a negative reverse Phalen's should not lead the therapist to rule out CTS. The **Carpal Compression Test (CCT)** is a test in which the examiner applies direct pressure to the median nerve at the carpal tunnel with both thumbs for as long as 30 seconds. A positive test is if the patient experiences sensory distribution changes in the median nerve distal to the carpal tunnel during the external compression of the carpal tunnel.[16] In 2004, MacDermid and Wessel[17] performed a systematic review of studies that utilized clinical tests to diagnose CTS. They found that the CCT had the highest sensitivity (64%) and specificity (83%) overall. When considering the diagnosis of CTS, the physical therapist must consider not only the results of special tests, but also the patient's overall clinical presentation such as where the sensory changes are occurring, complaints of night pain, and thenar weakness and/or atrophy.

Plan of Care and Interventions

Individuals with CTS generally have a good prognosis when presenting with a first-time episode.[18] Physical therapy is usually the patient's first choice of treatment. Duration of symptoms, previous treatment strategies, work and environmental factors, and patient compliance all play a role in prognosis. If the patient's symptoms reoccur after a period of having no symptoms, then the prognosis is more difficult to determine. Patient education and compliance is vital to a successful outcome. The primary physical therapy goals are to reduce pain, improve function, improve strength, increase flexibility, improve joint mobility, and improve soft tissue mobility. In the acute phases of treatment, therapy should focus on pain relief and edema control. **Resting nighttime hand splints** have been shown to be an effective adjunct to manage pain. A recent review of 21 trials involving 884 individuals concluded that splinting and ultrasound resulted in significant short-term benefits.[19] Patient education and activity modification are important during the early stages of management. In the subacute phases of management, interventions should focus on restoring flexibility, ROM, joint mobility, soft tissue mobility, nerve mobility, and initiation of gentle isometric exercises. Symptom provocation should be avoided during *all* exercises.[1] During later stages of management, more aggressive flexibility and strengthening exercises should be incorporated. Strength and endurance of the thenar muscles and lumbricals should improve during this time. The patient should be educated on upper extremity and wrist positioning during activities, and how to modify activities in the future if symptoms reoccur.

Interventions commonly used to meet the goals set forth in the plan of care consist of pain-free active and passive ROM of wrist movements in all planes as well as joint mobilization of the intercarpal joints, distal radioulnar joint, and the radiocarpal joint. Soft tissue mobilization should be directed at the flexor retinaculum and the flexor tendons of the wrist. Therapeutic exercise is directed at stretching any shortened forearm and hand muscles and strengthening wrist flexors and extensors and functional grip strength. The therapist should incorporate functional activities that the patient does day-to-day such as gripping, pinching, and fine motor skills such as twisting, turning, and manipulating small objects. Neuromuscular re-education includes postural training with avoidance of provocative joint positions. Ergonomic workstation design should be modified to limit neck and upper extremity stresses. The therapist may recommend a wrist splint to avoid increased pressure in the carpal tunnel. The therapist can advise the patient to wear the wrist splint during the day, at work (if the job allows), and/or at night. A study of 25 patients (47 affected hands) suggested that patients with less severe carpal tunnel symptoms may benefit more from nighttime splinting compared to patients with more severe symptoms.[20] Activity moderation, in which the patient avoids or modifies activities known to cause symptoms, is also part of conservative management.

Surgical treatment is reserved for those patients who have persistent symptoms for more than a year despite conservative management, experience sensation loss, thenar atrophy, and/or display fibrillation potentials on electromyograms.[18] Goals for carpal tunnel release surgery are to decompress the nerve, improve nerve excursion, and prevent progressive median nerve damage.[18] Because the patient's compliance plays a critical role in healing during both nonoperative and/or surgical management of CTS, the physical therapist must emphasize to the patient the necessity of active involvement in his rehabilitation.

Evidence-Based Clinical Recommendations

SORT: Strength of Recommendation Taxonomy

A: Consistent, good-quality patient-oriented evidence
B: Inconsistent or limited-quality patient-oriented evidence
C: Consensus, disease-oriented evidence, usual practice, expert opinion, or case series

1. Conservative management of carpal tunnel syndrome that includes physical therapy is effective for short-term management of mild symptoms. **Grade B**

2. Of the clinical special tests for diagnosing carpal tunnel syndrome, the Carpal Compression Test (CCT) has the highest sensitivity (64%) and specificity (83%). **Grade B**

3. Resting wrist splints worn at night are an effective tool to manage pain in CTS. **Grade B**

COMPREHENSION QUESTIONS

22.1 A 34-year-old patient who works as a paralegal complains of symptoms in her left hand suggestive of carpal tunnel syndrome. If the patient does indeed have CTS, which of the following muscles would *most* likely be weak?

   A. Extensor carpi radialis brevis
   B. Pronator teres
   C. Flexor carpi ulnaris
   D. Opponens pollicis

22.2 Phalen's test is the gold standard clinical test for identifying CTS.

   A. True
   B. False

ANSWERS

22.1 **D.** The opponens pollicis is a part of the thenar muscle group that is innervated by the median nerve distal to the carpal tunnel. The extensor carpi radialis brevis is innervated by the radial nerve (option A). While the median nerve innervates the pronator teres (option B), its innervation is proximal to the carpal tunnel; involvement of the pronator teres produces forearm symptoms and is part of the pronator teres syndrome, not CTS. The flexor carpi ulnaris is innervated by the ulnar nerve (option C).

22.2 **B.** There is no provocative clinical test that is considered a gold standard for diagnosis of CTS. The best option for clinically diagnosing CTS is compiling the results of the subjective and objective examination and those of a combination of clinical provocation tests.

REFERENCES

1. Kisner C, Colby LA. *Therapeutic Exercise: Foundations and Techniques*. 5th ed. Philadelphia, PA: F.A. Davis Company; 2007:594-638.

2. Kostopoulos D. Treatment of carpal tunnel syndrome: a review of the non-surgical approaches with emphasis on neural mobilization. *J Bodywork Movement Ther*. 2004;8:2-8.

3. Gelberman RH, Hergenroeder PT, Hargens AR, Lundborg GN, Akeson WH. The carpal tunnel syndrome. A study of carpal canal pressures. *J Bone Joint Surg Am*. 1981;63:380-383.

4. Silverstein B, Adams D. Work-related musculoskeletal disorders of the neck, back, and upper extremity in Washington State: state fund and self-insured workers' compensation claims. 1997-2005. In: Levy BS, Wegman DH, Baron SL, Sokas RK, eds. *Occupational and Environmental Health. Recognizing and Preventing Disease and Injury*. 6th ed. Oxford University Press, USA; 2011.

5. Silverstein BA, Fan ZJ, Bonauto DK, et al. The natural course of carpal tunnel syndrome in a working population. *Scan J Work Environ Health*. 2010;36:384-393.

6. Hertling D, Kessler RM. *Management of Common Musculoskeletal Disorders: Physical Therapy Principles and Methods*. 4th ed. Philadelphia, PA: Lippincott Williams & Wilkins; 2006:415-416.

7. Levine DW, Simmons BP, Koris MJ, et al. A self-administered questionnaire for the assessment of severity of symptoms and functional status in carpal tunnel syndrome. *J Bone Joint Surg Am*. 1993;75:1585-1592.

8. Rozmaryn LM, Dovelle S, Rothman ER, Gorman K, Olvey KM, Bartko JJ. Nerve and tendon gliding exercises and the conservative management of carpal tunnel syndrome. *J Hand Ther*. 1998;11:171-179.

9. Verdugo RJ, Salinas RA, Castillo JL, Cea JG. Surgical versus non-surgical treatment for carpal tunnel syndrome. *Cochrane Database Syst Rev*. 2008;8(4):CD001552.

10. Huisstede BM, Hoogvliet P, Randsdorp MS, Glerum S, Van Middelkoop M, Koes BW. Carpal Tunnel Syndrome. Part I: effectiveness of nonsurgical treatments—a systematic review. *Arch Phys Med Rehabil*. 2010;91:981-1004.

11. Dammers JW, Veering MM, Vermeulen M. Injection with methylprednisolone proximal to the carpal tunnel: randomized double blind trial. *BMJ*. 1999;319:884-886.

12. Marshall S, Tardif G, Ashworth N. Local corticosteroid injection for carpal tunnel syndrome. *Cochrane Database Syst Rev*. 2007 Apr 18;2:CD001554.

13. Magee DJ. *Orthopedic Physical Assessment*. 5th ed. St. Louis, MO: Saunders Elsevier; 2008:441-443.

14. Moldaver J. Tinel's sign: its characteristics and significance. *J Bone Joint Surg Am*. 1978;60:412-414.

15. Scifers JR. *Special Tests for Neurologic Examination*. Thorofare, NJ: Slack Incorporated; 2008:350-351.

16. Durkan JA. A new diagnostic test for carpal tunnel syndrome. *J Bone Joint Surg Am*. 1991;73:535-538.

17. MacDermid JC, Wessel J. Clinical diagnosis of carpal tunnel syndrome: a systematic review. *J Hand Ther*. 2004;17:309-319.

18. Brotzman SB, Robert CM. *Clinical Orthopaedic Rehabilitation: An Evidence-based Approach*. 3rd ed. Philadelphia, PA: Elsevier Mosby; 2011:18-22.

19. O'Connor D, Marshall S, Massy-Westropp N. Non-surgical treatment (other than steroid injection) for carpal tunnel syndrome. *Cochrane Database Syst Rev*. 2003;1:CD003219.

20. Boyd KU, Gan BS, Ross DC, Richards RS, Roth JH, MacDermid JC. Outcomes in carpal tunnel syndrome: symptoms severity, conservative management, and progression to surgery. *Clin Invest Med*. 2005;28:254-260.

Chronic Exertional Compartment Syndrome

Jon Warren

A 21-year-old rugby football player presents to an outpatient physical therapy clinic with a 4-month history of intermittent deep aching pain in his right antero-lateral lower leg and paresthesia in the first web space. The pain starts after 15 minutes of running. He can continue to run for about 30 minutes when he has to stop due to the pain intensity (9 on the 0-10 visual analog scale). He reports that this pain started after intense pre-season rugby training for 3 weeks. This training consisted of 5 sessions per week, each with an aerobic component and 3 with resistance training (gym program) incorporated. The running during this training was at faster speeds and for longer distances than he had previously done. He decided to seek professional treatment because a similar ache has been develop-ing in his left leg over the past few weeks. The pain is less severe and he has no paresthesia in the left leg. Except for self-administered ice and occasional oral anti-inflammatories (which he reported provided no pain relief), he has received no previous treatment. The physical therapy referral is for evaluation and treat-ment of his shin pain. No diagnostic imaging has been requested yet.

▶ Based on the patient's symptoms and history, what are the most appropriate tests and measures to help determine the etiology of his shin pain?
▶ Based on his suspected diagnosis, what do you anticipate may be the contrib-uting factors to the condition?
▶ What is his rehabilitation prognosis?
▶ Describe a physical therapy plan of care for this patient.

KEY DEFINITIONS

FASCIA: "Band" (derived from the Latin); superficial and deep connective tissue surrounding individual muscles, groups of muscles, blood vessels, and nerves; fascia binds some structures together while allowing others to glide smoothly over each other

PERIOSTITIS: Inflammation of the periosteum, the connective tissue layer surrounding bone

STRESS FRACTURE: Microfracture in bone caused by repetitive physical loading *below* the single cycle failure threshold due to redistribution of impact forces resulting in stress at focal points in the bone or the action of muscle pull across the bone[1]

Objectives

1. Describe chronic exertional compartment syndrome (CECS) and the potential risk factors for this condition.
2. Describe three main causes of lower leg or shin pain.
3. List the different compartments in the lower leg and the muscles, blood vessels, and nerves that each compartment contains.
4. Identify key questions to confirm a suspected diagnosis of CECS.
5. Describe the common impairments found with CECS and discuss the rationale of physical therapy.
6. Determine when a surgical consultation is appropriate for an individual with CECS.

Physical Therapy Considerations

PT considerations during management of the individual with suspected chronic exertional compartment syndrome:

▶ **General physical therapy plan of care/goals:** Improve neurologic symptoms; relieve leg pain during running; identify and treat musculoskeletal impairments and additional risk factors to prevent recurrence

▶ **Physical therapy interventions:** Patient education (regarding diagnosis, risk factors, prognosis, treatment expectations, potential orthotic application); manual therapy (myofascial mobilization, joint mobilization); dry needling; therapeutic exercise (progressive stretching, aerobic conditioning); home exercise program (HEP) prescription; return-to-sport program

▶ **Precautions during physical therapy:** Monitor application of deep myofascial techniques because these techniques can be uncomfortable and could potentially aggravate the condition; monitor patient's ability to adhere to a slowly progressive return-to-sport program

▶ **Complications interfering with physical therapy:** Patient/client who is unwilling or unable to alter training regimen; comorbidities (*e.g.*, hormonal status, nutritional status, overall health status); deterioration of health status

Understanding the Health Condition

Compartment syndrome is the increased pressure within a closed fibro-osseous space. The increased pressure causes reduced blood flow and tissue perfusion, which subsequently leads to ischemic pain and possible permanent damage to the tissues within the compartment.[2] Compartment syndrome is further defined as either acute or chronic (exertional). Acute compartment syndrome typically occurs as a complication following fractures, soft tissue trauma, and reperfusion after acute arterial obstruction.[3] Atraumatic compartment syndrome is rare, but has been described after horseback riding, prolonged walking, and soccer.[4,5] Atraumatic compartment syndrome can manifest insidiously and be missed on initial presentation—with severe consequences.[4] Early diagnosis and treatment are associated with better results. An emergency surgical fasciotomy must be performed to release pressure from the affected compartment to prevent tissue necrosis and functional loss.[6]

Chronic exertional compartment syndrome (CECS) differs from acute compartment syndrome in its association with repetitive physical activity and its reversible and recurrent nature. CECS becomes a neurologic condition when the pressure in the compartment is increased to a level at which nerve tissue is becoming compressed. This deterioration in the condition is significant due to the sensitivity of the nervous system. Symptoms of nerve compression are paresthesia and weakness distal to the compression. The pattern of sensation loss and muscle weakness indicates the involved compartment (Table 23-1).

CECS is most commonly seen in athletes, with a particularly high incidence in runners as well as athletes in jumping and cutting sports.[7] The condition is frequently bilateral. Elite and recreational athletes are affected equally and the median age of presentation is 20 years.[8] Although equal incidence has been reported in males and females, it is thought to be rising in females.[9] The anterior compartment is the most commonly involved compartment in 70% of cases.[9] Involvement of both anterior and lateral compartments accounts for 95% of cases.[10]

Table 23-1	COMPARTMENTS IN THE LEG			
Compartment	Muscles	Blood Vessels	Nerves	Sensation
Anterior	Tibialis anterior, extensor digitorum longus, extensor hallucis longus, fibularis tertius	Anterior tibial artery and vein	Deep fibular nerve	First web space
Superficial posterior	Gastrocnemius, soleus, plantaris	Branch of the tibial artery and vein	Sural nerve	Lateral side of foot
Deep posterior	Flexor hallucis longus, flexor digitorum longus, tibialis posterior, popliteus	Posterior tibial artery and vein	Tibial nerve	Plantar aspect of foot
Lateral	Fibularis longus, fibularis brevis	Branch of the anterior tibial artery and vein	Superficial fibular nerve	Dorsum of foot

The precise etiology of CECS is unclear. However, many precipitating factors have been identified. The intrinsic factors include bony malalignment of the knee (either valgus or varus deformities), leg length discrepancies,[11] and abnormal foot biomechanics. Decreased muscle capillary supply is a potential pathogenic factor. A study of muscle biopsies from individuals with CECS during fasciotomy and 1 year later found a lower muscle capillary supply in the tibialis anterior compared with muscles from unaffected individuals.[12] Extrinsic factors that may contribute to the development of CECS include decreased strength, flexibility, and endurance; poor or incorrect motor pattern and control, as well as a training regimen that is inappropriate in terms of volume, intensity, or frequency.[13] A training regimen that causes repetitive overuse can induce microtraumatic muscular injuries and inflammation, which may lead to fibrosis and subsequent reduced elasticity of the fascia surrounding the muscles.[14] Indeed, biopsies from individuals suffering from CECS have revealed stiffer and thicker muscle fascia surrounding the anterior compartment.[15] This lack of fascial compliance results in muscles that are unable to expand with exercise—resulting in increased pressure and pain.

At rest, individuals with CECS are often asymptomatic. However, immediately post-exercise, a palpable tenseness over the compartment can be felt and muscle bulges or herniations may be seen. Fascial thickening or scarring could be an explanation for these findings. The **gold standard for diagnosis of CECS** is direct measurement of elevated intracompartment pressures using a needle or catheter.[16] Intracompartment pressures are measured during activities such as running, jumping, and stair climbing for 5 minutes. To diagnose CECS, increased measurements must be accompanied by pain reproduction. Normal intracompartment pressures range between 0 and 10 mm Hg. The CECS diagnosis is confirmed with pain reproduction and either a maximal pressure of 35 mm Hg, 10 mm Hg elevation of pressure from baseline (no activity), or post-exercise resting pressure > 25 mm Hg.[14] When the patient's pain has been reproduced post-exertion, pressures are checked in all compartments. However, there is some debate about the necessity of measuring all compartments. Some physicians feel that only the involved compartment should be tested to prevent undue trauma from additional needle sticks.[7]

The lower leg is responsible for one-third of running injuries in long distance runners, second only to knee injures.[17] Because shin pain is a very common complaint in athletes (particularly runners), careful evaluation is necessary to ascertain the correct etiology of the shin pain. Patients and medical professionals commonly use the term 'shin splints.' However, 'shin splints' provide no indication regarding the pathogenesis of the pain and therefore should not be used as diagnostic terminology. The etiology of anterior tibial pain can be broadly divided into three main categories: CECS, tibial stress fractures, and medial tibial traction periostitis. Tibial stress fractures are characterized by gradual onset of pain with exercise, but pain can also be felt at rest and at night. This is often associated with over-training and poor sport-specific techniques. A key finding is localized tenderness over the tibia. There are frequently associated biomechanical abnormalities (e.g., rigid pes cavus, overpronating foot). A bone scan, magnetic resonance imaging, or computed tomography scan can be used to confirm

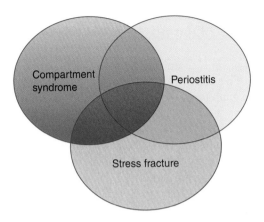

Figure 23-1. Potential overlap of anterior tibial pain conditions.

the diagnosis of tibial stress fracture. Medial tibial traction periostitis (sometimes termed medial tibial stress syndrome) results in more diffuse pain along the medial border of the tibia. This pain can be felt at rest and when initiating exercise, but the pain often decreases or is eliminated once the individual has warmed up. Pain often returns post-exercise and increases the following morning. Contributing factors to medial tibial traction periostitis also include pes planus and overpronation,[18] as well as inappropriate training regimens and muscle imbalances.

The differential diagnosis of anterior tibial pain incorporates the whole evaluation process starting with specific questioning and applying special tests to confirm or rule out differential diagnoses. It is important to remember that two or three conditions may also exist concurrently (Fig. 23-1). For example, periostitis or a stress fracture may lead to intracompartment swelling and cause an individual with asymptomatic exertional compartment syndrome to develop symptomatic CECS.[14]

Physical Therapy Patient/Client Management

A patient with CECS typically presents to an outpatient physical therapy clinic either via direct access (in states that allow this) or via referral by the primary physician. The typical main complaint is chronic exercise-induced anterior tibial pain (commonly bilateral) that may be accompanied by paresthesia and isolated weakness in the lower leg. Identification of the impairments requires a comprehensive examination including range of motion (ROM), flexibility, joint mobility and biomechanics, sports-specific function, and footwear assessment. The primary physical therapy goals are returning the individual to pain-free exercise, improving neurologic function, and preventing recurrence. Physical therapy interventions may include myofascial mobilizations, specific stretching and strengthening, dry needling, correction of any biomechanical abnormalities, and a modified sport-specific exercise regimen. The physical therapy episode of care should continue until resolution of the condition, the patient's improvement plateaus, or surgical referral is indicated.

Examination, Evaluation, and Diagnosis

It is important that a thorough examination is completed to accurately determine the etiology of the patient's shin pain. This starts with the history, which includes an accurate description of the patient's symptoms, and proceeds to specific clinical testing. Understanding how the symptoms are reproduced through questioning and testing is paramount.

The history needs to establish when symptoms were first perceived. Particular note is made of the specific sporting activity involved, any changes in exercise regimen including type of footwear, and the sports terrain or surface. The typical history of a patient with CECS includes no pain at rest and pain that develops with exercise at exactly the same time, distance, or with a particular increase in intensity.[9] The pain increases in intensity with continued exercise until the point at which the pain and muscle tightness become unbearable. Although the pain resolves with rest, the length of time before resolution increases with the severity of the condition. This pain is initially described as deep aching, progresses to burning over the whole compartment, and may include paresthesia related to the involved nerve. Table 23-2 lists several important questions that can help the therapist identify the causes as well as potential therapeutic interventions for anterior tibial pain.

The structural inspection is an important part of the objective examination. Particular attention is taken of the bony alignment. The physical therapist must check

Table 23-2 QUESTIONS TO AID IN DIFFERENTIATING THE PATHOGENESIS OF ANTERIOR TIBIAL PAIN	
Question	Rationale
Do you have a history of previous fractures or trauma to the leg?	Previous injuries can lead to scar tissue, tightness, and abnormal movement patterns.
Where is the pain? Is it localized or more diffuse? Is the pain superficial or deep?	A general deep, dull achy (cramping) pain could indicate CECS associated with one or more compartments. Localized pain (which may feel deep) over the bone is typically associated with stress fractures. If pain is more localized to soft tissue, this could indicate muscle strain or tendinopathy, which can be felt as either superficial or deep pain. Diffuse superficial pain over the medial tibial border would be more indicative of periostitis.
Do you have pain on loading, especially during impact when running?	Pain with CECS is often worse in soft underfoot conditions (e.g., off-road) due to the increased muscular effort required for control. Pain is often worse on impact with stress fractures and to a lesser extent, with periostitis.
Does the pain improve once you have warmed up?	Pain associated with CECS and stress fractures does *not* improve after an aerobic warm-up. In contrast, pain associated with periostitis and tendon injuries often improves after a warm-up.
Do you have any numbness and/or tingling?	These symptoms indicate neurologic involvement. Screening questions for the lumbar spine and the other potential sites of the potential neural irritation are necessary.

for leg length discrepancies, genu varus or valgus, pes planus or cavus, hypertrophy of the calf or anterior crural muscles. No edema or inflammatory signs are evident in CECS. The ROM of the knee, ankle, and foot is tested—noting any limitations as well as end feels. Pre-exercise, the expected end feels are normal with CECS. Tightness in both the posterior and anterior leg musculature may be found on flexibility testing. The **tightness of the plantarflexors** (particularly gastrocnemius and soleus) should be assessed because tightness could predispose the individual to anterior compartment syndrome.[14]

Because it is common for the physical examination to be unremarkable in the patient with CECS, key examination components should be performed post-exercise when the patient is symptomatic. Activities such as running, jumping, and stair climbing for at least 5 minutes may be necessary to reproduce the patient's symptoms. In the clinic, an easy way to recreate a patient's symptoms is to have the patient walk or run on an inclined treadmill, which particularly increases contraction of the anterior leg compartment (the most common compartment involved in CECS). Post-exercise, it may be possible to observe hypertrophy and pallor of the involved muscles.[9] When symptoms are reproduced, the anterior compartment muscles are firm with associated palpable tenderness and may have obvious muscle bulges or herniations. Muscle bulges or herniations are typically at the junction of the middle and distal one-third of the leg.[1] A **key diagnostic finding is increased pain with passive stretching of the gastrocnemius and soleus in the post-exercise state** (when intracompartment pressures are elevated).[19] Palpable tenderness in the calf musculature can also highlight any areas of localized muscle or fascial thickening. The neurovascular examination should include testing of sensation and strength and palpation of pulses (*e.g.*, dorsalis pedis). Sensory testing for light touch, hot/cold, and sharp/dull may reveal paresthesia or numbness in the first web space (with involvement of the anterior compartment). To assess for mechanosensitivity of neural tissues within the leg, neural tension tests such as the test for the tibial nerve (straight leg raise with ankle dorsiflexion and eversion) should be performed. Neural tension tests are considered positive when movement is limited by neural stretch pain and/or the test reproduces the patient's neural symptoms. In severe cases of anterior compartment involvement, weakness or atrophy may be noted in the anterior musculature (tibialis anterior, extensor digitorum longus, extensor hallucis longus, fibularis tertius). Typically, there is no change in distal pulses post-exercise.

Gait analysis should include a functional assessment of the patient's running technique. Close attention should be paid to cadence, stride length, foot pronation, and heel strike. Gait abnormalities like overpronation are common in patients with CECS.

Plan of Care and Interventions

While there are discrepancies regarding the efficacy of each type of conservative intervention for CECS,[11] it is agreed that conservative treatment is the first treatment choice and should be started as soon as possible once the condition has been diagnosed. The frequency and duration of treatment depends on the severity and chronicity of the condition and the sporting level of the patient. As with any condition, patient education and compliance is vital to the outcome. **Treatment success critically depends on rest and cessation or modification of the aggravating sporting activity.**[20] Treatment options include intermittent massage (myofascial mobilizations) with stretching, taping, orthotics, and nonsteroidal anti-inflammatory drugs (NSAIDs).[21] Taping is used to target any biomechanical foot/ankle impairments. Benefits from NSAIDs would only be gained when the compartment contents are inflamed. Other interventions such as dry needling, therapeutic exercise, and return-to-sport programs have minimal evidence to support their efficacy. There are no randomized controlled studies investigating the effectiveness of these conservative treatment interventions for CECS.[13] A number of authors have stated that conservative treatment will not result in full symptom relief, but it should be noted that most research on CECS has been conducted by surgeons investigating the efficacy of surgical interventions.[13] More research is needed into the efficacy of conservative interventions for CECS.

Prognosis is dependent on the patient's age and severity and duration of symptoms. The prescription of rest and exercise modification requires that the patient avoid any aggravating exercise, which typically means cessation of running and limiting walking duration. In the initial stages, the prime focus of interventions should be on attainment of musculoskeletal balance. The physical therapist must determine the source of any ROM abnormalities as either joint hypo- or hypermobility or muscle length (flexibility) discrepancies. Foot architecture dysfunctions and overpronation may cause subtalar joint and forefoot impairments, typically involving either hypo- or hypermobile subtalar or tarsal-metatarsal joints. Hypomobility is treated by appropriate accessory joint mobilizations and hypermobility is addressed with stability exercises including foot intrinsic musculature strengthening. Neurodynamic mobilizations that aim to improve the sliding of nerves and restore neural tissue mobility may be beneficial, particularly with posterior compartment involvement. Stretch pain or paresthesia are suggested to be a result of tension being placed on some component of the nervous system.[22]

Foot stability may also be augmented by orthotics that support the longitudinal arch of the foot. Before the application of any orthotic, appropriate footwear is necessary. The patient's footwear should be thoroughly assessed on one of the initial appointments. First, check for excessive wear: inadequate tread or uneven tread wear (which can confirm running problems) can indicate the necessity for new footwear. Second, the internal strength of the shoe is assessed by checking the longitudinal flex and noting whether the forefoot flexibility is adequate for toe-off. If the forefoot region of the shoe is too rigid, extra loading will be placed on the calf muscles. Last, the midsole should be firm enough to be a good shock absorber to provide a stable platform for running.

Myofascial mobilizations can be utilized to loosen the fascial sheath surrounding the gastrocnemius/soleus muscles and between the different compartments. Specific myofascial mobilization techniques such as transverse play of the gastrocnemius-soleus, cross frictions of the gastrocnemius-soleus junction, lateral fascial distraction of the tibia, lateral elongation of the peroneal tissue, and bone clearing of the tibia have all been suggested for treatment of lower leg compartment syndromes.[23]

Sustained myofascial techniques combined with passive and active plantarflexion have been shown to be effective in restoring fascial flexibility for anterior and lateral compartments.[14] Since these techniques may be quite painful in patients with very tight fascia, care should be taken to monitor the patient's reaction to prevent excessive pain and the potential for inflammation or aggravation of the affected tissues. To improve flexibility of tight musculature, the physical therapist must educate the patient in appropriate stretching techniques (sets of at least 5 stretches held for a minimum of 30 seconds) and incorporate stretching into a home exercise program. Tissue length increases may be augmented by heat applications and contract-relax techniques. Stretching may be important for return to sports to maintain flexibility, reduce the risk of injury, reduce soreness after exercise, and to enhance athletic performance despite evidence that clinically important changes have *not* been demonstrated.[24]

The final component of conservative treatment for CECS is a comprehensive return-to-sport training regimen. In the initial relative rest phase, cardiovascular fitness can be maintained by cross-training cycling or 'aqua jogging' with a buoyancy device to decrease weightbearing on the affected leg or legs. After biomechanical impairments have been addressed, weightbearing exercise can be introduced. A zero-gravity treadmill is an effective method to ease the transition to normal weightbearing running. At this time, any running technique issues should be addressed. During this conditioning phase, emphasis is placed on technique and duration with care to always avoid provoking any symptoms. There is some research that suggests that **forefoot running** (as opposed to typical heel strike running) may be beneficial in treatment of CECS, specifically for involvement of the anterior compartment.[25,26] A case series of ten patients with anterior compartment CECS found decreased post-running lower leg intracompartmental pressures after a 6-week forefoot strike running intervention. One year later, all ten patients experienced greatly reduced pain and disability and avoided surgical intervention.[26] Following 2 to 4 weeks of asymptomatic running on the treadmill, the patient can transition to training on a more sport-specific terrain. The intensity of all facets of fitness (aerobic, anaerobic, strength, flexibility, agility, speed, cross-training, sports-specific skill) should be monitored and progressed as tolerated within pain-free limits.

When the diagnosis of CECS is confirmed and there are no contributing factors (*e.g.*, biomechanical/training), conservative treatment often fails and surgical release of the affected compartment/s is required.[14] Individuals with anterior or lateral compartment symptoms had better surgical outcomes (> 80% success rate) compared to those with involvement of the deep posterior compartment (approximately 50% success rate).[20,27] Surgical intervention involves an endoscopic release of the anterior and lateral compartments with a minimal percutaneous incision. This procedure has an approximately 90% success rate with the anterior and lateral compartments; thus, a fasciotomy is rarely necessary.[14] Since serious complications post-fasciotomy such as infection or postoperative bleeding occur in 11.5% to 13% of cases, patients need to be adequately informed of the risks of this procedure.[27]

Physical therapy after surgical release is based on the scientific and clinical rationales of tissue healing, scar tissue formation, neurodynamic loading, muscle loading, and consideration of all the tissues within the involved compartment.[11] The postoperative rehabilitation is typically a 12-week program largely based on the specific surgeon's protocol. The protocol necessitates the use of crutches for 3 to 5 days with restricted weightbearing. The immediate treatment is focused on preventing or reducing edema by means of rest, ice, compression, and elevation. Treatment then focuses on improving soft tissue mobility and strength, and restoration or improvement of knee and ankle ROM. Postsurgical rehabilitation also includes myofascial mobilizations, ROM exercises, stretching, strengthening, sport-specific biomechanical analysis, and a comprehensive return-to-sports training regimen. The athlete should be pain-free with 90% strength prior to full sports participation.[21]

Evidence-Based Clinical Recommendations

SORT: Strength of Recommendation Taxonomy

A: Consistent, good-quality patient-oriented evidence
B: Inconsistent or limited-quality patient-oriented evidence
C: Consensus, disease-oriented evidence, usual practice, expert opinion, or case series

1. The gold standard diagnostic test for chronic exertional compartment syndrome is direct measurement of elevated intracompartmental pressure post-exercise with reproduction of the patient's pain. **Grade A**

2. Tightness of the plantarflexors predisposes individuals to CECS within the anterior compartment of the leg. **Grade B**

3. A key diagnostic finding in individuals with CECS is pain during passive stretching of the gastrocnemius and soleus in the post-exercise state. **Grade C**

4. Relative rest, which allows for pain-free activity only, and cessation or modification of the aggravating sporting activity are necessary for successful treatment of CECS. **Grade A**

5. Forefoot running may improve the prognosis in CECS specifically with involvement of the anterior compartment of the leg. **Grade C**

COMPREHENSION QUESTIONS

23.1 Subjective history is vital to generating a diagnostic hypothesis prior to the objective assessment. The answers to which of the following questions would be *most* indicative of CECS?
    A. Where is the pain or discomfort?
    B. Does your pain improve when you warm up prior to exercise?
    C. Does your pain or discomfort appear at the same time during exercise?
    D. Do you have any associated numbness, tingling, or muscular weakness?

23.2 Which of the following is *not* a contributing factor for CECS?

A. Leg length discrepancies

B. Abnormal foot biomechanics

C. Genetic predisposition

D. Inappropriate training regimen

ANSWERS

23.1 **D.** CECS is associated with an increased pressure in a specific muscular compartment. The typical history includes symptoms (pain, tightness, burning, etc) that appear at the same time or at a specific intensity during exercise. These symptoms resolve when the patient stops exercising.

23.2 **C.** There is no evidence for a genetic predisposition to CECS. In order for treatment to be successful, all contributing factors must be taken into account and appropriate interventions applied. All of the other factors (options A, B, and D) have been associated with an increased risk of CECS.

REFERENCES

1. Brukner PD, Khan K. *Clinical Sports Medicine*. Revised 3rd ed. Sydney, Australia: McGraw Hill; 2009.

2. Fraipont MJ, Adamson GJ. Chronic exertional compartment syndrome. *J Am Acad Orthop Surg.* 2003;11:268-276.

3. Frink M, Hildebrand F, Krettek C, Brand J, Hankemeier S. Compartment syndrome of the lower leg and foot. *Clin Orthop Relat Res.* 2010; 468:940-950.

4. Naidu KS. Bilateral peroneal compartment syndrome after horse riding. *Am J Emer Med.* 2009;27:901. e3-901.e5.

5. Rehman S, Joglekar SB. Acute isolated lateral compartment syndrome of the leg after a noncontact sports injury. *Orthopedics.* 2009;32:523.

6. Gorczyca JT, Roberts CS, Pugh KJ, Ring D. Review of treatment and diagnosis of acute compartment syndrome of the calf: current evidence and best practices. *Instr Course Lect.* 2011;60:35-42.

7. George CA, Hutchinson MR. Chronic exertional compartment syndrome. *Clin Sports Med.* 2012;31:307-319.

8. Hutchinson MR, Ireland ML. Common compartment syndromes in athletes: treatment and rehabilitation. *Sports Med.* 1994;17:200-208.

9. Shah SN, Miller BS, Kuhn JE. Chronic exertional compartment syndrome. *Am J Orthop.* 2004;33:335-341.

10. Verleisdonk E, Schmitz RF, van der Werken C. Long-term results of fasciotomy of the anterior compartment in patients with exercise-induced pain in the lower leg. *Int J Sports Med.* 2004;25:224-229.

11. Schubert AG. Exertional compartment syndrome: review of the literature and proposed rehabilitation guidelines following surgical release. *Int J Sports Phys Ther.* 2011;6:126-141.

12. Edmundsson D, Toolanen G, Thornell LE, Stal P. Evidence for low muscle capillary supply as a pathogenic factor in chronic compartment syndrome. *Scand J Med Sci Sports.* 2010;20:805-813.

13. Anuar K, Gurumoorthy P. Systematic review of the management of chronic compartment syndrome in the lower leg. *Physiotherapy Singapore.* 2006;9:2-15.

14. Bradshaw C, Hislop M, Hutchinson M. Shin pain. In: Brukner P, Khan K. *Clinical Sports Medicine*. Revised 3rd ed. Sydney, Australia: McGraw Hill; 2009:555-577.

15. Turnipseed WD, Hurschler C, Vanderby R, Jr. The effects of elevated compartment syndrome on tibial arteriovenous flow and relationship of mechanical and biochemical characteristics of fascia to genesis of chronic anterior compartment syndrome. *J Vasc Surg.* 1995;21:810-817.

16. Amendola A, Rorabeck CH, Vellett D, Vezina W, Rutt B, Nott L. The use of magnetic resonance imaging in exertional compartment syndromes. *Am J Sports Med.* 1990;18:29-34.

17. van Gent RN, Siem D, van Middlekoop M, van Os AG, Bierma-Zeinstra SM, Koes BW. Incidence and determinants of lower extremity running injuries in long distance runners: a systematic review. *Br J Sports Med.* 2007;41:469-480.

18. Bennett JE, Reinking MF, Pluemer B, Pentel A, Seaton M, Killian C. Factors contributing to the development of medial tibial stress syndrome in high school runners. *J Orthop Sports Phys Ther.* 2001;31:504-510.

19. Pedowitz RA, Hargens AR. Acute and chronic compartment syndromes. In: Garrett WE, Speer KP, Kirkendall DT, eds. *Principles and Practice of Orthopeadic Sports Medicine.* Philadelphia, PA: Lippincott Williams & Wilkins; 2001:87-89.

20. Blackman PG. A review of chronic exertional compartment syndrome in the lower leg. *Med Sci Sports Exerc.* 2000;32:S4-S10.

21. Brennan FH, Jr, Kane SF. Diagnosis, treatment options, and rehabilitation of chronic lower leg exertional compartment syndrome. *Curr Sports Med Rep.* 2003;2:247-250.

22. Butler DS. *Mobilisation of the Nervous System.* New York, NY: Churchill Livingstone; 1991.

23. Cantu RI, Grodin AJ, Stanborough RW. *Myofascial Manipulation: Theory and Clinical Application.* 3rd ed. Austin, TX: Pro-Ed; 2012.

24. Herbert RD, de Noronha M, Kamper SJ. Stretching to prevent or reduce muscle soreness after exercise. *Cochrane Database Syst Rev.* 2011: CD004577.

25. Diebal AR, Gregory R, Alitz C, Gerber JP. Effects of forefoot running on chronic exertional compartment syndrome: a case series. *Int J Sports Phys Ther.* 2011;6:312-321.

26. Diebal AR, Gregory R, Alitz C, Gerber JP. Forefoot running improves pain and disability associated with chronic exertional compartment syndrome. *Am J Sport Med.* 2012;40:1060-1067.

27. Howard JL, Mohtadi NG, Wiley JP. Evaluation of outcomes in patients following surgical treatment of chronic exertional compartment syndrome of the leg. *Clin J Sport Med.* 2000;10:176-184.

Thoracic Outlet Syndrome

Aimie F. Kachingwe

CASE 24

A 22-year-old collegiate swimmer presents to an outpatient physical therapy clinic with a primary complaint of right arm pain and numbness in his fourth and fifth fingers. The symptoms began insidiously approximately 6 months ago and have gradually worsened over the past month to the point where he is no longer able to practice with his team. He is right-hand dominant and swims the butterfly and freestyle strokes. He rates the worst pain as 3/10 to 5/10 and the lowest pain as 2/10 on the 0 to 10 visual analog scale. He describes the pain as "dull, deep, achy, and intermittent," and relates that the symptoms increase throughout the day and with overhead activities. He is occasionally awakened at night with his fingers feeling "numb." The numbness decreases when he shakes his hand. His goal is to return to competitive swimming in order to maintain his athletic scholarship.

▶ Based on this scenario, what diagnoses would you consider?
▶ What tests and measures could be performed to confirm or refute your suspected diagnosis?
▶ What is his rehabilitation prognosis?
▶ What are the most appropriate physical therapy interventions?

KEY DEFINITIONS

BRACHIAL PLEXUS: Major nerve plexus innervating the upper limb that consists of the ventral primary rami of the fifth cervical to first thoracic spinal nerves

POSTURAL SYNDROMES: Muscular imbalances of the cervical spine, shoulder, and scapular regions that can lead to thickening or fibrosis of certain muscle groups and potentially compress the brachial plexus

Objectives

1. Describe thoracic outlet syndrome (TOS).
2. Identify key signs and symptoms suggestive of TOS.
3. Identify constitutional red flag signs and symptoms suggesting systemic pathology.
4. Determine applicable tests and measures to examine a patient with suspected TOS.
5. Identify reliable and valid outcome tools to assess TOS.
6. Discuss possible postural impairments that could lead to TOS and how these impairments could be addressed with physical therapy interventions.
7. Describe the most effective evidence-based physical therapy interventions utilized to treat TOS.

Physical Therapy Considerations

PT considerations during management of the individual with thoracic outlet syndrome:

▶ **General physical therapy plan of care/goals:** Relieve symptoms, improve function, improve posture, prevent recurrence

▶ **Physical therapy interventions:** Postural education; activity modification; increase muscle length and strength impairments through passive and active techniques; improve joint hypomobility through mobilization techniques; restore upper limb neurodynamics

▶ **Precautions during physical therapy:** Presence of constitutional signs/symptoms; increased radicular signs and symptoms including reduced reflexes, sensation loss, or myotomal weakness

Understanding the Health Condition

TOS is a multifaceted musculoskeletal condition attributed to compression of neurovascular structures within the thoracic outlet. First coined by Peet[1] in 1956, TOS has a variable presentation due to the variety of tissues that can be involved and multiple sites where compression can occur.[2-4] The incidence of TOS is 3 to 80 cases/1000 individuals. The condition more commonly affects females, with an 8-9:1 female-to-male ratio.[3]

TOS can be divided into three categories depending on the structures compressed. Neurogenic TOS, which results from compression of the brachial plexus, has a very low incidence (and occurs primarily in females).[5] Vascular TOS, accounting for 5% to 10% of all TOS cases, is due to compression of the subclavian artery (1%-5% of cases) and/or vein (2%-3% of cases) and affects men more than women.[5,6] Nonspecific TOS is the most common form and accounts for 90% of all TOS surgeries.[7] Because nonspecific TOS has an unknown etiology and symptoms do not follow true neurologic patterns, there are no objective criteria for its diagnosis and little consensus for optimal conservative treatment. Other diagnoses that must be ruled out when evaluating a patient with suspected TOS include carpal tunnel syndrome (Case 22), cervical radiculitis, cervical disc disease, complex regional pain syndrome (Case 26), and systemic pathology including rheumatoid arthritis, multiple sclerosis, and vasculitis.[3]

Whether the pathophysiology of TOS involves compression of the brachial plexus, vascular bundle (arterial or venous), or both, there are typically three sites where these structures can be compressed: the interscalene triangle, the costoclavicular space, and the subpectoral space. Anatomic causes of compression in the interscalene triangle include morphological changes in the scalene muscles, a prominent C7 transverse process, malformation or elevation of the first rib, fibrous fasciculus (abnormal muscle fibers) between the scalene muscles, and/or the lower cervical transverse processes.[8-15] Entrapment may also result from the presence of a cervical rib, which occurs in 0.2% to 1% of the population.[16-18] The costoclavicular space may be constricted due to changes in the subclavian muscle, clavicular depression, first rib elevation, and/or callus formation of the clavicle or first rib.[8,11,19,20] The subpectoral space can be compressed by an abnormal chondrocoracoid (between the coracoid and underlying rib) and/or claviopectoral fasciculus or by pectoralis minor hypertrophy or shortening.[21] The neurovascular bundle may also be compromised in this area during shoulder abduction and external rotation, as the pectoralis minor and coracoid process act as a fulcrum about which neurovascular structures change direction from running medial-lateral to running superior-inferior.[11] Other potential entrapment sites where brachial plexus compression can occur have also been cited, including the region anterior to the humeral head and the axilla.[4,22]

True neurogenic TOS can be diagnosed via a nerve conduction velocity (NCV) test, electromyography (EMG), magnetic resonance imaging (MRI), or radiographs.[23] Vascular TOS can be diagnosed with a venogram, arteriogram, or MRI scan.[23] **Nonspecific TOS is diagnosed** by exclusion of true neurogenic or vascular TOS and any other condition that could account for the signs and symptoms; thus, NCV and EMG studies are normal.[11,15,24] Since there is no gold standard diagnostic test, diagnosis of nonspecific TOS requires performing a thorough history and examination.[3,6,7] Signs and symptoms typically indicative of nonspecific TOS include pain and paresthesia in the upper extremity, most often in the ulnar nerve distribution of the hand, insidious onset of symptoms, and the presence of anatomic and/or postural abnormalities that could compress the neurovascular bundle.[4,15,23]

Physical Therapy Patient/Client Management

A patient with TOS typically presents with insidious onset of symptoms including a report of "pain" and "heaviness" in the cervical region or shoulder, and pain and/or paresthesias in the fourth and fifth fingers of the hand. Symptoms are often aggravated by overhead positioning of the arm, especially abduction and external rotation. Identification of impairments includes the presence of anatomic or postural abnormalities that could compress the neurovascular bundle, an elevated first rib with inferior glide hypomobility, impaired upper extremity nerve mobility, supraclavicular tenderness over the interscalene triangle, and muscle tenderness and trigger points in the upper trapezius and anterior/middle scalene muscles. The results of diagnostic tests (e.g., radiographs, MRI, EMG, NCV) are typically negative in patients with nonspecific TOS. Physical therapy goals include relieving symptoms, improving neurologic function, and correcting the postural abnormalities and muscular imbalances of the neck, shoulder, and scapular region. Physical therapy interventions may include modalities for symptom relief, manual therapy techniques focusing on passive stretching and improving joint mobility, therapeutic exercise focusing on strengthening and active stretching, and patient education on correct posture and activity modifications. Surgical intervention, primarily first-rib resection, has been shown to have good outcomes, but should only be considered if physical therapy interventions have been unsuccessful.

Examination, Evaluation, and Diagnosis

The first component of the examination consists of taking a thorough, comprehensive subjective history. The guiding question "What is your chief complaint?" allows the patient to describe his symptoms in his own words. The visual analog scale (VAS) allows the patient to give a numeric rating of perceived pain on a 1 to 10 ordinal scale. The test-retest reliability of the VAS for measuring acute and chronic pain is 0.97.[25-27] The patient should be further prompted to describe the pain as dull/sharp, deep/superficial, constant/intermittent. Having the patient complete an anatomic pain drawing provides a visual documentation of his symptoms. Symptoms of TOS may include a report of "pain" and "heaviness" in the cervical region and arms that is thought to be associated with muscle imbalances in the neck, shoulders, and scapular region.[9,13,28,29] Patients may also complain of pain and/or paresthesias in the ulnar nerve distribution of the forearm and hand. Compression of the brachial plexus most often involves the lower trunk of the brachial plexus, consisting of the rami of the C8 and T1 nerve roots. Lower trunk compression can be more prevalent if the patient has a cervical rib or elevation of the first rib. Symptoms include pain and/or paresthesias into the fourth and fifth fingers of the hand. If the condition is serious enough, it can lead to motor involvement of the hand intrinsic muscles.[10,11,13,15,30-32] TOS symptoms are often aggravated by overhead positioning of the arm, especially when the upper extremity is in abduction and external rotation.[11,13,30] If there is a vascular component to the TOS, the patient may report fatigability, heaviness, edema, paleness, or coldness of the hand.[4,15,30,31] Patients may report waking from sleep with complaints of pain and hand numbness.[15,30]

Other information that must be gathered in the patient interview includes a thorough account of the present condition, aggravating and easing factors, the patient's past medical history, and current medications. A brief systems review should be conducted, including listening for any "red flag" signs or symptoms of a systemic condition warranting referral to a more appropriate healthcare professional. These constitutional symptoms include unexplained fever, diaphoresis, night sweats, nausea, vomiting, diarrhea, pallor, syncope, fatigue, and/or recent unintended weight loss.[33,34] Any diagnostic tests, including radiographs, MRI, EMG, and NCV, should be reviewed.

Objective tests and measures should begin with a postural assessment since abnormal posture can be a significant contributing factor in all three categories of TOS. Alignment of the head, cervical spine, shoulder, scapula, and humerus should be assessed from posterior (Fig. 24-1), lateral (Fig. 24-2), and anterior views. The patient in this case scenario had large, hypertrophied arms, rounded and internally rotated shoulders with the humeral heads sitting anterior in the glenoid fossas, and bilaterally overdeveloped latissimus dorsi. Anterior tipping of the right scapula, in which the superior border of the scapula is positioned anteriorly and the inferior

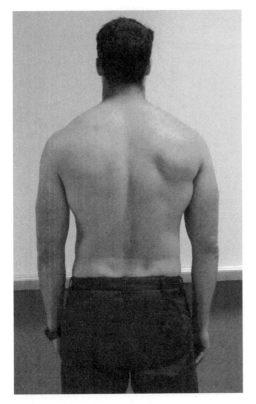

Figure 24-1. Posterior view of patient with right thoracic outlet syndrome. Note bilaterally lengthened upper trapezius muscles, low lateral acromions, overdeveloped latissimus dorsi, and the anterior tipping of the right scapula.

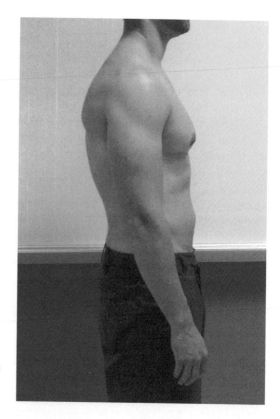

Figure 24-2. Lateral view of patient with right thoracic outlet syndrome. Note the rounded and internally rotated shoulder with the humeral head sitting anterior in the glenoid fossa.

angle is positioned posteriorly, was also evident. The patient had lengthened upper trapezius muscles with scapular depression. His lateral acromions were low, and his scapulae remained low during shoulder elevation. Sahrmann[35] describes this observed postural dysfunction as scapular depression and humeral medial rotation syndrome. Swift[36] coined this postural dysfunction "droopy shoulder syndrome," and found that it accounted for most cases of nonspecific TOS. Many of these postural abnormalities can be attributed to the patient's swimming career that requires repetitive overhead motion with humeral internal rotation.[35] Postural syndromes due to muscular imbalances of the cervical spine, shoulder, and scapular regions can lead to thickening or fibrosis of certain muscle groups that can potentially compress the brachial plexus.[3,13,23] Shortened and/or hypertrophied muscles can push on underlying structures. For example, a shortened pectoralis minor can push on the brachial plexus in the subpectoral region.[35]

Suspected muscle impairments should be confirmed by measuring muscle strength, muscle length, and joint range of motion (ROM). Dominance and shortening of the latissimus dorsi, teres major, pectoralis major, and pectoralis minor are common in patients who participate in work or sports requiring repetitive humeral internal rotation such as swimming.[35] Borstad[37] reported that the resting length of the pectoralis minor can be reliably measured (ICC of 0.96 for test-retest reliability) using a tape measure between the palpable landmarks of the coracoid process and fourth rib. Shortening of the pectoralis minor increases passive tension and results in anterior scapular tipping—both of which can lead to brachial plexus compression.[38,39] This patient had a shortened right pectoralis minor as evidenced by the anterior tip of his scapula (Fig. 24-2). Shortening of the internal rotators can lead to insufficient external humeral rotation during glenohumeral elevation. The therapist can ask the patient to flex his involved shoulder with the elbow flexed and observe whether the elbow moves laterally, which would indicate humeral internal rotation.[35] With the patient in the standing position, the therapist observed that when the patient flexed his shoulder, there was reduced humeral external rotation, a tendency to go into lumbar lordosis (indicating latissimus dorsi shortening), and rib cage elevation (indicating pectoralis major shortening). In supine with his lumbar spine flat on the table, the patient had only 160° of shoulder flexion, a finding that can indicate shortening of the latissimus dorsi and pectoralis major/minor.[35] Goniometric readings revealed only 80° of shoulder external rotation. The patient also presented with weakness of the humeral external rotators and the serratus anterior. Muscles that are stretched beyond their physiological limit disrupt the myofilament alignment, interfering with the tension-generating ability of the contractile elements and leading to weakness.[40] A lengthened upper trapezius may exert a constant tension on the cervical spine and this patient presented with limited cervical ROM. Shortening of the anterior and middle scalenes can lead to elevation of the first rib due to their distal attachment to the first rib.[14] This patient also presented with an elevated first rib. Although the patient did not have limited forearm, wrist, or grip strength, individuals with TOS may present with slight weakness of the musculature in the affected limb, including the hand intrinsic muscles.[30,31]

Since many patients with TOS complain of upper extremity numbness and/or tingling, a thorough neurologic screen should be conducted, including sensory testing and upper extremity deep tendon reflexes. Novak et al.[41] found that two-point discrimination was normal in 98% of TOS cases. Another component of the neurologic assessment is performance of Upper Limb Neurodynamic (tension) Testing (ULNT).[42] Patients with TOS may have mild increases in their symptoms with ulnar nerve ULNT and perhaps with median nerve bias.[15] Wainner et al.[43] reported a substantial kappa of 0.76 and 0.83, and a sensitivity of 97% and 72%, for median and radial nerve bias, respectively, when the ULNT was used as screening tool for ruling out radiculopathy. Coppieters et al.[44] found excellent intra- and inter-tester reliability when testing median nerve mobility within the same session (ICC = 0.98, 0.95) and a moderate ICC of 0.86 after 48 hours in asymptomatic subjects as well as patients with neurogenic TOS. During the performance of several variations of the neurodynamic tests for the median nerve, the authors measured elbow range at the "onset of pain" and when the subject reported "substantial discomfort," and found that improvements of 7.5° of increased elbow extension may be interpreted as meaningful improvements in nerve mobility. Given that concomitant neurologic dysfunction can also produce a positive result during neurodynamic testing, a positive ULNT should be correlated with a reproduction of the patient's symptoms and an asymmetrical response.[28] In TOS, deep tendon reflexes (DTRs) are normal and sensation to light touch is intact. The current patient had a mild reproduction of the paresthesias in his fourth and fifth fingers with ulnar nerve bias of the ULNT, and DTRs and sensation testing were normal.

Joint passive accessory motion testing revealed an elevated first rib with inferior glide hypomobility. Lindgren et al.[45] found that cervical rotation combined with lateral flexion is the direction most restricted by subluxation of the first rib; they reported excellent inter-rater reliability (kappa = 1) for detection of first rib inferior glide hypomobility as well as good agreement compared to radiologic examination of first rib position (kappa = 0.84). Smedmark et al.[46] examined the inter-rater reliability of two physical therapists for assessing first rib mobility graded as "stiff" or "not stiff" and found a moderate kappa coefficient of 0.43. The patient also exhibited hypomobility of the upper thoracic spine and hypermobility of the glenohumeral joint, especially with humeral anterior glide, which was likely associated with his decreased scapular mobility.[39]

Individuals with TOS may present with supraclavicular tenderness over the brachial plexus in the interscalene triangle.[15,30] Palpation of soft tissues typically reveals tenderness of strained muscles due to stretching of muscle filaments beyond their physiologic limit.[40] This patient presented with muscle tenderness most notable in the upper trapezius and anterior/middle scalene muscles. Muscles that are shortened and/or continually mechanically stimulated by poor posture should be palpated for trigger points; this patient exhibited trigger points over his upper trapezius and anterior scalenes. These hypersensitive nodules in the muscles can cause a local twitch response and referred pain patterns.[47] One course of treatment for myofascial trigger points is direct compression (ischemic pressure). There is some evidence that trigger points in the upper trapezius and cervical spine musculature can be treated effectively with manual pressure.[48,49]

There are many provocation tests for TOS, but unfortunately most are unreliable and invalid. The Adson's, Roos, hyperabduction, Wright, and Allen tests are all considered positive if the radial pulse is decreased or obliterated and/or the patient's symptoms are reproduced during the performance of these maneuvers. These tests have been shown to have fair predictive value for any type of TOS; the average individual sensitivities and specificities are 72% and 53%, respectively, when compared to Doppler ultrasonography showing vascular compression.[50] Nord et al.[51] reported that many special tests for TOS have low specificity and thus a high false-positive rate in normal subjects. Rayan and Jensen[14] have suggested that these special tests can also be positive for a vascular response in *asymptomatic* populations. The brachial plexus compression test, in which the examiner applies a compressive traction force to the brachial plexus bundle superior to the clavicle, is considered positive if there is a reproduction of radicular symptoms.[28] Uchihara et al.[52] reported that this test had a sensitivity of 69% and specificity of 83%. Plewa and Delinger[53] reported that the brachial plexus compression test had different specificities, depending on what was considered a positive test. The specificity was 79%, 85%, and 98% for vascular changes, paresthesia, and pain, respectively. Thus, the brachial plexus compression test has a reasonably low false-positive rate when the positive outcome was defined as a report of pain in the upper extremity, neck, or head. However, it is still questionable whether the brachial plexus compression test can discriminate between

TOS and cervical radiculopathy, and thus the patient's clinical presentation must be thoroughly considered in determining the diagnosis.

It is good practice to include a functional activity survey in order to document improvement in activities and function. The **Disability of the Arm, Shoulder, and Hand (DASH) Questionnaire** is a 30-item, self-report questionnaire designed to measure upper extremity function and symptoms. The DASH is scored from 0 (no disability) to 100 (highest disability). The DASH has good construct validity, as shown by a positive correlation with the health-related quality of life Short-Form (SF)-12 score.[54] The test-retest reliability of the DASH has an ICC of 0.92 to 0.96[2] and there are a fair number of studies utilizing the DASH to document patient outcomes following surgical and conservation treatment of TOS.[55-57]

Plan of Care and Interventions

Specific treatment interventions for TOS depend on the TOS type, but conservative treatment is recommended as the first course of management for all types of TOS. The focus of **physical therapy interventions for nonspecific TOS** should be on correcting postural abnormalities and muscular impairments of the neck, shoulder, and scapular regions.

Stretching of shortened muscles can be accomplished with manual stretching and self-stretching techniques.[4,11,15,24,35] The patient can be instructed to perform a corrected movement pattern frequently throughout the day that addresses both the shortened muscles and the impaired muscle performance. For the patient in this case study, three stretches can be prescribed: (1) for the latissimus dorsi and humeral internal rotators, the patient stands with the lumbar spine flat against a wall, elbows at 90° and forearms in supination and then repetitively flexes the shoulders, allowing the elbows to extend but keeping them in the sagittal plane, and finally retracting both scapulae at end of range, (2) for the pectoralis major, this movement is repeated, but with the arms in the coronal plane, and (3) for the latissimus dorsi and pectoralis muscles, the patient lies supine with a flat lumbar spine and elevates his arms overhead.[24,35] In human cadavers, Muraki et al.[58] found that the greatest increase in muscle length of the pectoralis minor occurred with a stretch at 30° of shoulder flexion with passive scapular retraction (while in the sitting position).

Weakened muscles that occur due to a postural abnormality must be selectively strengthened with therapeutic exercise. Strengthening the infraspinatus and teres minor can be accomplished with prone humeral external rotation that simultaneously strengthens the external rotators while stretching the internal rotators. In the prone position, the patient should be taught to stabilize the scapulae by contracting the scapular adductors and serratus anterior before contracting the external rotators.[35] Reinold et al.[59] found that the highest EMG activity of the infraspinatus and teres minor occurred while performing sidelying external rotation with a towel roll under the elbow.

Patient education includes instructing the patient with TOS to minimize glenohumeral internal rotation during shoulder flexion and to effectively recruit the upper trapezius to elevate the shoulder girdle during shoulder elevation. He must be taught activity modification strategies such as sitting with his arms supported on armrests and avoiding carrying heavy objects.[35] Studies with subjects wearing shoulder retraction orthoses designed to decrease the downward pull of the shoulders in order to relieve TOS symptoms have been inconclusive.[12,60]

A recent systematic review found two prospective studies supporting the effectiveness of physical therapy intervention in reducing TOS symptoms.[61] Hanif et al.[62] conducted a prospective study of 50 adults with neurogenic TOS (confirmed with positive Roos test and NCV/EMG). The subjects took anti-inflammatory medication and participated in a supervised therapeutic exercise program every 2 weeks for 6 months and daily active strengthening and stretching as part of a home exercise program (HEP). At 6 months, there was a statistically significant mean decrease in pain and improvement in NCV. Kenny et al.[63] prospectively evaluated eight patients with vascular TOS (positive Adson's test and negative NCV) who were treated for 3 weeks with repetitive shoulder shrugging progressed daily (in repetitions) and weekly (with resistance by holding weights in the hands). All subjects reported a statistically significant reduction in pain and had normal cervical and shoulder ROM after treatment. There are multiple case studies of patients with TOS reporting relief of pain and symptoms after physical therapy interventions.[23,31,64-66] While there have been no randomized controlled trials assessing the efficacy of physical therapy interventions for TOS, several prospective cohort studies have reported favorable, yet modest, results with supervised exercises and a HEP focusing on stretching and strengthening.[63,67,68] It is paramount that the patient is compliant with prescribed activity modifications and HEP for long-term results.

Joint mobilization/manipulation techniques can be utilized to address any capsular hypomobility in the patient with TOS. First rib mobilization can be very beneficial if an elevated or hypomobile first rib is thought to be contributing to TOS.[15,67] For pain control, modalities such as heat and transcutaneous electrical nerve stimulation (TENS) may be helpful.[4] Mechanical traction has not been shown to be beneficial.[15,69]

Treatment of adverse neural tension is challenging because neural tissue is highly sensitive and easily irritated. Thus, symptom irritability must be assessed to determine the degree of aggressiveness with which physical therapy techniques can be applied.[15] The goal of neural mobilization techniques is to decrease symptoms and improve functional mobility of the neural structures.[15] Butler[42] suggests neural tissue mobilization can be accomplished by either direct mobilization of the neural tissues through neural tension techniques and/or joint mobilization techniques. Coppieters et al.[44] documented a case study in which a patient with TOS had successful outcomes after receiving lateral glide mobilizations to his cervical spine. Neural mobilization can also be indirectly accomplished by treating related tissue including joints, muscles, fascia, and skin through soft tissue mobilization, joint mobilization, modalities and exercise, and by postural advice and ergonomic modifications.

Surgical intervention for treating neurogenic and vascular TOS typically involves resecting the first rib. Outcomes from surgical interventions vary, but there are many studies documenting successful surgical outcomes for treating neurogenic TOS.[2,10,57,70-74] Other studies cite less than favorable outcomes.[12,75-78] Given the invasive nature of surgery and the risk for potential complications, surgical intervention for treating TOS is generally a viable option only when conservative interventions have failed. Although first-rib resection has been shown to produce favorable outcomes in the treatment of neurogenic TOS, outcomes for treating nonspecific TOS have not been documented.

Evidence-Based Clinical Recommendations

SORT: Strength of Recommendation Taxonomy
A: Consistent, good-quality patient-oriented evidence
B: Inconsistent or limited-quality patient-oriented evidence
C: Consensus, disease-oriented evidence, usual practice, expert opinion, or case series

1. Diagnosis of nonspecific thoracic outlet syndrome (TOS) is based on exclusion: negative NCV and EMG studies, presence of pain and/or paresthesias in the upper extremity (most notably in the ulnar distribution of the hand), and anatomic or postural abnormalities that could compress the brachial plexus. **Grade B**

2. Physical therapists can use the **Disability of the Arm, Shoulder, and Hand (DASH)** questionnaire to reliably measure changes in upper extremity symptoms and function following surgical or conservation treatment of TOS. **Grade A**

3. A multimodal treatment program including correcting postural dysfunction by muscle stretching and strengthening, manual therapy (soft tissue techniques, joint mobilizations, neural tissue mobilization), and education on correct posture and activity modifications improves outcomes in patients with nonspecific TOS. **Grade B**

COMPREHENSION QUESTIONS

24.1 A physical therapist is working with a patient with a diagnosis of nonspecific TOS. Which of the following test results are *most* likely?

　　A. Abnormal nerve conduction velocity (NCV) test

　　B. Shortened pectoralis minor muscle

　　C. Abnormal two-point discrimination

　　D. Positive Adson's test

24.2 Which outcome tool provides a reliable and valid measurement of improved upper extremity function and symptoms?

　　A. Adson's test

　　B. Oswestry Disability Questionnaire

　　C. Brachial plexus compression test

　　D. Disability of the Arm, Shoulder, and Hand (DASH) Questionnaire

ANSWERS

24.1 **B.** Patients with true neurogenic TOS present with abnormal NCV and two-point discrimination sensation tests (options A and C). Patients with vascular TOS may present with a positive Adson's test (option D), although the test has only fair predictive value and a high false-positive rate. A diagnosis of nonspecific TOS is based on exclusion. Usually, the patient presents with abnormal posture from muscle length and strength impairments including a shortened pectoralis minor.

24.2 **D.** The DASH has excellent test-retest reliability and good construct validity compared with the SF-12. The Adson's and brachial plexus compression tests are both provocation tests utilized to diagnose TOS (options A and C). The Oswestry Disability Questionnaire is utilized to assess disability from low back pain (option B).

REFERENCES

1. Peet RM, Henriksen JD, Anderson TP, Martin GM. Thoracic-outlet syndrome: evaluation of the therapeutic exercise program. *Proc Staff Meet Mayo Clin.* 1956;31:281-287.

2. Athanassiadi K, Kalavrouziotis G, Karydakis K, Bellenis I. Treatment of thoracic outlet syndrome: long-term results. *World J Surg.* 2001;25:553-557.

3. Huang JH, Zager EL. Thoracic outlet syndrome. *Neurosurgery.* 2004;55:897-903.

4. Vanti C, Natalini L, Romeo A, Tosarelli D, Pillastrini P. Conservative treatment of thoracic outlet syndrome: a review of the literature. *Eura Medicophys.* 2007;43:55-70.

5. Wilbourn AJ. The thoracic outlet syndrome is overdiagnosed. *Arch Neurol.* 1990;47:328-330.

6. Fechter JD, Kuschner SH. The thoracic outlet syndrome. *Orthopedics.* 1993;16:1243-1251.

7. Poole GV, Thomae KR. Thoracic outlet syndrome reconsidered. *Am Surg.* 1996;62:287-291.

8. Atasoy E. Thoracic outlet compression syndrome. *Orthop Clin North Am.* 1996;27:265-303.

9. Atasoy E. Thoracic outlet syndrome: anatomy. *Hand Clin.* 2004;20:7-14.

10. Balci AE, Balci TA, Cakir O, Eren S, Eren MN. Surgical treatment of thoracic outlet syndrome: effect and results of surgery. *Ann Thorac Surg.* 2003;75:1091-1096.

11. Dutton M. *Orthopaedic Examination, Evaluation, and Intervention.* New York, NY: McGraw-Hill; 2004.

12. Mailis A, Papagapiou M, Vanderlinden RG, Campbell V, Taylor A. Thoracic outlet syndrome after motor vehicle accidents in a Canadian pain clinic population. *Clin J Pain.* 1995;11:316-324.

13. Novak CB, Mackinnon SE. Thoracic outlet syndrome. *Orthop Clin North Am.* 1996;27:747-762.

14. Rayan GM, Jensen C. Thoracic outlet syndrome: provocative examination maneuvers in a typical population. *J Shoulder Elbow Surg.* 1995;4:113-117.

15. Saunders HD, Ryan RS. *Evaluation, Treatment and Prevention of Musculoskeletal Disorders.* Vol. 1: Spine. 4th ed. Chaska, MN: The Saunders Group; 2004.

16. Brewin J, Hill M, Ellis H. The prevalence of cervical ribs in a London population. *Clin Anat.* 2009;22:331-336.

17. King TC, Smith CR. Chest wall, pleura, lung, and mediastinum. In: Schwartz SI, Shires GT, Spencer FC, eds. *Principles of Surgery.* New York, NY: McGraw-Hill; 1989:627.

18. Roos DB. The place for scalenectomy and first-rib resection in thoracic outlet syndrome. *Surgery.* 1982;92:1077-1085.

19. Kitsis CK, Marino AJ, Krikler SJ, Birch R. Late complications following clavicular fractures and their operative management. *Injury*. 2003;34:69-74.

20. Lindgren KA, Leino E. Subluxation of the first rib: a possible thoracic outlet syndrome mechanism. *Arch Phys Med Rehabil*. 1988;69:692-695.

21. Sanders RJ, Rao NM. The forgotten pectoralis minor syndrome: 100 operations for pectoralis minor syndrome alone or accompanied by neurogenic thoracic outlet syndrome. *Ann Vasc Surg*. 2010;24:701-708.

22. Poitevin LA. Proximal compressions of the upper limb neurovascular bundle. An anatomic research study. *Hand Clin*. 1988;4:575-584.

23. Bargar CJ, DeRienzo V, George SZ. Treatment of a young, male patient with left upper arm pain and left arm numbness: A case report. *Orthop Practice*. 2007:19:25-32.

24. Magee DJ. *Orthopedic Physical Assessment*. 5th ed. St. Louis, MO: Saunders; 2008.

25. Beaton DE, Katz JN, Fossel AH, Wright JG, Tarasuk V, Bombardier C. Measuring the whole or the parts? Validity, reliability, and responsiveness of the Disabilities of the Arm, Shoulder and Hand outcome measure in different regions of the upper extremity. *J Hand Therapy*. 2001;14:128-146.

26. Bijur PE, Silver W, Gallagher EJ. Reliability of the visual analog scale for measurement of acute pain. *Acad Emerg Med*. 2001;8:1153-1157.

27. Price DD, McGrath PA, Raffi A, Buckingham B. The validation of visual analog scales as ratio scale measures for chronic and experimental pain. *Pain*. 1983;17:45-56.

28. Cook CE, Hegedus EJ. *Orthopedic Physical Examination Tests: An Evidence-Based Approach*. Upper Saddle River, NJ: Pearson-Prentice Hall; 2008.

29. Mackinnon SE, Novak CB. Clinical commentary: pathogenesis of cumulative trauma disorder. *J Hand Surg Am*. 1994;19:873-883.

30. Cooke RA. Thoracic outlet syndrome—aspects of diagnosis in the differential diagnosis of hand-arm vibration syndrome. *Occup Med (Lond)*. 2003;53:331-336.

31. Ozçakar L, Inanici F, Kaymak B, Abali G, Cetin A, Hasçelik Z. Quantification of the weakness and fatigue in thoracic outlet syndrome with isokinetic measurements. *Br J Sports Med*. 2005;39:178-181.

32. Rayan GM. Thoracic outlet syndrome. *J Shoulder Elbow Surg*. 1998;7:440-451.

33. Boissonnault WG. *Primary Care for the Physical Therapist: Examination and Triage*. St. Louis, MO: Elsevier; 2005.

34. Goodman CC, Snyder TEK. *Differential Diagnosis in Physical Therapy*. 3rd ed. Philadelphia, PA: WB Saunders Co; 2000.

35. Sahrmann SA. *Diagnosis and Treatment of Movement Impairment Syndromes*. St. Louis, MO: Mosby; 2002.

36. Swift TR, Nichols FT. The droopy shoulder syndrome. *Neurology*. 1984;34:212-215.

37. Borstad JD. Measurement of pectoralis minor muscle length: validation and clinical application. *J Orthop Sports Phys Ther*. 2008;38:169-174.

38. Borstad JD. Resting position variables at the shoulder: evidence to support a posture-impairment association. *Phys Ther*. 2006;86:549-557.

39. Borstad JD, Ludewig PM. The effect of long versus short pectoralis minor resting length on scapular kinematics in healthy individuals. *J Orthop Sports Phys Ther*. 2005;35:227-238.

40. Lieber RL, Woodburn TM, Friden J. Muscle damage induced by eccentric contractions of 25% strain. *J Appl Physiol*. 1991;70:2498-2507.

41. Novak CB, Mackinnon SE, Patterson GA. Evaluation of patients with thoracic outlet syndrome. *J Hand Surg Am*. 1993;18:292-299.

42. Butler D. *The Sensitive Nervous System*. Adelaide, Australia: NOI Group Publications; 2000.

43. Wainner RS, Fritz JM, Irrgang JJ, Boninger ML, Delitto A, Allison S. Reliability and diagnostic accuracy of the clinical examination and patient self-report measures for cervical radiculopathy. *Spine*. 2003;28:52-62.

44. Coppieters M, Stappaerts K, Janssens K, Jull G. Reliability of detecting 'onset of pain' and 'sub-maximal pain' during neural provocation testing of the upper quadrant. *Physiother Res Int*. 2002; 7:146-156.

45. Lindgren KA, Leino E, Hakola M, Hamberg J. Cervical spine rotation and lateral flexion combined motion in the examination of the thoracic outlet. *Arch Phys Med Rehabil*. 1990;71:343-344.

46. Smedmark V, Wallin M, Arvidsson I. Inter-examiner reliability in assessing passive intervertebral motion of the cervical spine. *Man Ther*. 2000;5:97-101.

47. Simons DG, Travell JG, Simons LS. Myofascial pain and dysfunction. *The Trigger Point Manual*. Vol 1. *Upper Half of Body*. 2nd ed. Philadelphia, PA: Lippincott, Williams & Wilkins; 1999.

48. Hanten WP, Olson SL, Butts NL, Nowicki AL. Effectiveness of a home program of ischemic pressure followed by sustained stretch for treatment of myofascial trigger points. *Phys Ther*. 2000;80:997-1003.

49. Itoh K, Katsumi Y, Hirota S, Kitakoji H. Randomised trial of trigger point acupuncture compared with other acupuncture for treatment of chronic neck pain. *Complement Ther Med*. 2007;15:172-179.

50. Gillard J, Perez-Cousin M, Hachulla E, et al. Diagnosing thoracic outlet syndrome: contribution of provocation tests, ultrasonography, electrophysiology, and helical computed tomography in 48 patients. *Joint Bone Spine*. 2001;68:416-424.

51. Nord KM, Kapoor P, Fisher J, et al. False positive rate of thoracic outlet syndrome diagnostic maneuvers. *Electromyogr Clin Neurophysiol*. 2008;48:67-74.

52. Uchihara T, Furukawa T, Tsukagoshi H. Compression of brachial plexus as a diagnostic test of cervical cord lesion. *Spine*. 1994;19:2170-2173.

53. Plewa MC, Delinger M. The false-positive rate of thoracic outlet syndrome shoulder maneuvers in healthy subjects. *Acad Emerg Med*. 1998;5:337-342.

54. Atroshi I, Gummesson C, Andersson B, Dahlgren E, Johansson A. The disabilities of the arm, shoulder, and hand (DASH) outcome questionnaire: reliability and validity of the Swedish Version evaluated in 176 patients. *Acta Orthop Scand*. 2000;71:613-618.

55. Chang DC, Rotellini-Coltvet LA, Mukherjee D, De Leon D, Freischlag JA. Surgical intervention for thoracic outlet syndrome improves patient's quality of life. *J Vasc Surg*. 2009;49:630-637.

56. Dubuisson A, Lamotte C, Foidart-Dessalle M, et al. Post-traumatic thoracic outlet syndrome. *Acta Neurochir*. 2012;154:517-526.

57. Glynn RW, Tawfick W, Elsafty Z, Hynes N, Sultan S. Supraclavicular scalenectomy for thoracic outlet syndrome: functional outcomes assessed using the DASH scoring system. *Vasc Endovascular Surg*. 2012;46:157-162.

58. Muraki T, Aoki M, Izumi T, Fujii M, Hidaka E, Miyamoto S. Lengthening of the pectoralis minor muscle during passive shoulder motion and stretching techniques: a cadaveric biomechanical study. *Phys Ther*. 2009;89:333-341.

59. Reinold MM, Wilk KE, Fleisig GS, et al. Electromyographic analysis of the rotator cuff and deltoid musculature during common shoulder external rotation exercises. *J Orthop Sports Phys Ther*. 2004;34:385-394.

60. Nakatsuchi Y, Saitoh S, Hosaka M, Matsuda S. Conservative treatment of thoracic outlet syndrome using an orthosis. *J Hand Surg Br*.1995;20:34-39.

61. Christopher C, Musc M, Bukry SA, Alsuleman S, Simon JV. Systematic review: the effectiveness of physical treatments on thoracic outlet syndrome in reducing clinical symptoms. *Hong Kong Physiotherapy J*. 2011;29:53-63.

62. Hanif S, Tassadaq N, Rathore MF, Rashid P, Ahmed N, Niazi F. Role of therapeutic exercises in neurogenic thoracic outlet syndrome. *J Ayub Med Coll Abbottabad*. 2007;19:85-88.

63. Kenny RA, Traynor GB, Withington D, Keegan DJ. Thoracic outlet syndrome: a useful exercise treatment option. *Am J Surg*. 1993;165:282-284.

64. Aydog ST, Ozcakar L, Demiryurek D, Bayramoglu A, Yorubulut M. An intervening thoracic outlet syndrome in a gymnast with levator claviculae muscle. *Clin J Sport Med*. 2007;17:323-325.

65. Robey JH, Boyle KL. Bilateral function thoracic outlet syndrome in a collegiate football player. *N Am J Sports Phys Ther.* 2009;4:170-181.

66. Singh VK, Singh PK, Balakrishnan SK. Bilateral coracoclavicular joints as a rare cause of bilateral thoracic outlet syndrome and shoulder pain treated successfully by conservative means. *Singapore Med J.* 2009;50:214-217.

67. Lindgren KA. Conservative treatment of thoracic outlet syndrome: a 2-year follow-up. *Arch Phys Med Rehab.* 1997;78:373-378.

68. Novak CB, Collins ED, Mackinnon SE. Outcome following conservative management of thoracic outlet syndrome. *J Hand Surg Am.* 1995;20:542-548.

69. Cuetter AC, Bartoszek DM. The thoracic outlet syndrome: controversies, overdiagnosis, overtreatment, and recommendations for management. *Muscle Nerve.* 1989;12:410-419.

70. Hempel GK, Shutze WP, Anderson JF, Bukhari HI. 770 consecutive supraclavicular first rib resections for thoracic outlet syndrome. *Ann Vasc Surg.* 1996;10:456-463.

71. McGough EC, Pearce MB, Byrne JP. Management of thoracic outlet syndrome. *J Thorac Cardiovasc Surg.* 1979;77:169-172.

72. Samarasam I, Sadhu D, Agarwal S, Nayak S. Surgical management of thoracic outlet syndrome: a 10-year experience. *ANZ J Surg.* 2004;74:450-454.

73. Sanders RJ, Hammond SL. Management of cervical ribs and anomalous first ribs causing neurogenic thoracic outlet syndrome. *J Vasc Surg.* 2002;36:51-56.

74. Takagi K, Yamaga M, Morisawa K, Kitagawa T. Management of thoracic outlet syndrome. *Arch Orthop Trauma Surg.* 1987;106:78-81.

75. Cuypers PW, Bollen EC, van Houtte HP. Transaxillary first rib resection for thoracic outlet syndrome. *Acta Chir Belg.* 1995;95:119-122.

76. Franklin GM, Fulton-Kehoe D, Bradley C, Smith-Weller T. Outcome of surgery for thoracic outlet syndrome in Washington state workers' compensation. *Neurology.* 2000;54:1252-1257.

77. Landry GL, Moneta GL, Taylor LM, Edwards JM, Porter JM. Long-term functional outcome of neurogenic thoracic outlet syndrome in surgically and conservatively treated patients. *J Vasc Surg.* 2001;33:312-319.

78. Lindgren KA, Oksala I. Long-term outcome of surgery for thoracic outlet syndrome. *Am J Surg.* 1995;169:358-360.

Suprascapular Neuropathy

Margaret A. Wicinski

CASE 25

A 17-year-old right-hand dominant high school female volleyball player presents to an outpatient physical therapy clinic with complaints of diffuse right posterior shoulder pain and weakness. Weakness is most prominent with shoulder external rotation. She reports gradual weakness and pain over the last month and notes that her shoulder blades no longer look symmetrical. She denies a single specific mechanism of injury. Past medical history is unremarkable for systemic complaints, previous surgeries, or previous shoulder injuries. Impairments revealed on initial physical therapy examination include supraspinatus and infraspinatus weakness and decreased active shoulder external rotation and abduction. Passive horizontal shoulder adduction reproduces the patient's pain with a muscle guarding end feel.

▶ What examination signs may be associated with the suspected diagnosis?
▶ What are the examination priorities?
▶ What is her rehabilitation prognosis?
▶ What are the most appropriate physical therapy interventions?

KEY DEFINITIONS

ATROPHY: Wasting or loss of muscle tissue

ENTRAPMENT: Direct pressure on a single nerve due to intrinsic (*e.g.*, bony abnormalities) and/or extrinsic factors (*e.g.*, repetitive overhead activities)

GANGLION CYST: Abnormal fluid-filled sac-like structure surrounding a joint or covering a tendon

SUPRASCAPULAR NEUROPATHY: Damage to the suprascapular nerve that results in decreased sensation and strength of the structures innervated by the suprascapular nerve

Objectives

1. Describe examination findings that would lead to a suspected diagnosis of suprascapular neuropathy or a suprascapular nerve entrapment.
2. Identify mechanisms of entrapment of the suprascapular nerve.
3. Discuss the differential diagnosis process to differentiate between rotator cuff pathology and suprascapular neuropathy.
4. Identify differential diagnoses for a suprascapular neuropathy.
5. Identify diagnostic tests for suprascapular neuropathy.
6. Describe physical therapy interventions to address impairments present in a patient with a suprascapular neuropathy.

Physical Therapy Considerations

PT considerations during management of the individual with muscle weakness, scapular dyskinesia, and posture impairments due to suprascapular neuropathy:

▶ **General physical therapy plan of care/goals:** Increase muscle strength; increase muscular flexibility; restore normal joint and soft tissue mechanics

▶ **Physical therapy interventions:** Muscular strengthening, scapular stabilization, soft tissue and/or joint mobilization

▶ **Precautions during physical therapy:** Monitor patient's physiological response to treatment

▶ **Complications interfering with physical therapy:** Repetitive overhead activities required for recreational or occupational activities; noncompliance with home exercise program and activity modification

Understanding the Health Condition

The suprascapular nerve is derived from the C5 and C6 nerve roots[1-8] and has a variable contribution from C4.[3-5,9] The suprascapular nerve innervates the infraspinatus and supraspinatus muscles[1,3,5,10-12] and provides sensory fibers to the coracoacromial ligament, acromioclavicular and glenohumeral joints,[3-5,8,10-13] subacromial bursa,[10] the scapula,[8] and shoulder joint capsule.[1,6,8,13,14] It is estimated that 15% of individuals have a cutaneous branch of the suprascapular nerve supplying sensation to the lateral arm.[4,5,10,15]

To understand injuries to the suprascapular nerve, a review of the anatomical course of the nerve is helpful. The suprascapular nerve runs parallel to the omohyoid beneath the trapezius to the superior edge of the scapula and then through the suprascapular notch,[3,6,14] which is a bony depression medial to the base of the coracoid process. The transverse scapular ligament encloses the superior aspect of the nerve.[1,10,14] Once the suprascapular nerve passes through the notch, a branch innervates the supraspinatus muscle and the nerve continues to the supraspinous fossa and to the spinoglenoid notch at the lateral edge of the scapular spine, where it innervates the infraspinatus muscle. An articular branch splits off of the suprascapular nerve after it passes the supraspinous fossa and travels to the acromioclavicular and glenohumeral joints.[1,3] It also innervates the coracoclavicular and coracohumeral ligaments as well as the subacromial bursa.[3] There are two *fixed* points along the course of the suprascapular nerve: the origin in the upper trunk of C5 and the termination in the infraspinatus muscle. Two critical points for potential injuries include the lateral edge of the spine of the scapula and the suprascapular notch.[2] Normally, the suprascapular nerve moves in parallel with scapular movements. However, the nerve can become injured due to repetitive stresses.[2]

The incidence and prevalence of suprascapular neuropathy is unknown. The prevalence has been reported as rare,[11,13] uncommon,[8] largely unknown,[13,16] misdiagnosed,[6,8] and infrequently considered and therefore underdiagnosed.[17] Some authors have stated that 1% to 2% of all shoulder pain can be attributed to a neuropathy of the suprascapular nerve.[5,8,9,11,13] In the athletic population, reported prevalence is higher—ranging from 12% to 33%[4] and 8% to 100% in patients with massive rotator cuff tears.[5] One physician with an exclusive shoulder practice reported a 4% incidence of suprascapular neuropathy (92/937 patients) in a 1-year period.[5] Suprascapular neuropathies typically occur in the dominant upper extremity of individuals ranging from 20 to 50 years of age.[3] These neuropathies mainly occur in individuals under 40 years of age[11] and result from a traction or compression injury to the nerve by itself or in conjunction with other impairments.[13]

There are multiple mechanisms or factors that can cause neuropathy of the suprascapular nerve, including anatomical variations, space-occupying lesions, and overuse injuries of the upper extremity. Anatomical structures and mechanisms of injury can lead to compression of the suprascapular nerve. Stretch and/or compression of any peripheral nerve can result in ischemia, edema, micro-environmental changes, and conduction impairments.[3] While the suprascapular nerve can become compressed or tethered at any point along its course, the two most common areas are the spinoglenoid notch and the suprascapular notch.[13] An individual's clinical presentation may vary depending on the entrapment site. For example, if the nerve compression is more distal, only the infraspinatus may be affected. It has been reported that some entrapments affecting only the infraspinatus are painless.[8]

Anatomical variations of bone and ligament structures can lead to impairments of the suprascapular nerve.[9,10,12] Certain suprascapular notch configurations may predispose individuals to suprascapular nerve injury or irritation.[6,11,12] The bony position of the suprascapular notch has been described as having six possible morphological variations.[4,6,10,11] The suprascapular notch can be depressed, shallow v-shaped, u-shaped, or deep v-shaped and the transverse scapular and spinoglenoid ligaments can be partially or completely ossified.[4,5] Space-occupying lesions (soft tissue or bone) can compress the suprascapular nerve.[4,5,8,10,13] Lesions can be located at the suprascapular or spinoglenoid notches or along the path of the nerve itself. In males, a ganglion cyst is more likely to compress the suprascapular nerve than in females.[11] Other structures that can compress the suprascapular nerve include the anterior coracoscapular ligament, the edge of a hypertrophic infrascapular ligament, or the spinoglenoid septum.[9]

Suprascapular nerve injuries can also be associated with fractures of the shoulder girdle/scapula,[3-5,10,12,14] humerus, and clavicle,[3] as well as with shoulder dislocations[3,4,8,10,15] and rotator cuff tears.[4,10,16] Malunion or hardware involvement can irritate, stretch, or compress the nerve.[10] A retracted supraspinatus or infraspinatus muscle due to a massive rotator cuff tear, especially in older patients, can traction branches of the suprascapular nerve.[5,6,10,12-14,16] Trauma and penetrating injuries can compromise the suprascapular nerve.[3-6,8,16] During surgery at the shoulder region using a posterior approach, nerve injuries can also occur.[3-5,8]

Overuse of the extremity with repetitive overhead activities can lead to traction of the suprascapular nerve and microtraumas at the suprascapular or spinoglenoid notch.[3-6,8,13,16] Table 25-1 lists professions and sports that have been identified in the literature to promote suprascapular nerve impairment. Repetitive scapular movements may cause traction and tethering because the nerve is fixed proximally at the cervical spine and distally at the scapula as it passes through the suprascapular notch and around the spinoglenoid notch.[8] Overdevelopment of the subscapularis muscle can also contribute to suprascapular nerve impairment. The subscapularis is a medial rotator and adductor of the glenohumeral joint and the muscle often becomes hypertrophied in volleyball and baseball players due to the requisite repetitive overhead activities. Compression of the suprascapular nerve takes place when the hypertrophied subscapularis covers the anterior surface of the suprascapular notch.[12] Prolonged overhead repetitive or sustained activity can compromise the suprascapular nerve either by compressing or by tractioning the nerve. When the shoulder is in a position of overhead throwing (with extreme abduction with external rotation and into the follow-through), the spinoglenoid ligament becomes tightened, which increases the pressure on the suprascapular nerve.[3-5,10,15] This can occur with volleyball players during overhand serving or with baseball pitchers during overhand hitting of the ball. The tension against the suprascapular nerve leads to increased friction and the potential for tractioning the nerve.[10,15] Combined scapular protraction and infraspinatus contraction during the follow-through of throwing

Table 25-1   PROFESSIONS AND SPORTS THAT CAN LEAD TO SUPRASCAPULAR NERVE IMPAIRMENT
Baseball pitchers[3,10,12,18]
Boxers[15]
Dancers[3,15]
Electricians[15]
Figure skaters[2,3]
Hunters[3]
Painters[15]
Patients in cardiac rehabilitation[15]
Photographers[2]
Skeet shooters[18]
Swimmers[8,19]
Tennis players[2,8,15]
Throwing (general)[8]
Throwing javelin[19]
Volleyball players[8,10,12,15,19]
Weightlifters[2,3,8,15,18]
Workers on a conveyor line[2]

may bowstring (pull taut) the nerve against the scapular spine along with a traction neuropathy that may occur with the excessive nerve excursion.[10]

Movement combinations at the glenohumeral joint increase the risk of injury to the suprascapular nerve. First, the combination of cross-body adduction, flexion, and external rotation pulls the nerve against the medial wall of the notch or ligament and external rotation of the humerus pulls the nerve against the lateral margin of the notch.[2,15] Second, combined elevation and rotation of the glenohumeral joint stretches the suprascapular nerve.[15]

Physical Therapy Patient/Client Management

Physical therapists identify impairments that limit an individual's functional status. The primary goal is to identify the reason/s for the neuropathy and develop a plan to maximize the individual's ability to return to her prior level of function. In the absence of a space-occupying lesion, most sources recommend an undefined course and duration of conservative treatment before any surgical intervention. Conservative treatment for most cases of suprascapular neuropathy includes activity modification (avoiding overhead activities), nonsteroidal anti-inflammatory drugs (NSAIDs), and physical therapy. The success rate of nonoperative treatment is unclear. However, some physical therapy interventions to address impairments due to suprascapular neuropathy have proven beneficial for nonoperative cases.[3,5,7-10,13,15,20]

Examination, Evaluation, and Diagnosis

The subjective history includes questions regarding the patient's mechanism of injury and pain, including aggravating and relieving factors. The patient may or may not be aware of any specific mechanism of injury. It is important for the physical therapist to ask about recent trauma or other injuries, work and recreational activities, past medical history, systemic complaints, and changes in functional use of the involved extremity. Pain that is described as a dull ache in the posterior and/or superior aspect of the shoulder that increases with overhead activities is consistent with suprascapular neuropathy.[3,5,6,9,11,13,16] The patient may also report weakness or fatigue with overhead activities.[5,13] The pain may be described as deep and diffuse[9,11] or burning[10] at the posterior lateral shoulder. Occasionally, pain radiates to the neck or lateral arm.[10] Pain at night and with sleeping is variable due to the patient's preferred sleep position.[5,16] Pain is often exacerbated with sleeping on the affected side.[9]

The physical examination includes observing the patient's structure and movement patterns, palpation, assessing active and passive range of motion (ROM), assessing accessory passive motion, testing strength, and performing special tests. The physical therapist begins by observing the patient from the posterior view to enable inspection of scapular landmarks for symmetry and to appreciate atrophy of the supraspinatus and/or infraspinatus, which is evident if the scapular spine is visible. From the lateral view, the physical therapist notes the position of the head and shoulders to determine if a forward head posture is present. From the anterior view, symmetry of the clavicles and shoulder heights along with the position of the head should be determined.

Next, the physical therapist observes and palpates the shoulder for warmth, edema, atrophy, bruising, change in skin texture, and/or scarring from previous injuries or surgeries. If a suprascapular neuropathy has been present for a long period of time, atrophy of supraspinatus and/or infraspinatus may be present.[3-7,13-17] Atrophy of both the supraspinatus and infraspinatus indicates a more proximal injury of the nerve,[1] typically at the suprascapular notch.[10] Isolated infraspinatus atrophy suggests a spinoglenoid notch entrapment that usually causes pain at the posterior-superior joint line[10] and is typically the result of ganglion cysts.[11]

With a suprascapular neuropathy, glenohumeral active ROM is limited and painful in abduction and external rotation; flexion may also be limited.[5] Scapular motion can increase pain.[6] During active ROM, scapular rhythm must be carefully observed. At > 30° of shoulder flexion, the scapula abducts and upwardly rotates in a 1:2 ratio to the glenohumeral joint; once glenohumeral flexion achieves 90°, the ratio changes to 1:1. The scapular rhythm influences the length-tension relationship of the rotator cuff muscles.[20] In suprascapular neuropathy with associated weakness of the supraspinatus and/or infraspinatus, increased scapular elevation may be noted when the patient elevates her arm.[21] Passive glenohumeral adduction typically increases discomfort due to tightening of the spinoglenoid ligament.[4,5,13] Limitations in joint accessory mobility at the glenohumeral and scapulothoracic joints may be present, depending on the mechanism of injury. If the patient has infraspinatus weakness or paralysis, the therapist may perceive a hypomobile inferior glide of the humeral head. This results from the decreased function of this major humeral head depressor and a potential imbalance in the force couple formed by the deltoid and short rotators.[2]

Strength testing of the muscles innervated by the suprascapular nerve (supraspinatus and infraspinatus) is a priority, followed by testing of the remaining rotator cuff muscles. Depending on the extent and duration of the neuropathy, the patient may present with weakness in external rotation, abduction, extension,[3-7,9-11,13-15,17] and/or flexion.[5] If the neuropathy causes only isolated infraspinatus impairment, strength deficits may not be as prominent due to the function of the teres minor, which is innervated by the axillary nerve.[9,10] Assessing strength of the scapular stabilizers, including the rhomboids, trapezius (upper, middle, and lower portions), and serratus anterior allows the physical therapist to identify muscle imbalances that may alter the static and dynamic movements of the scapula.

Next, the therapist carefully palpates the shoulder and scapula with the intent to elicit tenderness. The patient may experience tenderness around and/or deep to the suprascapular notch,[1,6,9,13,14,17] or within the supraspinatus fossa.[10] Depending on the site of the suprascapular nerve injury, tenderness may also be present posterior to the acromioclavicular joint,[4,14] at the posterior clavicle between the clavicle and scapular spine (in a proximal nerve lesion),[3,4] or at the spinoglenoid notch.[13]

There are few special tests for suprascapular nerve injuries. The most frequently recommended test is the **cross-body adduction test**.[1,3,18] For this test, the therapist passively moves the involved arm into adduction across the midline of the chest. If pain is elicited in the posterior aspect of the shoulder region, then it is a positive test.[1] Performance of the cross-body adduction test tenses the suprascapular nerve by levering the scapula away from the thorax. Another provocation test for suprascapular neuropathy is the scapular traction test in which the patient places the hand of her affected arm on the opposite shoulder and actively lifts the elbow to the horizontal plane.[22] Next, the examiner pulls the elbow toward the uninvolved side. If there is a compression neuropathy of the suprascapular nerve, pain will be elicited. Sahu et al.[23] have recently described another clinical test to detect a suprascapular neuropathy. With the patient seated, the examiner laterally rotates the patient's head *away* from the affected shoulder while simultaneously retracting the affected shoulder. A positive test is increased pain in the posterior aspect of the scapula. Butler[24] describes another test to determine the physical "health" of the suprascapular nerve. For this test, the therapist stands in front of the patient on the opposite side of the painful shoulder. The therapist places the patient's arm into horizontal adduction with the patient's elbow resting on the therapist's sternum. The patient is asked to laterally flex her neck away from the painful shoulder and the therapist pushes through the patient's humeral shaft, depressing the shoulder girdle and rotating the scapula. It is assumed that pain and/or reproduction of the patient's symptoms may indicate an injury to or entrapment of the suprascapular nerve.

It is critical for the physical therapist to rule out other conditions causing the patient's impairments. The therapist should perform a thorough assessment of the shoulder girdle, glenohumeral joint, and cervical and upper thoracic spinal regions. Suprascapular nerve impairment can be mistaken for more common pathologies and needs to be differentiated from shoulder, cervical, and thoracic pathologies (Table 25-2).

Table 25-2   DIFFERENTIAL DIAGNOSES FOR SUPRASCAPULAR NEUROPATHY

Acromioclavicular arthritis[6,10,14]
Adhesive capsulitis[6,10,14]
Brachioplexopathy[8,9]
Bursitis[6,9,10,14,17]
Cervical radiculopathy[10,18]
Cervical spine and/or disc disease[6,9,14,15,17]
Degenerative joint disease[6,14,17]
Diffuse peripheral neuropathy[6,14,17]
Glenohumeral arthritis[10]
Joint instability[9]
Labral pathology[4,10]
Musculoskeletal strain[10]
Pancoast tumor[6,14,17]
Parsonage-Turner syndrome[4,5,10,15,18]
Rotator cuff tears and/or injury[4,6,8-11,14,15,17-19]
Scapulocostal syndrome[15]
Subacrominal impingement[8,11]
Tendonitis[6,9,14,17,19]
Thoracic outlet syndrome[17]

Differentiating between suprascapular neuropathy and rotator cuff impairment is clinically relevant. Both conditions present with muscle dysfunction, but key findings of rotator cuff pathology are important to recognize for accurate diagnosis and treatment. With a tendinopathy of a rotator cuff muscle, pain is present with contraction of the muscle and palpation. Lengthening the tendon increases symptoms. With a partial tear of a rotator cuff tendon, pain and weakness of the involved muscle are present along with tenderness to palpation of the involved tendon; lengthening the tendon also increases symptoms. If a full rotator cuff tendon tear is present, weakness (0/5 manual muscle testing grade) without pain predominates.

Patients may have had diagnostic imaging performed prior to consultation with the physical therapist. If available, the therapist should review imaging to help determine whether the neuropathy is caused by intrinsic factors and to help determine the anticipated duration and extent of the condition. If the neuropathy is due to a bony abnormality or anatomical variation, physical therapy interventions may not be effective. Diagnostic testing includes plain film radiographs, magnetic resonance imaging (MRI), computed tomography (CT), ultrasonography, suprascapular nerve block, and electromyographic and nerve conduction velocity studies. Plain film radiographs can be used to rule out osseous causes of suprascapular neuropathies. A Stryker notch view that allows visualization of the suprascapular notch is especially helpful.[10] While CT scans can evaluate soft tissue masses, MRI is the best modality to assess soft tissue.[3] MRI can identify ganglion cysts[3] and changes in supraspinatus and infraspinatus muscles due to denervation (muscle atrophy and fatty infiltration).[3,4,13] Besides identifying soft tissue lesions, MRI can be used to identify other sources of pathology[4] and to visualize the course of the nerve.[10] Ultrasonography can be used to identify ganglion cysts or other masses at the shoulder.[3,9] Ultrasound is inexpensive; however, its sensitivity and specificity are highly dependent on the individual performing the study.[3] A nerve block procedure—in which an anesthetic agent is injected into the suprascapular notch—is a valuable tool in diagnosing suprascapular nerve neuropathy.[1,10,22] A positive sign of suprascapular neuropathy is if pain decreases[1,10,17,22] or scapular motion with horizontal adduction increases after the injection.[1,10,17] However, a negative test does not definitively rule out a suprascapular neuropathy since it can be difficult to confirm that the injection was at the suprascapular notch.[22] In a series of 27 cases, Callahan et al.[17] reported that the nerve block was the most sensitive diagnostic test in their patients. The **gold standards for diagnosis of suprascapular neuropathy are electromyography (EMG) and nerve conduction velocity (NCV) studies.**[4,5,13] EMG can demonstrate increased spontaneous activity,[3,9] fibrillations,[3,9,10,23] and positive sharp waves in denervated muscles.[3] Other changes include polyphasic activity with a reduction in the amplitude of evoked potentials.[3,6,9,10,13,22,23] NCV studies may show increased latencies.[3,10,14,22]

Plan of Care and Interventions

Except in cases of space-occupying lesions, persistent pain, and/or when nonoperative management has failed, nonoperative treatment is recommended for neuropathies.[9,13] Physical therapy goals should be based on the results of the initial examination, the individual's current status, daily functional requirements, recreational activities, and the patient's goals. Identification of impairments, dysfunction, and functional limitations such as presence of weakness, decreased shoulder ROM, posture impairments, and/or pain in daily, recreational, or functional activities assists the therapist in determining appropriate goals and interventions. Common interventions include **patient education, activity modification, therapeutic exercises, and functional mobility training.**

Rehabilitation of the shoulder involves activity modification and strengthening of the scapular stabilizing muscles and rotator cuff.[9] Interventions should focus on maintaining and/or improving ROM of the shoulder, strengthening scapular stabilizers, and avoidance of aggravating overhead exercises and activities.[5] Exercises are specifically directed toward scapular retraction with maintenance of good postural alignment, and strengthening of the trapezius, rhomboids, and serratus anterior.

With an overhead athlete, addressing scapular impairments is the typical starting point in rehabilitation. Exercises to remedy scapular muscle imbalances must be performed *before* any interventions to address mobility of the suprascapular nerve are initiated. Strengthening and increasing the endurance of the scapular stabilizers to promote depression and retraction of the scapula allows increased scapular dynamic rhythm and potentially reduces the stress being placed on the suprascapular nerve, which may decrease nerve irritation and allow healing prior to strengthening the supraspinatus and infraspinatus. Strengthening starts with increasing the endurance of musculature surrounding the shoulder and then progressing to sport-specific, high speed, and power motions. Generally, this progression begins with isometrics for neuromuscular control and moves to closed chain activities. From closed chain activities, the patient starts with concentric exercises using light hand-held weights and resistance bands, moves to eccentric exercises, and then to explosives and plyometrics, focusing on activities that are sport specific.

The therapist instructs the patient to start with isometric exercises to improve neuromuscular control of the serratus anterior and lower trapezius. Two exercises that focus on these muscles are: (1) isometric holds of shoulder adduction while sitting with the arm abducted to 90° and fist clinched against a stable surface and inferiorly depressing the scapula for 5 seconds, and (2) standing with the elbow fully extended, forearm pronated, and palm of the hand pressing against a stable surface, ask the patient to extend her trunk and push her hand into the stable surface while depressing and retracting the scapula holding for 5 seconds.[25] Next, closed chain activities should be incorporated to promote scapular depression and retraction. With the patient in the quadruped position, the therapist provides verbal and/ or tactile cues to maintain the scapula in a neutral position. Static activities are progressed to dynamic exercises in which the proximal segment is stabilized and the distal segment (the hand) is moving on a fixed surface. For example, the patient could be instructed to move a towel placed under her hand in small circles on the plinth with emphasis on neutral scapular positioning (not overly protracted). As the patient's neuromuscular control improves, the angle of the arm can be increased by changing the height of the high-low table and then progressing to a wall. Depending on the patient's functional demand requirements, ranges can vary. Besides circles, the patient can work with medial-lateral strokes as well as vertical strokes.

Gliding (or flossing) the suprascapular nerve is indicated only after any inflammatory process that was initially present has decreased and the strength of the scapular stabilizers has improved. The goal of nerve gliding is to facilitate movement of the suprascapular nerve, which needs to pass through the scapular notch with ease. To glide the suprascapular nerve, the physical therapist horizontally adducts the glenohumeral joint with internal rotation along with scapular protraction and asks the patient to perform contralateral cervical sidebending to pull the nerve through the scapular notch. Another way to glide the suprascapular nerve is to horizontally adduct the patient's arm while protracting and retracting the scapula to allow the nerve to glide through the notch.[24] While gliding the nerve, the therapist continuously assesses the patient's and tissue's response to this maneuver. Based on the patient and tissue response, this maneuver can be held for a brief period of time (15-20 seconds) and repeated several times. Symptoms should *not* increase after the intervention.

Once scapular stabilizing muscles have increased strength and endurance and nerve gliding interventions have improved the mobility of the suprascapular nerve, strengthening exercises for the supraspinatus and infraspinatus muscles can commence. These should begin with isometrics by performing resisted external rotation with the glenohumeral joint in approximately 20° of shoulder abduction (positioned with a towel roll under the arm). Shoulder external rotation strengthening can be progressed by using a resistance band in the same manner. The position of the gleno-humeral joint can increase from 20° to 90° of abduction to target the rotators at increasing angles. At 90° of abduction, proper patient position is essential to avoid shoulder impingement between the glenohumeral joint and the acromion. The supraspinatus muscle can be more specifically strengthened by placing the arm in scaption with shoulder internal rotation.[26] When beginning this exercise, the use of a t-bar (any lightweight pole configured to look like a "T") can guide the movement pattern. This exercise can be progressed by moving the arm through scaption with the glenohumeral joint in internal rotation without the use of the t-bar and then eventually adding a weight or resistance band. Performing a military press[26] and prone horizontal abduction at 100° with full external rotation are two additional exercises that have been shown to activate the supraspinatus muscle. Exercises for strengthening the infraspinatus include performing prone horizontal abduction with the glenohumeral joint in external rotation and progressed by adding a hand-held weight or resistance band.[20,26]

Looking at the requirements of a volleyball player's dominant upper extrem-ity, this patient must be able to perform high speed and power movements with the shoulder above 90° of abduction in various angles of shoulder rotation. It is important to train at these levels using concentric exercises with the progression to eccentric exercises and eventually to plyometrics. Resisted band concentric and eccentric internal and external rotation at arm angles greater than 90° should be implemented. Resisted bands can be used for loading during activities that mimic passing, setting, spiking, or serving the volleyball. Plyometric training can be incor-porated by throwing/catching weighted medicine balls overhead and side throwing to another individual or at a mini-trampoline that can be fixed at varying angles.

Evidence-Based Clinical Recommendations

A: Consistent, good-quality patient-oriented evidence
B: Inconsistent or limited-quality patient-oriented evidence
C: Consensus, disease-oriented evidence, usual practice, expert opinion, or case series

1. The cross-body adduction special test can identify suprascapular neuropathy. **Grade C**

2. Electromyography (EMG) and nerve conduction velocity (NCV) tests are the gold standards for diagnosing suprascapular neuropathy. **Grade A**

3. Patient education, activity modification, and exercises designed to strengthen scapular stabilizers and increase the mobility of the glenohumeral joint and supra-scapular nerve are effective interventions for suprascapular neuropathy. **Grade C**

COMPREHENSION QUESTIONS

25.1 A physical therapist is treating a patient with a diagnosed suprascapular neuropathy and consequent infraspinatus weakness. During overhead function movement, which of the following arthrokinematic impairments would be *most* likely?

A. Decreased anterior gliding of the humeral head on the glenoid fossa

B. Decreased interior rotation of the humeral head on the glenoid fossa

C. Decreased inferior gliding of the humeral head on the glenoid fossa

D. Decreased posterior gliding of the humeral head on the glenoid fossa

25.2 A physical therapist is working with an athlete who has been diagnosed with suprascapular neuropathy. Which muscle stretch should *not* be performed in order to avoid increased tension on the suprascapular nerve?

A. Infraspinatus

B. Latissmus dorsi

C. Pectoralis major, sternal portion

D. Serratus anterior

ANSWERS

25.1 **C.** The infraspinatus is responsible for gliding the humeral head inferiorly. An impairment of the infraspinatus will allow the humeral head to remain superior in the glenoid causing possible impingement between the acromion and the humeral head that may lead to supraspinatus tendinopathy.

25.2 **A.** A common method of stretching the infraspinatus is by assuming a cross-body horizontal adduction position with external pressure provided from the opposite arm into further adduction. This position reproduces a position of traction on the supraspinatus nerve.

REFERENCES

1. Kopell HP, Thompson WA. *Peripheral Entrapment Neuropathies*. 2nd ed. Malabar, FL: Robert E. Krieger Pub. Co; 1976:146-159.

2. Black KP, Lombardo JA. Suprascapular nerve injuries with isolated paralysis of the infraspinatus. *Am J Sports Med*. 1990;18:225-228.

3. Cummins CA, Messer TM, Nuber GW. Suprascapular nerve entrapment. *J Bone Joint Surg Am*. 2000;82:415-424.

4. Boykin RE, Friedman DJ, Higgins LD, Warner JJ. Suprascapular neuropathy. *J Bone Joint Surg Am*. 2010;92:2348-2364.

5. Freehill MT, Shi LL, Tompson JD, Warner JJ. Suprascapular neuropathy: diagnosis and management. *Phys Sportsmed*. 2012;40:72-83.

6. Post M, Mayer J. Suprascapular nerve entrapment. Diagnosis and treatment. *Clin Orthop Relat Res*. 1987;223:126-136.

7. Drez D. Suprascapular neuropathy in the differential diagnosis of rotator cuff injuries. *Am J Sports Med*. 1976;4:43-45.

8. Walsworth MK, Mills JT, III, Michener LA. Diagnosing a suprascapular neuropathy in patients with shoulder dysfunction: a report of 5 cases. *Phys Ther*. 2004;84:359-372.

9. Gosk J, Urban M, Rutowski R. Entrapment of the suprascapular nerve: anatomy, etiology, diagnosis, treatment. *Ortop Traumatol Rehabil*. 2007;9:68-74.

10. Piasecki DP, Romeo AA, Bach BR, Jr, Nicholson GP. Suprascapular neuropathy. *J Am Acad Orthop Surg*. 2009;17:665-676.

11. Zehetgruber H, Noske H, Lang T, Wurnig C. Suprascapular nerve entrapment. A meta-analysis. *Int Orthop*. 2002;26:339-343.

12. Bayramoğlu A, Demiryürek D, Tüccar E, et al. Variations in anatomy at the suprascapular notch possibly causing suprascapular nerve entrapment: an anatomical study. *Knee Surg Sports Traumatol Arthrosc*. 2003:11:393-398.

13. Boykin RE, Friedman DJ, Zimmer ZR, Oaklander AL, Higgins LD, Warner JJ. Suprascapular neuropathy in a shoulder referral practice. *J Shoulder Elbow Surg*. 2011;20:983-988.

14. Post M. Diagnosis and treatment of suprascapular nerve entrapment. *Clin Orthop Relat Res*. 1999;368:92-100.

15. Pecina MM, Markiewitz AD, Krmpotic-Nemanic J. *Suprascapular Nerve Syndrome: Tunnel Syndromes: Peripheral Nerve Compression Syndromes*. 3rd ed. Boca Raton, FL: CRC Press LLC; 2001:49-55,284.

16. Shah AA, Butler RB, Sung SY, Wells JH, Higgins LD, Warner JJ. Clinical outcomes of suprascapular nerve decompression. *J Shoulder Elbow Surg*. 2011:20;975-982.

17. Callahan JD, Scully TB, Shapiro SA, Worth RM. Suprascapular nerve entrapment. A series of 27 cases. *J Neurosurg*. 1991;74:893-896.

18. Liveson JA, Bronson MJ, Pollack MA. Suprascapular nerve lesions at the spinoglenoid notch: report of three cases and review of the literature. *J Neurol Neurosurg Psychiatry*. 1991;54:241-243.

19. Fabre T, Piton C, Leclouerec G, Gervais-Delion F, Durandeau A. Entrapment of the suprascapular nerve. *J Bone Joint Surg Br*. 1999:81:414-419.

20. Martin SD, Warren RF, Martin TL, Kennedy K, O'Brien SJ, Wickiewicz TL. Suprascapular neuropathy. Results of non-operative treatment. *J Bone Joint Surg Am*. 1997;79:1159-1165.

21. Miller T. Peripheral nerve injuries at the shoulder. *J Manual Manipulative Ther*. 1998;6:170-183.

22. Osterman AL, Babhulkar S. Unusual compressive neuropathies of the upper limb. *Orthop Clin North Am*. 1996;27:389-408.

23. Sahu D, Fullick R, Lafosse L. Arthroscopic treatment of suprascapular nerve neuropathy. In: Steele C, ed. *Applications of EMG in Clinical and Sports Medicine*. www.miotec.com.br/pdf/Applications_of_EMG_in_Clinical_and_Sports_Medicine.pdf. Accessed May 22, 2013.

24. Butler D. *The Neurodynamic Techniques: A Definitive Guide from the Noigroup Team*. Adelaide City West, South Australia: Noigroup Publications; 2005.

25. Kibler WB, Sciascia AD, Uhl TL, Tambay N, Cunningham T. Electromyographic analysis of specific exercises for scapular control in early phases of shoulder rehabilitation. *Am J Sports Med*. 2008;36:1789-1798.

26. Townsend H, Jobe FW, Pink M, Perry J. Electromyographic analysis of the glenohumeral muscles during a baseball rehabilitation program. *Am J Sports Med*. 1991;19:264-272.

Complex Regional Pain Syndrome

Beth Phillips

A 27-year-old right-hand dominant female presents with a history of uncompli-cated well-healed right Colles' fracture without overt insult to the peripheral nerves 10 weeks ago. Now, 4 weeks after cast removal, she reports burning pain in her right hand and distal forearm, pain with movement of wrist and digits, and hyper-sensitivity to touch and temperature. When the patient enters the physical therapy clinic, she is holding her right arm rigidly away from her body and her shoulder is shrugged. On examination, she is reluctant to allow any palpation or contact on the right extremity. Her right forearm and hand are swollen, red and blotchy, and the skin appears thin and shiny on the hand with slightly more hair growth on the right forearm compared to the left.

▶ What are the most appropriate examination tests to determine whether this patient has complex regional pain syndrome (CRPS)?

▶ What are the most appropriate physical therapy interventions given the patient's type and stage of CRPS?

▶ What precautions should be taken during physical therapy?

▶ Identify the other medical team members typically included in management of this diagnosis.

KEY DEFINITIONS

ALLODYNIA: Perception of pain from a normally nonpainful stimulus

CAUSALGIA: Previous term for CRPS type II; symptoms and signs include burning pain and trophic changes to skin and nails, resulting from injury to nerve fibers

REFLEX SYMPATHETIC DYSTROPHY: Previous term for CRPS when it was presumed that symptoms were primarily caused and/or maintained by hyperactivity of the sympathetic nervous system (SNS)

SUDOMOTOR: Relating to nerves that stimulate sweat gland activity

TROPHIC CHANGES: Changes in skin and nails (hair loss, cracked nails, etc.) typically seen with declining nourishment; due to impaired function of efferent nerves that control growth and nourishment of structures they innervate

Objectives

1. Describe CRPS type I and type II and the criteria outlined by the International Association for the Study of Pain (IASP) for diagnosis.

2. Identify trophic changes typically associated with CRPS.

3. Identify demographic, medical, and psychosocial predisposing factors that have the strongest association with CRPS.

4. Identify at least one outcome measure used to assess functional improvement in CPRS.

5. Discuss appropriate physical therapy interventions for preventing and treating CRPS.

Physical Therapy Considerations

PT considerations during management of the individual with CRPS:

▶ **General physical therapy plan of care/goals:** Decrease pain, swelling, and allodynia; restore range of motion (ROM), strength, and functional use of involved extremity

▶ **Physical therapy interventions:** Passive range of motion (PROM) progressing through active assisted range of motion (AAROM) and active ROM to resisted ROM and proprioceptive neuromuscular facilitation (PNF); sensory bombardment; joint mobilizations; hold-relax techniques to relieve guarding initially and then for increasing ROM; gradual progression of strengthening and endurance training; modalities (transcutaneous electrical stimulation, biofeedback); neuromuscular re-education including mirror therapy/motor imagery; patient education on mechanisms and purpose of pain, perception of pain and progression of condition, overall wellness, health and stress management/relaxation practices

▶ **Precautions during physical therapy**: Monitor pain carefully and frequently; interventions may cause pain at onset, but should diminish pain quickly and not result in post-intervention increases in pain

▶ **Complications interfering with physical therapy**: Fear of movement and pain may require substantial education; certain pre-existing psychological conditions may interfere with progress (prior life events within past year have highest correlation[1]); psychological factors should not be used to determine the patient's potential for healing or to predict development of CRPS[2-4]

Understanding the Health Condition

CRPS is a painful, debilitating condition of the extremities that has uncertain pathophysiology, unclear diagnostic criteria, and inconsistently defined intervention strategies without predictable outcomes.[5] Categorized as either type I (without injury to a nerve) or type II (with direct injury to a nerve), CRPS symptoms include severe burning, swelling, sweating, disproportionate pain and sensitivity to touch and temperature, and discolorations or other trophic changes in the skin.[6] CRPS type I or II may be observed poststroke, postamputation, or following major or even minor orthopaedic traumas, particularly fractures.[7] Precise reporting of the incidence of CRPS is difficult because symptoms vary widely and misdiagnoses are frequent.[8] CRPS afflicts all ages with highest occurrence between the ages of 50 and 70 years; females are more frequently affected than males, and the upper extremity is more often involved than the lower extremity.[9] In an epidemiological study in the Netherlands, the annual incidence was between 16.8 new cases per 100,000 (when a detailed specialist evaluation was required for diagnosis) and 26.2 new cases per 100,000 (when diagnosed by clinical findings alone). These authors found that the occurrence was three times higher in females than in males.[7] If a similar incidence were assumed in the United States, this could mean tens of thousands of new cases annually.

CRPS type I (CRPS1) was previously called reflex sympathetic dystrophy because of observations of SNS regulation problems in this condition. In the 1990s, the name was changed by the International Association for the Study of Pain (IASP) due to the lack of evidence that the syndrome is caused or solely maintained by sympathetic deregulation and the observations that, in some cases, no sympathetic involvement was noted.[6] The IASP ascribes specific criteria for diagnosing CRPS. The individual may report a noxious event or causative factor (with or without nerve lesion) and any other condition that might otherwise account for the level of pain and dysfunction must be ruled out.[10] The IASP criteria further specify that all individuals must present with a combination of the following to be diagnosed with CRPS: (1) a level and constancy of pain, hyperalgesia, or allodynia disproportionate to the injury event; (2) some period of edema, blood flow changes to skin, or abnormal sweating in the painful extremity. Since the first description of the IASP criteria, other authors have modified or further delineated objective inclusion criteria for research subjects that are also used in the diagnosis of CRPS. These include the Veldman criteria and the Harden and Bruehl criteria.[11,12] To date, a rationale to use one set of criteria over another has not been established.[8]

The National Institute of Neurological Disorders and Stroke discusses three stages associated with the progression of CRPS.[13] Due to the widely varying presentations and durations of symptoms in any phase of CRPS, the three-stage model is not closely adhered to for diagnosis but may be valuable for defining severity or planning therapeutic intervention.[14] Stage 1 (acute phase lasting 1-3 months) is characterized by severe burning pain, muscle spasm, joint stiffness, rapid hair growth in affected area, and blood vessel alterations that result in increased skin temperature and color changes. Stage 2 (dystrophic phase; from months 3-6) is characterized by intensified swelling, pain, joint stiffness, decline in hair growth, weakness, trophic changes to nails (grooved, brittle/cracked, or spotty), and softening of bones. In Stage 3 (chronic/atrophic phase), the individual experiences unyielding pain possibly involving the whole limb, marked atrophy, dystonia, contorted limbs, coldness of skin, and severe loss of mobility.[13]

Attempts to identify factors that predict the likelihood of CRPS have not produced consistently reproducible results. However, after evaluating data on 600,000 CRPS cases, de Mos et al.[7] found fractures to be the most common precipitating event and two studies showed postmenopausal females are at greater risk.[7,15] Post-stroke development of CRPS has been reported as occurring in 1.5% to 12.5% of stroke cases.[16] In a prospective cohort study of 596 patients with a single fracture, investigators found that a subsequent CRPS diagnosis was more likely with lower extremity fractures, where ankle fracture, dislocation fracture, and intra-articular fracture significantly contributed to the likelihood of CRPS development.[11] While there are some associations with psychological conditions arising *after* the development of CRPS—such as depression, anxiety, expressed helplessness[4,17]—there is no evidence suggesting a causative relationship with the exception of significant life events occurring in the year prior to injury, which has demonstrated a strong predictive value.[1,2]

Pathophysiological explanations for CRPS are elusive. In recent years, much more has become clear about the neurological, cortical, and chemical changes involved with the condition. There appears to be a strong involvement of the small diameter C-fibers that have a slow conduction speed and respond to both mechanical and thermal stimuli. In addition, there may be abnormally high concentrations of neuropeptides such as calcitonin and substance P.[14] In some adults with neuropathic pain, disrupted C-fibers became hypersensitive to vasoconstricting catecholamines and contributed to their altered pain perception without any evidence of an overactive SNS in maintaining pain symptoms.[18] In fact, following sympathetic denervation, tissues can have increased sensitivity to circulating catecholamines.[19] Regardless of these results, the practice of sympathetic nerve blocks is still used in an attempt to "re-set" the system and quench the pain thought to be due to SNS involvement.[13] C-fibers have also been implicated in sensitizing and influencing nociceptive and non-nociceptive information processing in the dorsal horn of the spinal cord. Implantation of stimulating electrodes next to the spinal cord to inhibit afferent input from C-fibers helps some patients with their pain, but is recommended as a treatment strategy only in severe chronic stages.[20]

Central motor processing disturbances,[21-24] reduced somatosensory cortex representation of the affected limb,[22] altered body schemas,[25] and dysregulation of autonomic responses[26] have been demonstrated in individuals with CRPS. Schilder and colleagues[27] found that CRPS patients had impaired voluntary motor control during a finger tapping task in both the involved and noninvolved extremity. Subjects with CRPS display altered somatomotor pathways and autonomic responses.[26] Within seconds of viewing an ambiguous visual stimulus, subjects with CRPS demonstrated heightened pain compared to healthy controls. In addition, they experienced asymmetrical autonomic vasomotor response in the affected limb compared to the unaffected limb, suggesting an overflow of symptoms to the uninvolved extremity.[26]

Certain biomarkers have been identified in patients with CRPS. These biomarkers may contribute to the current understanding of the pathophysiology and may lead to novel treatment approaches. A comparison of 148 subjects with CRPS to sex- and age-matched healthy controls revealed increased plasma levels of neurogenic inflammatory and immune system cytokines, chemokines, and their associated soluble receptors.[28] Accumulated plasma concentrations of these substances correlated with severity and duration of CRPS, which could become useful as a marker of disease progression. Another chemical change demonstrated in CRPS that may have value for diagnostic confirmation and understanding of the pathophysiologic disease process is substance P released from primary afferent neurons.[29] Substance P mediates accumulation of mast cells and the degranulation processes; it has been noted to be abnormally high in CRPS, which contributes to nociceptor hyperactivity.[29] A rat-model study evaluated the potential for a substance P receptor antagonist to inhibit this process. The investigators found positive results that may hold some promise for treatment of these neurochemically induced symptoms in patients with CRPS.[29]

While the role of neurologic and chemical changes is evident in the presentation and maintenance of CRPS symptoms, it is unclear why these responses are triggered in some individuals and not others—that is, why some individuals develop CRPS while others heal without complication is still largely a mystery. There may be a genetic predisposition to the development of CRPS.[30] Increased fear during periods of sustained pain can contribute to the functional limitations in CRPS.[31] Levels of stress and the presence or absence of stress-reducing habits (e.g., relaxation techniques, meditation) may help explain why some individuals develop or maintain pain syndromes[32,33] and others manage to avoid being affected so adversely by similar precipitating events. The complexity and multisystem involvement of CRPS necessitates a multimodal treatment approach including physical therapy and medical management as well as the need for additional investigation and testing of alternative therapies that show promise in the treatment of CRPS.

Prognosis varies by individual and severity of dysfunction. While large-scale research is needed to develop clear prognostic indicators, earlier identification and intervention may help limit the severity of the disorder.[13] Symptoms of CRPS may spontaneously resolve or progress to unrelenting irreversible and crippling pain despite treatment.

Physical Therapy Patient/Client Management

An individual with a diagnosis of CRPS typically presents with significant pain, loss of ROM, weakness, joint hypomobility, and skin sensory disturbances possibly involving an entire extremity. There may or may not be a recent history of a noxious precipitating event (*e.g.*, stroke, fracture, tissue trauma) and there may or may not be an injury to a nerve. This information should be thoroughly explored in the subjective examination as it helps in determining whether the patient is presenting with type I or type II CRPS. It is important for physical therapists in all practice areas to be educated on the potential for the development of CRPS, its signs and symptoms, and on the crucial nature of intervening with restorative therapy and preventative measures prior to the full development of the condition.[17] Because CRPS can be such a debilitating condition, it might be a beneficial practice to include education and some simple preventative interventions (*e.g.*, sensory bombardment) to all patients who have suffered a stroke, amputation, fracture, or trauma, even in the absence of apparent signs.

The plan of care to manage CRPS includes interventions to control pain, decrease swelling, restore normal sensory responses, and increase joint mobility and strength to maintain or regain functional use of the involved extremity. Long-term goals should be set according to the patient's functional recovery needs, but incremental short-term goals are helpful to demonstrate step-wise changes that can maintain the patient's confidence and sense of progress. **Multidisciplinary care** with medical prescription of analgesics or neural blocks, psychological support and complementary approaches (acupuncture, meditation) may assist in recovery. The primary goal of medical, psychological, and complementary interventions is to improve the patient's tolerance for physical therapy, which is the essential component for addressing impairments and improving functional restoration.[5,14]

Examination, Evaluation, and Diagnosis

The patient examination requires a thorough subjective history and review of the medical chart, when available. Without a gold standard diagnostic test,[34] diagnosis depends on a meticulous subjective and objective examination.[8] The patient interview should include details of any precipitating event (*e.g.*, prior injury or stroke), progression of current symptoms, details of functional activity impairment, psychosocial impact, and previous and current medical management including medications and use of sympathetic nerve blocks or spinal cord stimulator implants.

Several assessments of pain have been used to evaluate and monitor changes in symptom severity. The McGill Pain Questionnaire is a commonly used pain questionnaire employed in research with individuals with CRPS.[35,36] Another useful tool during the examination and throughout interventions is the visual analog scale (VAS) that allows the patient to give a numeric rating of perceived pain on a 1 to 10 ordinal scale. The test-retest reliability of the VAS for measuring acute and chronic pain is 0.97.[37,38] Because absence of pain is not likely for quite some time in persons with CRPS, it is vital to include a functional activity survey to document improvement in activities and function. The **Disability of the Arm, Shoulder, and Hand Questionnaire (DASH)** is a 30-item, self-report questionnaire designed to measure upper extremity function and symptoms. The DASH is scored on a 0 (no disability) to 100 (highest disability) scale. The test-retest reliability is excellent (ICC = 0.92-0.96).[37,39] The DASH demonstrates good construct validity, as indicated by positive correlations with the health-related quality of life Short-Form (SF)-12 scores.[39]

Objective examination includes measurements of swelling (pitting or nonpitting edema), ROM, and strength, as tolerated. A thorough examination of the sensory system is prudent and serves to document both severity and progression. It is also imperative to rule out other conditions or diagnoses before making the diagnosis of CRPS.[10] Differential diagnoses include nerve entrapment, post-herpetic neuralgia, plexopathy, connective tissue disease, vascular disorders, rheumatic or inflammatory arthritis, migratory osteoporosis, or other delayed-healing orthopaedic conditions.[14] The patient may present with hypersensitivity to light touch and two-point discrimination tests, but the sensation changes do not conform to a dermatomal or peripheral sensory nerve distribution.[40] Deep tendon reflexes may or may not be normal, but typically are *not* found to be hyper-reactive.[40] During sensory testing and palpation, the therapist should observe for abnormal hair loss or excessive growth, trophic changes in the nails (grooves, cracking), and skin changes. Changes in skin temperature, texture, sweating, or color should be noted. Warm, red skin may indicate sympathetic hypoactivity and cold, mottled, pale, or blue skin may reflect hyperactive sympathetic function.[12] If available to the therapist, thermosensitive tape or a spot-temperature device is an objective means of documenting vasomotor autonomic problems.[41] Assessing the patient's reaction to cold and warm temperatures placed on the skin of the involved extremity compared to that on the uninvolved extremity may help determine the presence of hypersensitivity or allodynia. A simple, though not quantifiable, means of assessing increased sweating is to drag a smooth-handled instrument across the involved extremity and the uninvolved extremity—the instrument will slide easily across sweaty skin compared to normal dry skin.[41] Because of the central processing disturbances often seen in individuals with chronic CRPS, motor control testing may be useful in documenting a diagnosis of CRPS. Simple activities like finger tapping may demonstrate impaired movement, speed, and time-to-fatigue in both the involved and uninvolved extremities.[27]

A diagnosis of CRPS may be suspected by the physical therapist when clinical examination findings of loss of ROM and strength, swelling, pain, trophic changes, and sensory or motor disturbances are of a greater magnitude and duration than reasonably anticipated given the history of injury and if other differential diagnoses have been ruled out.[10] Medical diagnostic tests may help confirm CRPS, but these are debated in the literature. The reliability of any one test as an absolute confirmation of a CRPS diagnosis has not been substantiated. In certain stages of CRPS, three-phase bone scans have sometimes demonstrated structural and blood flow changes in bones. However, the current literature suggests the diagnostic value of these scans is low[42] and sometimes confusing.[12] Nerve conduction velocity testing is not useful because of its limited sampling of large myelinated nerve fibers, which are not usually involved in CRPS.[14] Quantitative Sensory Testing for heat sensitivity and reduced pain thresholds may demonstrate positive findings, since these tests measure activity of the small diameter C-fibers that are implicated in CRPS.[43,44]

Plan of Care and Interventions

The plan of care and goals depend on findings from the examination, which illuminate the severity and duration of the patient's CRPS symptoms. Interventions must focus on pain control, managing edema, reducing sensory disturbances, and gentle progression of regaining ROM and strength to restore functional use of the involved extremity. Significant ongoing patient education on the physiologic processes of the condition and mechanisms of pain response is necessary as well as training in stress-reducing positive health behaviors to manage pain and stress appropriately. Due to varying pathophysiologic mechanisms, symptom presentations, and intervention protocols, no single treatment strategy has been unequivocally proven to be effective. Multiple healthcare professionals are typically involved in the management of CRPS in order to address various aspects of the condition. Physical therapy is always a primary treatment component.[5,14]

Physical therapy was found to be effective for reducing pain and improving mobility in patients with CRPS in two studies by Oerlemans and colleagues.[36,45] These studies compared three groups that received either physical therapy (PT), occupational therapy (OT), or social work support (control group). All subjects continued with medical management, consistent pharmacological regimen, and received general information about their condition. The PT group received education, relaxation techniques, connective tissue massage, transcutaneous electrical stimulation, exercises aimed at reducing pain by mechanoreceptor stimulation, and activity corrections or modifications (e.g., instruction in proper form and skill training). The OT group received inflammation control and protection of the extremity through splinting and positioning, tactile and proprioceptive activities to normalize sensation, and use of devices and/or training in normal movement or alternatives for completing activities. One study demonstrated that the PT group experienced faster pain reduction than the social work control group.[36] In addition, the PT group demonstrated greater mean improvement on McGill Pain Questionnaire (MPQ) outcomes than either the OT or the control group.[36] The control group showed significantly slower improvement in impairments than the PT group. The PT group also showed more rapid improvement on MPQ outcomes than the OT group and was also more cost-effective.[45] However, long-term impairment (> 1 year duration) was not significantly different between PT, OT, or control groups when measured with the American Medical Association's Guides to the Evaluation of Permanent Impairment.[36] A nonrandomized study by Kemler et al.[46] found no functional status improvements in 54 subjects in the chronic stages of CRPS who had received 6 months of physical therapy after they had previously undergone a trial of spinal cord stimulation. The authors pointed out that subjects with less severe baseline symptoms improved the most, but overall improvements at 12 months for all subjects was not large enough to demonstrate significant change, particularly in the absence of a control group. Frequency of physical therapy is not consistently mentioned in research protocols. However, one study in a pediatric population found that subjects improved significantly on five measures of pain and function whether they received one therapy session per week or three sessions per week.[47]

In the early stages of CRPS, physical therapy interventions should initially focus on relieving pain and swelling and normalizing sensation. Elevation of the involved extremity may reduce the hydrostatic pressure caused by venoconstriction and capillary membrane leakage. When combined with manual lymphatic drainage, these strategies may help reduce pain and restore normal sensation.[48] Other pain management and sensory desensitization techniques include carbon dioxide baths with cool temperatures[49] and contrast baths in which the temperature differences are gradually broadened.[12] To help restore appropriate central processing responses to touch and proprioceptive stimuli, several sensory bombardment techniques may be useful. These include exposing the skin to light and deep pressure, vibration, or varying and alternating textures of cloth (e.g., silk, dry towel, cotton, wet and dry sponge, etc.).[14] If tolerated, cryotherapy may assist with controlling swelling and pain. Care must be taken to avoid lowering the skin temperature by > 16°C (60.8°F) because when tissue temperature reaches 2°C (35.6°F), vasodilation occurs.[50] Heat modalities should be avoided as they may increase swelling.[12]

Transcutaneous electrical nerve stimulation (TENS) has frequently been used for pain control in CRPS research studies. Some evidence suggests possible benefits,[47,51-53] while some authors caution that TENS might aggravate pain, particularly for patients who have central pain mechanisms activated.[54,55] Parameters such as high-frequency short pulse and low-frequency with slower pulse (acupuncture-like) can be attempted.[5,56] However, low-frequency TENS with its bias for C-fiber stimulation might be more effective in treating CRPS.[43,44] A rat-model study determined that a combination of both high- and low-frequency TENS most comprehensively controlled allodynia in CRPS type II.[57] Electrode placement should progressively move toward the most painful region. First, the physical therapist should place the electrodes along the spinal segments supplying the involved area, then proximally on the extremity with pain, then superior and inferior to the painful area, and eventually directly on the hyperaesthetic portion.[5]

The physical therapist must remain in close contact with the physician to determine if and when the implementation or alteration of analgesic medications, neural blockades, or psychological support might be useful for promoting pain relief, encouragement, and confidence in the overall effort to avoid complications resulting from anxiety and fear.[31] The goal of medical measures such as drugs and neural blocks is to make continuation of physical therapy possible.[17] The combination of medical and therapy interventions is more effective to potentially reset abnormal central pain processing and re-establish normal perception in the extremity so movement and functional use may be regained.[5,14]

As pain begins to be controlled, interventions to regain ROM and strength become an essential component of patient management. Progression starts with very gentle passive ROM, active assisted ROM (AAROM), resisted ROM, PNF, functional strengthening, and eventually to gentle weightbearing activities.[58] Examples of load-bearing for patients with upper extremity involvement include carrying increasingly heavier bags and scrubbing activities as described by Carlson and

Watson Stress-Loading Program[59] and partial weightbearing gait activities moving toward full weightbearing for lower extremity involvement. Biofeedback has been included as a component of treatment protocols for patients with CRPS to help retrain normal motor patterns and functional awareness of movement.[13,60] Immobilizing splints have been found to be counterproductive, but dynamic splinting may be useful for achieving complete ROM in later phases of intervention.[58] Caution must be taken in implementing strength training since aggressive approaches may aggravate stiffness and reduce ROM.[56] Progression should be slow, with eventual focus on functional use, endurance, and work hardening activities.[17] Joint passive accessory mobilizations may help reduce pain (grades I or II) and restore motion (grades III or IV) when immobility has led to capsular tightening that is affecting proper arthrokinematics.[61]

Attention to overall wellness habits are important considerations in managing CRPS including the need for aerobic activity,[12] avoidance of smoking,[62] stress management/relaxation techniques,[14] and possible referral for proper nutrition counseling (e.g., 500 mg daily intake of vitamin C has been shown to possibly prevent postfracture CRPS).[8] The negative effects of stress on health are widely known.[63-67] A healthy stress management technique deserving serious attention is **meditation**. Use of transcendental meditation (TM) and mindfulness meditation has demonstrated efficacy for managing a variety of signs and symptoms associated with CRPS including decreasing chronic pain,[32,33,68] reducing sympathetic system activity,[69,70] enhancing immune function,[71] decreasing levels of stress hormones,[72] and preventing disease.[63,73] In normal young adults, a 20-minute twice daily TM practice was associated with a reduction in adrenocortical hormones, which are elevated during both acute and chronic stress.[72] Practice of this type of meditation has important implications for counteracting the stress-related complications experienced by patients with CRPS.

The effect of meditation on the SNS and the brain's perception of pain merits further discussion with regards to CRPS. David Orme-Johnson[70] measured galvanic skin responses (GSR) in non-meditators compared to meditators. GSR measures the sympathetic-mediated response of sweating (sudomotor activity), one diagnostic sign of CRPS. He found longer galvanic skin response (GSR) in non-meditators following a startling noise; non-meditators also demonstrated more "false-alarm" increases in GSR that occurred in the absence of an additional stimulus. Functional magnetic resonance imaging (fMRI) of long-term TM meditators demonstrated less activity (40%-50%) in areas of the brain associated with pain (e.g., thalamus) than in non-meditators when their fingers were placed in extremely hot water even though both groups *rated* the pain level similarly.[33] The authors of this study postulated that meditators have a more relaxed SNS and therefore pay less attention to pain. Of even greater interest is that non-meditators who later learned to meditate demonstrated a 45% to 50% decrease in brain response to pain after only 5 months of meditation. Zeidan and colleagues[74] found that mindfulness meditation decreased pain and anxiety in experimentally induced pain. A large-scale investigation of meditation in patients with CRPS may confirm the beneficial effects of meditation on pain[68,74] and possibly validate the use of meditation for this patient population.

Psychological testing and counseling may become necessary because certain mental or emotional conditions may develop if patients become fearful or anxious about not getting well as their condition progressively worsens.[17] In a study by de Jong et al.[31], pain-related fear was found to impair function in early CRPS and perceived harmfulness of movement significantly predicted limitations in function (beyond level of pain contribution) for those with chronic CRPS. These findings support de Jong's suggestion that a pain exposure treatment program may be associated with functional restoration in patients with pain-related fear. A case series by Ek and colleagues[75] reports success using graded pain exposure in physical therapy interventions to "over-ride" the false warning type of pain found in CRPS.

Pain in the absence of true tissue damage or danger is a reflection of the adaptive ability of the brain to create, sustain, or ignore pain (or perception of pain). The use of **mirror therapy** and motor imagery to override central nervous system processes arose via the potential to reconcile sensory feedback and motor output[76,77] and premotor cortex activation.[78] Mirror therapy involves movement of the unaffected extremity reflected in a mirror to appear as movement of the involved extremity which is hidden behind the mirror. Motor imagery involves mental thoughts of movement in the absence of actual movement, which activates similar cortical areas.[79] Several case series studies have demonstrated successful trends in treating early stages of CRPS with mirror therapy and motor imagery for decreasing pain, stiffness, and movement impairments.[79-81] However, a systematic review by Ezendam et al.[76] points to the weak methodological quality of mirror studies. In tandem with therapeutic approaches to modify perceptions and brain responses, it is vital that the physical therapist educate the patient about the mechanisms and purpose of pain and help her understand that pain is a complex consciousness experience which thereby requires the patient to participate actively in rehabilitation with both physical and mental effort.[79]

Last, there is some promising research on **acupuncture** in the treatment of CRPS.[82,83] Although the evidence is currently from case studies, the reported outcomes are impressive and worth exploring for this difficult diagnosis. In one case, a 34-year-old female with chronic CRPS demonstrated marked improvement in disability, pain, and depression following acupuncture interventions. She improved from a score of 17 down to 4 on the Sheehan Disability Scale; 67 down to 10 on the McGill Pain Questionnaire; and 12 down to 0 on the Beck Depression Inventory.[83] In another study, two out of the three pediatric patients with CRPS undergoing acupuncture demonstrated 100% resolution of pain and the third patient showed a significant 80% reduction.[84] Large-scale studies are needed to substantiate the benefit of acupuncture as part of a comprehensive intervention plan for CRPS.

It is important for all physical therapists to be educated on signs and symptoms to observe and measure and to be familiar with a plethora of intervention strategies to try with this patient population, while keeping in mind that a multidisciplinary team approach is often required to be most effective.[5,12,14,20] This syndrome can be quite challenging for the physical therapist to understand and treat. Early detection and intervention, especially after fractures in females over 50 years of age (a population at higher risk[7]) may help prevent a minor orthopaedic injury or stroke from progressing to a complex chronic pain problem.[14,20] Adjunctive alternative approaches, particularly meditation, deserve attention and further investigation not simply for acute and chronic pain populations but perhaps for wellness and prevention of disease in all individuals.

Evidence-Based Clinical Recommendations

SORT: Strength of Recommendation Taxonomy

A: Consistent, good-quality patient-oriented evidence
B: Inconsistent or limited-quality patient-oriented evidence
C: Consensus, disease-oriented evidence, usual practice, expert opinion, or case series

1. Use of a multidisciplinary treatment program including physical therapy is appropriate for complex regional pain syndrome (CRPS). **Grade A**

2. In individuals with CRPS affecting the upper extremity, the Disability of the Arm, Shoulder, and Hand (DASH) questionnaire is a reliable outcome measure for demonstrating change in upper extremity function and symptoms. **Grade A**

3. Mirror therapy is an effective technique for increasing functional use of the involved extremity in CRPS. **Grade C**

4. Acupuncture and meditation may be helpful in treatment of chronic pain in CRPS. **Grade C for acupuncture and Grade B for meditation**

COMPREHENSION QUESTIONS

26.1 All of the following signs and symptoms are indicative of CRPS type I in the upper extremity except:
   A. Brittle cracked fingernails
   B. Abnormal sweating
   C. Hypersensitivity to touch
   D. Injury to one of the peripheral nerves

26.2 Which of the following medical or psychological factors has the highest correlation with development of CRPS?
   A. Intra-articular fracture
   B. History of depression
   C. History of prior life events
   D. Both A and C

ANSWERS

26.1 **D.** Brittle fingernails, abnormal sweating, and hypersensitivity to touch are all indicative of CRPS type I. Direct injury to a nerve is the one distinctive feature of CRPS type II.

26.2 **D.** From this list, intra-articular fracture and history of significant life events in the year preceding development of CRPS have statistical support as being predictive of acquiring CRPS.

REFERENCES

1. Beerthuizan A, van't Spijker A, Huygen FJ, Klein J, de Wit R. Is there an association between psychological factors and the complex regional pain syndrome type I (CRPS1) in adults? A systematic review. *Pain*. 2009;145:52-59.

2. Beerthuizen A, Stronks DL, Huygen FJ, Passchier J, Klein J, Spijker AV. The association between psychological factors and the development of complex regional pain syndrome type I (CRPS1)—a prospective multicenter study. *Eur J Pain*. 2011;15:971-975.

3. Geertzen JH, de Bruijin-Kofman AT, de Bruijin HP, van de Wiel HB, Dijkstra PU. Stressful life events and psychological dysfunction in complex regional pain syndrome type I. *Clin J Pain*. 1998;14:143-147.

4. Turners-Stokes L. Reflex sympathetic dystrophy—a complex regional pain syndrome. *Disabil Rehabil*. 2002;24:939-947.

5. Berger P. The role of the physiotherapist in the treatment of complex peripheral pain syndromes. *Pain Reviews*. 1999;6:211-232.

6. Stanton-Hicks M, Janing W, Hassenbusch S, Haddox JD, Boas R, Wilson P. Reflex sympathetic dystrophy: changing concepts and taxonomy. *Pain*. 1995;63:127-133.

7. de Mos M, de Bruijn AG, Huygen FJ, Dieleman JP, Stricker BH, Sturkenboom MC. The incidence of complex regional pain syndrome: a population-based study. *Pain*. 2007;129:12-20.

8. Quisel A, Gill JM, Witherell P. Complex regional pain syndrome underdiagnosed. *J Fam Pract*. 2005;54:524-532.

9. Bruehl S, Chung OY. How common is complex regional pain syndrome—type I? *Pain*. 2007;129:1-2.

10. Wilson PR. Taxonomy. Newsletter of the IASP special interest group on pain and the sympathetic nervous system. 2004:4-6.

11. Beerthuizen A, Stronks DL, Van't Spijker A, et al. Demographic and medical parameters in the development of complex regional pain syndrome type I (CRPS1): prospective study of 596 patients with a fracture. *Pain*. 2012;153:1187-1192.

12. Harden RN. Complex regional pain syndrome. *Brit J Anaesth*. 2001;87:99-106.

13. National Institutes of Health, National Institute of Neurological Disorders and Stroke. Complex regional pain syndrome fact sheet. http://www.ninds.nih.gov/disorders/reflex_sympathetic_dystrophy. Accessed June 25, 2012.

14. Vacariu G. Complex regional pain syndrome. *Disabil Rehabil*. 2002;24:435-442.

15. Sandroni P, Benrud-Larson LM, McClelland RL, Low PA. Complex regional pain syndrome type I: incidence and prevalence in Olmsted county, a population-based study. *Pain*. 2003;103:199-207.

16. Petchkrua W, Weiss DJ, Patel RR. Reassessment of the incidence of complex regional pain syndrome type I following stroke. *Neurorehabil Neural Repair*. 2000;14:59-63.

17. Stanton-Hicks M, Baron R, Boas R, et al. Complex regional pain syndrome: guidelines for therapy. *Clin J Pain*. 1998;14:155-166.

18. Torebjork E, Wahren L, Wallin G, Hallin R, Koltzenburg M. Noradrenaline-evoked pain in neuralgia. *Pain.* 1995;63:11-20.

19. Sato J, Perl ER. Adrenergic excitation of cutaneous pain receptors induced by peripheral nerve injury. *Science.* 1991;251:1608-1610.

20. Birklein F. Complex regional pain syndrome. *J Neurol.* 2005;252:131-138.

21. Janig W, Baron R. Complex regional pain syndrome is a disease of the central nervous system. *Clin Auton Res.* 2002;12:150-164.

22. Juottonen K, Gockel M, Silen T, Hurri H, Hari R, Forss N. Altered central sensorimotor processing in patients with complex regional pain syndrome. *Pain.* 2002;98:315-323.

23. Rommel O, Gehling M, Dertwinkel R, et al. Hemisensory impairment in patients with complex regional pain syndrome. *Pain.* 1999;80:95-101.

24. Thimineur M, Sood P, Kravitz E, Gudin J, Kitaj M. Central nervous system abnormalities in complex regional pain syndrome: clinical and quantitative evidence of medullary dysfunction. *Clin J Pain.* 1998;14:256-267.

25. Schwoebel J, Friedman R, Duda N, Coslett HB. Pain and the body schema: evidence for peripheral effects on mental representations of movement. *Brain.* 2001;124:2098-2104.

26. Cohen HE, Hall J, Harris N, McCabe CS, Blake DR, Janig W. Enhanced pain and autonomic responses to ambiguous visual stimuli in chronic Complex Regional Pain Syndrome (CRPS) type I. *Eur J Pain.* 2012;16:182-195.

27. Schilder JM, Schouten AC, Perez RM, et al. Motor control in complex regional pain syndrome: a kinematic analysis. *Pain.* 2012;153:805-812.

28. Alexander GM, Peterlin BL, Perreault MJ, Grothusen JR, Schwartzman RJ. Changes in plasma cytokines and their soluble receptors in complex regional pain syndrome. *J Pain.* 2012;13:10-20.

29. Li WW, Guo TZ, Liang DY, Sun Y, Kingery WS, Clark JD. Substance P signaling controls mast cell activation, degranulation, and nociceptive sensitization in a rat fracture model of complex regional pain syndrome. *Anesthesiology.* 2012;116:882-895.

30. Huhne K, Leis S, Schmelz M, Rautenstrauss B, Birklein F. A polymorphic locus in the intron 16 of the human angiotensin-converting enzyme (ACE) gene is not correlated with complex regional pain syndrome I (CRPS I). *Eur J Pain.* 2004;8:221-225.

31. de Jong JR, Vlaeyen JW, de Gelder JM, Patijn J. Pain-related fear, perceived harmfulness of activities, and functional limitations in Complex regional pain syndrome. *J Pain.* 2011;12:1209-1218.

32. Astin JA. Mind-body therapies for the management of pain. *Clin J Pain.* 2004;20:27-32.

33. Orme-Johnson DW, Schneider RH, Son YD, Nidich S, Cho ZH. Neuroimaging of meditaiton's effect on brain reactivity to pain. *Neuroreport.* 2006;17:1359-1363.

34. Hsu ES. Practical management of complex regional pain syndrome. *Am J Ther.* 2009;16:147-154.

35. Lagueux E, Charest J, Lefrancois-Caron E, et al. Modified graded motor imagery for complex regional pain syndrome type I of the upper extremity in the acute phase: a patient series. *Int J Rehabil Res.* 2012;35:138-145.

36. Oerlemans HM, Oostendorp RA, de Boo T, Goris RJ. Pain and reduced mobility in complex regional pain syndrome I: outcome of a prospective randomized controlled clinical trial of adjuvant physical therapy versus occupational therapy. *Pain.*1999;83:77-83.

37. Beaton DE, Katz JN, Fossel AH, Wright JG, Tarasuk V, Bombardier C. Measuring the whole or the parts? Validity, reliability, and responsiveness of the Disabilities of the Arm, Shoulder, and Hand outcome measure in different regions of the upper extremity. *J Hand Ther.* 2001;14:128-146.

38. Bijur PE, Silver W, Gallagher EJ. Reliability of the visual analog scale for measurement of acute pain. *Acad Emerg Med.* 2001;8:1153-1157.

39. Atroshi I, Gummesson C, Andersson B, Dahlgren E, Johansson A. The disabilities of the arm, shoulder and hand (DASH) outcome questionnaire: reliability and validity of the Swedish Version evaluated in 176 patients. *Acta Orthop Scand.* 2000;71:613-618.

40. Mugge W, Schouten AC, Bast GJ, Schurmans J, van Hilten JJ, van der Helm FC. Stretch reflex responses in Complex Regional Pain Syndrome-related dystonia are not characterized by hyperreflexia. *Clin Neurophysiol.* 2012;123,569-576.

41. Bruehl S, Lubenow TR, Nath H, Ivankovich O. Validation of thermography in the diagnosis of reflex sympathetic dystrophy. *Clin J Pain.* 1996;12:316-25.

42. Moon JY, Park SY, Kim YC, et al. Analysis of patterns of three-phase bone scintigraphy for patients with complex regional pain syndrome diagnosed using the proposed research criteria (the 'Budapest Criteria'). *Br J Anaesth.* 2012;108:655-661.

43. Veldman PH, Reynen HM, Arntz IE, Goris RJ. Signs and symptoms of reflex sympathetic dystrophy: prospective study of 829 patients. *Lancet.* 1993;342:1012-1016.

44. Yarnitsky D. Quantitative sensory testing. *Muscle Nerve.* 1997;20:198-204

45. Oerlemans HM, Oostendorp RA, de Boo T, van der Laan L, Severens JL, Goris JA. Adjuvant physical therapy versus occupational therapy in patients with reflex sympathetic dystrophy/complex regional pain syndrome type I. *Arch Phys Med Rehabil.* 2000;81:49-56.

46. Kemler MA, Rijks CP, de Vet HC. Which patients with chronic reflex sympathetic dystrophy are most likely to benefit from physical therapy? *J Manipulative Physiol Ther.* 2001;24:272-278.

47. Lee BH, Scharff L, Sethna NF, et al. Physical therapy and cognitive-behavioral treatment for complex regional pain syndromes. *J Pediatr.* 2002;141:135-140.

48. Blumberg H, Griesser HJ, Hornyak M. Das distal posttraumatische Odem: symptom einer sympathischen reflexdystrophie? *Zeitschrift fur Orthopadie.* 1992;130:9-15.

49. Mucha C. Einflub von CO_2-Badern im fruhfunktionellen therapiekonzept der algodystrophie. *Physikalische Medizin und Kur Medizin.* 1992;2:173-178.

50. Lehmann JF, de Lateur BJ. Ultrasound, shortwave, microwave, superficial hot and cold in the treatment of pain. In: Wall PD, Melzack R, eds. *Textbook of Pain.* 3rd ed. Edinburgh: Churchill Livingstone; 1994:717-724.

51. Greipp ME, Thomas AF, Renkun C. Children and young adults with reflex sympathetic dystrophy syndrome. *Clin J Pain.* 1988;4:217-221.

52. Jenker FL. Die elektrische blockade von sympathischen und somatischen nerven von der haut aus. *Wierier Klinische Wochens-chrift.* 1980;92:233-239.

53. Robaina FJ, Rodriquez JL, de Vera JA, Martin MA. Transcutaneous electrical nerve stimulation and spinal cord stimulation for pain relief in reflex sympathetic dystrophy. *Stereotact Funct Neurosurg.* 1989;52:53-62.

54. Beric A. Central pain: "new" syndromes and their evaluation. *Muscle Nerve.* 1993;16:17-24.

55. Leijon G, Boivie J. Central post-stroke pain—the effect of high and low frequency TENS. *Pain.* 1989;38:187-191.

56. Bengtson K. Physical modalities for complex regional pain syndrome. *Hand Clin.* 1997;13:443-454.

57. Somers DL, Clemente FR. Transcutaneous electrical nerve stimulation for the management of neuropathic pain: the effects of frequency and electrode position on prevention of allodynia in a rat model of complex regional pain syndrome type II. *Phys Ther.* 2006;86:698-709.

58. Sadil V. Reflex sympathetic dystrophy management in physical medicine and rehabilitation. *Eur J Physical Medicine Rehab.* 1992;2:55-57.

59. Carlson LK, Watson HK. Treatment of reflex sympathetic dystrophy using the stress-loading program. *J Hand Ther.* 1998;1:149-154.

60. Husslage P. Physiotherapy and its regimen in the treatment of reflex sympathetic dystrophy. *Pain Clin.* 1995;8:77-79.

61. Kisner C, Colby L. *Therapeutic Exercise: Foundation and Techniques.* 5th ed. Philadelphia, PA: F.A. Davis Company; 2007.

62. Lee SS, Kim SH, Nah SS, et al. Smoking habits influence pain and functional and psychiatric features in fibromyalgia. *Joint Bone Spine.* 2011;78:259-265.

63. Schneider RH, Alexander CN, Staggers F, et al. A randomized controlled trial of stress reduction in African Americans treated for hypertension over one year. *Am J Hypertens.* 2005;18:88-98.

64. Anderson JW, Liu C, Kryscio RJ. Blood pressure response to transcendental meditation: a meta-analysis. *Am J Hypertens.* 2008;21:310-316.

65. Bairey Merz CN, Dwyer J, Nordstrom CK, Walton KG, Salerno JW, Schneider RH. Psychosocial stress and cardiovascular disease. *Behav Med.* 2002;27:141-147.

66. Schneider RH, Alexander CN, Staggers F, et al. Long-term effects of stress reduction on mortality in persons ≥ 55 years of age with systemic hypertension. *Am J Cardiol.* 2005;95:1060-1064.

67. Webster Marketon JI, Glaser R. Stress hormones and immune function. *Cellular Immunol.* 2008;252:16-26.

68. Kabat-Zinn J, Lipworth L, Burncy R, Sellers W. Four-year follow-up of a meditation-based program for the self-regulation of chronic pain: treatment outcomes and compliance. *Clin J Pain.* 1986;143-205.

69. Goleman DJ, Schwartz GE. Meditation as an intervention in stress reactivity. *J Counseling Clin Psych.* 1976;44:456-466.

70. Orme-Johnson DW. Autonomic stability and transcendental meditation. *Psychosom Med.* 1973;35:341-349.

71. Davidson RJ, Kabat-Zinn J, Schumacher J, et al. Alterations in brain and immune function produced by mindfulness meditation. *Psychosom Med.* 2003;65:564-570.

72. Jevning R, Wilson AF, Davidson JM. Adrenocortical activity during meditation. *Horm Behav.* 1978;10:54-60.

73. Orme-Johnson D. Medical care utilization and the transcendental meditation program. *Psychosomatic Med.* 1987;49:493-507.

74. Zeidan F, Gordon NS, Merchant J, Goolkasian P. The effects of brief mindfulness meditation on experimentally induced pain. *J Pain.* 2010;11:199-209.

75. Ek JW, van Gijn JC, Samwel H, van Egmond J, Klomp F, van Dongen RT. Pain exposure physical therapy may be a safe and effective treatment for longstanding complex regional pain syndrome type I: a case series. *Clin Rehabil.* 2009;23:1059-1066.

76. Ezendam D, Bonger RM, Jannink MJ. Systematic review of the effectiveness of mirror therapy in upper extremity function. *Disabil Rehabil.* 2009;31:2135-2149.

77. Ramachandran VS, Rogers-Ramachandran D, Cobb S. Touching the phantom limb. *Nature.* 1995;337:489-490.

78. Seitz RJ, Hoflich P, Binkofski F, Tellmann L, Herzog H, Freund HJ. Role of the premotor cortex in recovery from middle cerebral artery infarction. *Arch Neurol.* 1998;55:1081-1088.

79. Moseley GL. Graded motor imagery is effective for long-standing complex regional pain syndrome: a randomised controlled trial. *Pain.* 2004;108:192-198.

80. McCabe CS, Haigh RC, Ring EF, Haligan PW, Wall PD, Blake DR. A controlled pilot study of the utility of mirror visual feedback in the treatment of complex regional pain syndrome (type I). *Rheumatology.* 2003;42:97-101.

81. Tran de QH, Duong S, Bertini P, Finlayson RJ. Treatment of complex regional pain syndrome: a review of the evidence. *Can J Anaesth.* 2010;57:149-166.

82. Kho KH. The impact of acupuncture on pain in patients with reflex sympathetic dystrophy. *Pain Clin.* 1995;8:59-61.

83. Sprague M, Chang JC. Integrative approach focusing on acupuncture in the treatment of chronic complex regional pain syndrome. *J Altern Complement Med.* 2011;17:67-70.

84. Kelly A. Treatment of reflex sympathetic dystrophy in 3 pediatric patients using 7 external dragons and devils acupuncture. *Med Acupuncture.* 2004;15:29-30.

Statin-Induced Myopathy

Annie Burke-Doe

CASE 27

A 68-year-old obese female was referred to outpatient physical therapy for lower extremity pain and weakness. She is employed as a school teacher and recently fell on her knees while trying to lift a heavy box. She treated her knees with ice, elevation, compression, and an over-the-counter pain reliever, but she has continued to have weakness and generalized pain in her lower extremities for the last several weeks. Her primary care physician referred her to physical therapy for her persistent symptoms. The patient takes gemfibrozil, niacin, and atorvastatin calcium (Lipitor; 40 mg) to lower her cholesterol and LDL plasma levels. She has also been taking red yeast rice, which her herbalist recommended as a natural remedy to decrease "bad cholesterol." During the second week of physical therapy treatment, her bilateral lower extremity muscle and joint pain had not changed and she felt that her arms were becoming weak. She also complained of increased exertion while performing her activities of daily living—a symptom she had not previously experienced. Given the patient's progressive pain and weakness, new report of dyspnea on exertion, and current medication and supplement use, the physical therapist referred the patient back to her primary care physician for further evaluation. Laboratory values revealed elevated creatine kinase (isoenzyme CK-MM) in the blood and myoglobinuria. She was diagnosed with medication-induced myopathy.

▶ What examination signs may be associated with this diagnosis?
▶ What are the most appropriate examination tests?
▶ What are the most appropriate physical therapy outcome measures for pain and functional change?
▶ What is her rehabilitation prognosis?
▶ What are possible complications interfering with physical therapy?

KEY DEFINITIONS

GEMFIBROZIL: Antihyperlipidemic agent used in the treatment of very high serum triglyceride levels

MYOGLOBINURIA: Reddish urine caused by excretion of myoglobin, a breakdown product of muscle

MYOPATHY: Any abnormal condition or disease of (skeletal) muscle tissue

NIACIN: Water-soluble B-complex vitamin important in carbohydrate metabolism; niacin supplements reduce serum triglyceride and LDL cholesterol concentrations and increase HDL cholesterol concentration

RED YEAST RICE: Dietary supplement that is a fungus grown on rice; it contains monacolin K, which is identical to the cholesterol-lowering agent lovastatin

Objectives

1. Describe statin-induced myopathy.
2. Identify the signs, symptoms, and risk factors of statin-induced myopathy.
3. Discuss appropriate components of the physical therapy examination as it relates to identification of medication-induced myopathy versus exercise-induced myopathy.
4. Identify key referrals for the client suspected of statin-induced myopathy.

Physical Therapy Considerations

PT considerations during management of the individual with statin-induced myopathy:

▶ **General physical therapy plan of care/goals:** Identification of risk factors for statin-induced myopathy; assess range of motion (ROM), strength, tone, sensation, reflexes; functional testing

▶ **Physical therapy interventions:** Referral to physician for further evaluation to determine cause of myopathy after other potential explanations are ruled out; modification of exercise routines; regular reassessment of functional measures and strength

▶ **Precautions during physical therapy:** Report signs/symptoms suggesting statin-induced myopathy to the primary care provider

▶ **Complications interfering with physical therapy:** Muscle pain and weakness, generalized fatigue, psychosocial factors, comorbidities, adverse drug reactions (ADRs) of statins

Understanding the Health Condition

Approximately 33.6 million Americans have hyperlipidemia, defined as a total blood cholesterol level of 240 mg/dL or higher.[1] Hyperlipidemia increases the risk of atherosclerosis, stroke, and heart disease. Treatment includes dietary changes, increased physical activity, and the use of several classes of antihyperlipidemic medications. The most commonly prescribed antihyperlipidemic drug class is the HMG-CoA reductase inhibitors, or—the statins.[2,3] Statins inhibit the activity of HMG-CoA reductase, a key enzyme in the liver involved in the production of cholesterol. On average, statins reduce LDL cholesterol levels by 20% to 40%. An estimated 94.1 million American adults have been prescribed statins.[3] In properly selected patients, statins decrease cardiovascular disease morbidity and mortality by about 25%.[4,5] This has prompted recommendations for over-the-counter sale of statins in the United States.[6-8] Observational studies indicate a higher frequency of muscle complaints occurring in statin-taking groups than in control groups.[4,9] These studies suggest that the frequency of statin-induced myopathy is between 9% and 20%.[10-12] However, statin-related myopathy is thought to be even more prevalent than reported in controlled clinical trials because patients who are prone to this complication are often excluded from clinical trials.[4]

There is little consensus on the definition of statin-induced myopathy,[13] which may contribute to underdiagnosis of this complication.[14-16] The American Heart Association, American College of Cardiology, National Heart Lung and Blood Institute,[17] National Lipid Association,[18] and United States Food and Drug Administration[19] each include slightly different terms encompassing the range of signs and symptoms of statin-induced pathology. These include myalgia, myopathy, myositis, and rhabdomyolysis.[2,4] Myalgia, which can affect up to 10% of individuals taking prescribed statins,[2,4] is described as muscle ache, pain, or weakness *without* elevation in plasma creatine kinase (CK), a marker of muscle breakdown. Myopathy is a general term referring to any muscle disease with symptoms of myalgia, weakness, or cramps, plus an otherwise unexplained elevation in CK ≥ 10 times the upper limit of normal (ULN).[4] Myositis is defined as muscle symptoms *with* plasma CK elevation.[4] Rhabdomyolysis is the rarest and most severe adverse effect of statins. This condition results from acute necrosis of skeletal muscle fibers with subsequent leakage of their cellular contents into the circulation and urine (myoglobinuria). Rhabdomyolysis can produce asymptomatic illness with elevation of CK or a life-threatening condition associated with extreme elevations in CK, electrolyte imbalances, acute renal failure, and disseminated intravascular coagulation.[13] Rhabdomyolysis usually resolves after statin use is stopped, unless it is severe enough to cause death.[18] In a large observational study in France of almost 8000 hyperlipidemic patients receiving high-dosage statin therapy for at least 3 months prior to the study, 10.5% reported muscle-related symptoms over 12 months, with a median symptom onset time of 1 month following initiation of taking statins.[20] Among those who developed myopathy, major sites of pain were thighs and calves (or both), although about 25% of affected patients had generalized myalgia. Statin-related myalgia and myopathy typically resolve within a few weeks after statin therapy is discontinued.

Risk factors for statin-induced myopathy and rhabdomyolysis include (but are not limited to) high dosage of statin, polypharmacy, impaired hepatic and renal function, diabetes mellitus, untreated hypothyroidism, advanced age (> 65 years) and frailty, small body frame, infection, female sex, recent surgery, consumption of interacting drugs, and excessive alcohol intake.[4,16,18] Physical exercise appears to increase the likelihood for developing myopathy in patients taking statins.[20,21] As many as 25% of statin users who exercise may experience muscle fatigue, weakness, aches, and cramping that is attributed to exercise alone by both the patient and physician.[21,22] In a retrospective review of 22 elite professional athletes, Sinzinger and O'Grady[23] found that the majority did not tolerate statins because of exacerbated exercise-induced muscle pain.

Physical Therapy Patient/Client Management

Individuals with statin-induced myopathy may present to a physical therapist with pain, weakness, and complaints of functional difficulties. There may be a history of a precipitating event (surgery) or the patient may have risk factors and/or concomitant use of other cholesterol-lowering medications (fibrates, nicotinic acid), drugs that interact with statins such as azole antifungal agents, macrolide antibiotics, HIV protease inhibitors, antidepressants (nefazodone), immunosuppressants (cyclosporine), antiarrhythmics (amiodarone), calcium channel blockers (verapamil), and/or consumption of > 1 L of grapefruit juice per day (which contains a substance that inhibits statin metabolism).[24,25] Recognition of medication-induced muscle symptoms is critical, since all physical therapists screen and treat patients with musculoskeletal complaints. The physical therapist needs to be able to distinguish between exercise-induced muscle pain and drug-induced myopathy. Exercise that causes unaccustomed loads on muscle may cause delayed onset muscle soreness (DOMS). Exercise-induced muscle soreness typically does not occur immediately after exercise. Instead, progressive muscle pain with restricted range of motion of the affected muscle groups develops 12 to 48 hours after exercise and subsides within 96 hours.[26,27] In contrast, **individuals with statin-induced myopathy often describe their symptoms as muscle aches, pain, soreness, cramps, stiffness, weakness, or early muscle fatigue with exercise.**[25] Statin-induced muscle symptoms often involve large symmetrical[28] proximal muscle groups, with lower extremity or calf muscles affected more often than upper extremities.[20,29] Myopathy caused by statins most commonly occurs within the first 6 weeks of statin initiation, when the statin dose is increased, and/or when another medication that affects the metabolism of statins is initiated.[20]

Examination, Evaluation, and Diagnosis

The patient examination requires a thorough subjective history and careful questioning about all prescriptions and over-the-counter medication use, physical activity (regular activity and any increase in exercise frequency, intensity, or type), occupation, alcohol consumption, and recreational drug use.[25] Information about the use of dietary and sports supplements is also important because rhabdomyolysis has been reported in association with the use of some supplements (*e.g.*, anabolic steroids, caffeine, guarana, and other stimulants), especially when their use is combined with strenuous muscle exertion.[30-33] Alcohol consumption and vitamin E use can also be occasional causes of muscle symptoms falsely attributed to statin therapy.[9] In the case of this patient, she reported taking the "natural" cholesterol-lowering agent red yeast rice. Red yeast rice is lovastatin. Thus, she is at an increased risk of statin-induced myopathy because she is consuming a higher statin dose—from the Lipitor and the red yeast rice—than was intended by her prescriber. To facilitate the differential diagnosis, additional questions should be asked related to the patient's onset, pattern, and duration of muscle weakness and her current exercise regimen. Complaints of muscle-specific weakness (*e.g.*, DOMS) or fatigue because of strength training affected muscles should resolve in 48 to 72 hours after the exercise bout,[27] allowing the therapist to potentially rule out exercise-induced muscle pain if complaints persist beyond this timeframe.

The examination should include testing ROM, strength, flexibility, sensation, reflexes, and functional testing as well as palpation of symptomatic muscles. The musculoskeletal examination focuses on excluding other conditions that cause muscle pain such as tendinopathies, arthropathies, fibromyalgia, and myofascial pain syndromes. A muscle dynamometer and handgrip strength dynamometer (*e.g.*, Jamar) should be used for **quantitative and precise strength measurements** that can be tracked over subsequent visits. These measurements can be helpful when referring the patient back to the physician because measurements of muscle strength assist with tracking recovery from myopathy as well as during subsequent statin rechallenges (*i.e.*, when the individual takes a statin again after 6 weeks of discontinuation of a statin).[9] During the evaluation, the therapist should identify the pattern of weakness. Although important exceptions exist, weakness that is predominantly proximal (shoulder and hip girdle) is usually indicative of a myopathic disorder whereas weakness that is predominantly distal (extremities) may indicate a neuropathic condition. Segmental weakness involving selected myotomes in a multifocal distribution may implicate a motor neuropathy (disorder of anterior horn cells). Task-specific fatigable weakness raises suspicion of a disorder of neuromuscular transmission.[34] Statin-induced weakness may involve muscles not recently exercised and symptoms may progress or fail to show signs of improvement even after several days of rest.[35] Statin-induced muscle symptoms often involve large symmetrical[28] proximal muscle groups, with major sites of pain in the thighs, calves, or both.[20,25]

Functional assessments can include a stair climbing test and the Six-Minute Walk Test, which may identify performance levels below those of age-matched norms or unexpected declines in the patient's functional status.[35,36] These tests have the advantage of functionally measuring the clinical presentation of statin-associated myopathies that include lower extremity pain and weakness as well as proximal muscle weakness.[37,38]

In the current case, the patient's pain began in her lower extremities and progressed to her upper extremities despite not having exercised her arms. Thus, she presented with a pattern of generalized weakness. She also complained of generalized fatigue with activities of daily living. Exercise-induced muscle fatigue and soreness would be limited to muscles previously exercised and should have resolved within a few days, which was not the case. Key risk factors for statin-induced myopathy in this patient's case include combined use of statins (red yeast rice and Lipitor), concomitant use of additional other cholesterol-lowering agents (gemfibrozil, niacin), sex (female), and older age.

Plan of Care and Interventions

Patient education on signs and symptoms that may indicate adverse effects of statin use is appropriate. The physical therapist must notify the physician regarding results of the physical therapy evaluation and request that the patient have further evaluation for her symptoms.[35] If medical examination confirms statin-related myopathy, both the treating physician and the physical therapist should devise a plan of care suitable for the patient's recovery from the adverse effects. Counseling regarding therapeutic lifestyle changes, including reduction of saturated fat and cholesterol, increased physical activity, and weight control, should be part of the management of all patients with hypercholesterolemia or cardiovascular disease. Since millions of Americans are prescribed statins to reduce hyperlipidemia, physical therapists will play an increasingly important role in detecting statin-induced myopathy, providing more complete information to patients regarding identification and prognosis of the condition, and reducing the likelihood of serious disability.

Evidence-Based Clinical Recommendations

SORT: Strength of Recommendation Taxonomy
A: Consistent, good-quality patient-oriented evidence
B: Inconsistent or limited-quality patient-oriented evidence
B: Consensus, disease-oriented evidence, usual practice, expert opinion, or case series

1. The risk of myopathy and rhabdomyolysis is increased by high doses of statins. **Grade A**

2. Clinical presentation of statin-induced myopathy often occurs within the first 6 weeks of statin initiation as muscle aches, pain, cramps, stiffness, or weakness in large symmetrical proximal muscle groups with lower extremity or calf muscles affected more often than upper extremities. **Grade B**

3. Quantitative strength measurements assist with tracking recovery from myopathy as well as during subsequent statin rechallenges. **Grade C**

COMPREHENSION QUESTIONS

27.1 Statin-related myopathy is associated with which of the following risk factors?
   A. Advanced age
   B. Female sex
   C. High dosage of statin
   D. All of the above

27.2 Which of the following serum cholesterol levels would be considered hyper-lipidemia?
   A. 120 mg/dL
   B. 180 mg/dL
   C. 200 mg/dL
   D. 240 mg/dL

ANSWERS

27.1 **D.** The Muscle Expert Panel[39] affirms that the frequency of statin-associated muscle complaints has been documented to increase with increasing statin serum concentration in humans and in animal models. Factors that elevate statin concentrations in blood, and possibly in muscle, are likely to increase statin-related muscle complaints. These include the statin dose and use of concomitant medications interfering with statin metabolism via either the cytochrome P450 (CYP) or glucuronidation processes. Advanced age is a risk factor, likely due to the decreased elimination of drugs in older adults. Female sex is also a risk factor for statin-induced myopathy.

27.2 **D.** Total blood cholesterol levels of ≥240 mg/dL result in the diagnosis of hyperlipidemia.[1]

REFERENCES

1. Roger VL, Go AS, Lloyd-Jones DM, et al. Executive summary: heart disease and stroke statistics—2012 update: a report from the American Heart Association. *Circulation.* 2012;125:188-197.

2. Bays H. Statin safety: an overview and assessment of the data—2005. *Am J Cardiol.* 2006;97:6C-26C.

3. The Use of Medicines in the United States: Review of 2010 Report. 2010. http://www.imshealth.com/portal/site/ims/menuitem.856807fe5773bfb9ec895c973208c22a/?vgnextoid=5687ce9e0a99f210VgnVCM10000071812ca2RCRD&vgnextfmt=default. Accessed February 14, 2013.

4. Joy TR, Hegele RA. Narrative review: statin-related myopathy. *Ann Intern Med.* 2009;150:858-868.

5. Baigent C, Keech A, Kearney PM, et al. Efficacy and safety of cholesterol-lowering treatment: prospective meta-analysis of data from 90,056 participants in 14 randomised trials of statins. *Lancet.* 2005;366:1267-1278.

6. Kraft S. Pfizer seeks to develop OTC Lipitor product as patent runs out. *Medical News Today.* August 5, 2011. http://www.medicalnewstoday.com./articles/232357.php. Accessed February 15, 2013.

7. Brass EP, Allen SE, Melin JM. Potential impact on cardiovascular public health of over-the-counter statin availability. *Am J Cardiol.* 2006;97:851-856.

8. Gemmell I, Verma A, Harrison RA. Should we encourage over-the-counter statins? A population perspective for coronary heart disease prevention. *Am J Cardiovasc Drugs.* 2007;7:299-302.

9. Fernandez G, Spatz ES, Jablecki C, Phillips PS. Statin myopathy: a common dilemma not reflected in clinical trials. *Cleve Clin J Med.* 2011;78:393-403.

10. de Sauvage Nolting PR, Buirma RJ, Hutten BA, Kastelein JJ. Two-year efficacy and safety of simvastatin 80 mg in familial hypercholesterolemia (the Examination of Probands and Relatives in Statin Studies With Familial Hypercholesterolemia [ExPRESS FH]). *Am J Cardiol.* 2002;90:181-184.

11. Franc S, Dejager S, Bruckert E, Chauvenet M, Giral P, Turpin G. A comprehensive description of muscle symptoms associated with lipid-lowering drugs. *Cardiovasc Drugs Ther.* 2003;17:459-465.

12. Kashani A, Phillips CO, Foody JM, et al. Risks associated with statin therapy: a systematic overview of randomized clinical trials. *Circulation.* 2006;114:2788-2797.

13. Huerta-Alardin AL, Varon J, Marik PE. Bench-to-bedside review: rhabdomyolysis—an overview for clinicians. *Crit Care.* 2005;9:158-169.

14. Tomlinson SS, Mangione KK. Potential adverse effects of statins on muscle. *Phys Ther.* 2005;85:459-465.

15. Thompson PD, Clarkson P, Karas RH. Statin-associated myopathy. *JAMA.* 2003;289:1681-1690.

16. Hansen KE, Hildebrand JP, Ferguson EE, Stein JH. Outcomes in 45 patients with statin-associated myopathy. *Arch Intern Med.* 2005;165:2671-2676.

17. Pasternak RC, Smith SC, Jr., Bairey-Merz CN, Grundy SM, Cleeman JI, Lenfant C. ACC/AHA/NHLBI Clinical Advisory on the Use and Safety of Statins. *Stroke.* 2002;33:2337-2341.

18. McKenney JM, Davidson MH, Jacobson TA, Guyton JR. Final conclusions and recommendations of the National Lipid Association Statin Safety Assessment Task Force. *Am J Cardiol.* 2006;97:89C-94C.

19. Sewright KA, Clarkson PM, Thompson PD. Statin myopathy: incidence, risk factors, and pathophysiology. *Curr Atheroscler Rep.* 2007;9:389-396.

20. Bruckert E, Hayem G, Dejager S, Yau C, Begaud B. Mild to moderate muscular symptoms with high-dosage statin therapy in hyperlipidemic patients—the PRIMO study. *Cardiovasc Drugs Ther.* 2005;19:403-414.

21. Dirks AJ, Jones KM. Statin-induced apoptosis and skeletal myopathy. *Am J Physiol Cell Physiol.* 2006;291:C1208-C1212.

22. Sinzinger H, Wolfram R, Peskar BA. Muscular side effects of statins. *J Cardiovasc Pharmacol.* 2002;40:163-171.

23. Sinzinger H, O'Grady J. Professional athletes suffering from familial hypercholesterolaemia rarely tolerate statin treatment because of muscular problems. *British J Clin Pharmacol.* 2004;57:525-528.

24. Egan A, Colman E. Weighing the benefits of high-dose simvastatin against the risk of myopathy. *N Engl J Med.* 2011;365:285-287.

25. Buettner C, Lecker SH. Molecular basis for statin-induced muscle toxicity: implications and possibilities. *Pharmacogenomics.* 2008;9:1133-1142.

26. American College of Sports Medicine. *Delayed Onset Muscle Soreness (DOMS),* 2011. http://www.acsm.org/docs/brochures/delayed-onset-muscle-soreness-(doms).pdf. Accessed February 14, 2013.

27. Connolly DA, Sayers SP, McHugh MP. Treatment and prevention of delayed onset muscle soreness. *J Strength Cond Res.* 2003;17:197-208.

28. Spatz ES, Canavan ME, Desai MM. From here to JUPITER. Identifying new patients for statin therapy using data from the 1999-2004 National Health and Nutrition Examination Survey. *Circ Cardiovasc Qual Outcomes.* 2009;2:41-48.

29. Buettner C, Davis RB, Leveille SG, Mittleman MA, Mukamal KJ. Prevalence of musculoskeletal pain and statin use. *J Gen Intern Med.* 2008;23:1182-1186.

30. Kamijo Y, Soma K, Asari Y, Ohwada T. Severe rhabdomyolysis following massive ingestion of oolong tea: caffeine intoxication with coexisting hyponatremia. *Vet Hum Toxicol.* 1999;41:381-383.

31. Mansi IA, Huang J. Rhabdomyolysis in response to weight-loss herbal medicine. *Am J Med Sci.* 2004;327:356-357.

32. Braseth NR, Allison EJ, Jr., Gough JE. Exertional rhabdomyolysis in a body builder abusing anabolic androgenic steroids. *Eur J Emergency Med.* 2001;8:155-157.

33. Donadio V, Bonsi P, Zele I, et al. Myoglobinuria after ingestion of extracts of guarana, Ginkgo biloba and kava. *Neurol Sci.* 2000;21:124.

34. David WS, Chad DA, Kambadakone A, Hedley-Whyte ET. Case records of the Massachusetts General Hospital. Case 7-2012. A 79-year-old man with pain and weakness in the legs. *N Engl J Med.* 2012;366:944-954.

35. Di Stasi SL, MacLeod TD, Winters JD, Binder-Macleod SA. Effects of statins on skeletal muscle: a perspective for physical therapists. *Phys Ther.* 2010;90:1530-1542.

36. Kennedy DM, Stratford PW, Wessel J, Gollish JD, Penney D. Assessing stability and change of four performance measures: a longitudinal study evaluating outcome following total hip and knee arthroplasty. *BMC Musculoskelet Disord.* 2005;6:3.

37. Phillips PS, Haas RH, Bannykh S, et al. Statin-associated myopathy with normal creatine kinase levels. *Ann Intern Med.* 2002;137:581-585.

38. Bennett WE, Drake AJ, 3rd, Shakir KM. Reversible myopathy after statin therapy in patients with normal creatine kinase levels. *Ann Intern Med.* 2003;138:436-437.

39. Thompson PD, Clarkson PM, Rosenson RS. An assessment of statin safety by muscle experts. *Am J Cardiol.* 2006;97:69C-76C.

Cerebral Palsy

Sheryl A. Low

CASE 28

A 5-year-old girl was referred to the school district physical therapist for an evaluation before she enrolls in kindergarten. Her medical and physical therapy records document a diagnosis of cerebral palsy—spastic diplegia. She has received Early Intervention (EI) services (physical, occupational, and speech therapy) at home for 3 years. The child wears an articulating lightweight ankle-foot orthosis (AFO) and ambulates at a very slow speed with a handheld posterior walker for distances of up to 30 ft. She is able to sit in a chair for activities, but her postural control is only fair. She requires extra time to move from a chair to standing in the walker, and has difficulty negotiating her walker around obstacles. The physical therapist is asked to evaluate the child and develop the physical therapy plan for achieving functional mobility outcomes in the school setting in consultation with her family and teachers. The report will be part of the Individualized Education Plan (IEP). Along with the IEP team, the physical therapist will determine what level of physical therapy services she will receive as part of her educational plan.

▶ Based on her health condition, what do you anticipate will be the contributors to activity limitations?
▶ What are the examination priorities?
▶ What are the most appropriate physical therapy outcome measures for functional mobility for children with spastic diplegia cerebral palsy in the school setting?
▶ What are possible secondary impairments for children with cerebral palsy?

KEY DEFINITIONS

CEREBRAL PALSY (CP): Group of permanent activity-limiting disorders of movement and posture development that are attributed to nonprogressive disturbances that occurred in the developing fetal or infant brain; motor disorders are often accompanied by disturbances of sensation, cognition, communication, perception, behavior, and/or by epilepsy, and by secondary musculoskeletal problems

INDIVIDUALIZED EDUCATION PLAN (IEP): Plan mandated under federal law called the Individuals with Disabilities Education Act (IDEA); developed annually by the family, school personnel and occupational, physical, and speech therapists, as indicated by the child's level of functioning; plan may include provision of physical therapy in the school setting, if the team determines it is needed to help the child achieve his/her educational goals[1]

Objectives

1. Describe the impairments and functional and activity limitations affecting children with cerebral palsy.
2. Identify key questions to determine the priorities of the child and family in the physical therapy plan of care.
3. Identify reliable and valid outcome tools to measure a child's mobility and level of functioning in school.
4. Discuss appropriate components of the examination for the child with cerebral palsy.

Physical Therapy Considerations

PT considerations during management of the child with mobility, activity, and participation limitations in the school setting due to cerebral palsy—spastic diplegia:

▶ **General physical therapy plan of care/goals:** Assess gait and mobility in the school setting including transitions to and from classroom seating, bathroom/toileting, and meal/snack times; assessment of necessary equipment and adaptations; maximize child's ability to participate in school-related activities with functional independence and safety while minimizing secondary impairments

▶ **Physical therapy interventions:** Patient/teacher/family education on level of assistance required for safe execution of tasks; strengthening, home stretching program, balance and postural control activities, functional mobility training, partial weightbearing treadmill training for endurance conditioning; coordination and communication with the IEP team

▶ **Precautions during physical therapy:** Possible comorbidities (e.g., seizure disorders); secondary impairments such as muscle contractures, hip subluxation, bony deformities, and poor cardiovascular endurance due to lower activity levels

▶ **Complications interfering with physical therapy:** Child's cognitive level and motivation; family's priorities and cultural understanding of child's disorder and potential; growth spurts require frequent checking of proper fit of equipment and orthotics and changes in muscle length affecting range of motion

Understanding the Health Condition

Cerebral palsy (CP) is a comprehensive term describing a cluster of disorders involving nervous system and brain functions including movement, learning, hearing, seeing, and thinking.[2] People with CP have motor disabilities linked to early damage in brain areas responsible for motor behaviors, which influences movement, muscle control, coordination, tone, reflexes, posture and balance, gross and fine motor skills, and oral motor performance.[3] While the posture and movement disorders can change and progress over time, the original insult to the brain is nonprogressive.[2] Even though the degree of the lesion remains unchanged, the sequelae vary with increased age due to abnormal motor patterns the child utilizes to compensate for decreased motor and postural control and deficiencies in motor learning. The patterns of abnormal movement are highly variable and largely dependent on the etiology, site, and degree of the initial damage.[3]

CP is the result of damage to specific parts of the developing brain, and can occur in utero or within the first few years of life while the brain is still developing. It can be caused by a variety of factors occurring prenatally, perinatally, or postnatally. Risk factors for CP include low birth weight, infection of the mother during pregnancy, premature birth, insufficient oxygen or blood flow to the brain in the womb, Rh disease, multiparity, head trauma (such as shaken baby syndrome), complications during labor and delivery, low Apgar score, seizures, and jaundice in the infant.[4] Recent literature has shown the risk factors of greatest importance are low birth weight, intrauterine infections, and multiple gestations.[3] In a literature review spanning the past 40 years, Odding et al.[4] found that infants born at 32 to 42 weeks with birth weights below the 10th percentile were as much as six times more likely to have CP than infants with birth weights in the 25th to 75th percentile. Infants that are carried to full-term but have been exposed to intrauterine infections have a 4.7% risk of having CP and if there is an intrauterine infection in an infant with low birth weight, the risk increases four times.[4] Multiparity increases the risk of CP as well; the prevalence is 12.6 per thousand with twins, and 44.8 per thousand with triplets.[5]

In the United States, about 2 to 3 children per thousand have CP. The United Cerebral Palsy Foundation estimates that there are 800,000 people living with CP in the United States.[6] There is no correlation in the prevalence of CP with gender, ethnicity, or socioeconomic status. Currently, the life expectancy for individuals with CP is between 29 and 37 years.[7] Life expectancy varies depending on severity as well as the person's level of mobility. The incidence of CP has increased significantly over the last 40 years, which can be partially attributed to advances in neonatal medical services leading to an increased survival rate of premature infants.[8]

There is a wide variety of impairments and functional limitations specific to CP. Common impairments include decreased range of motion (ROM), strength deficits, decreased motor control, abnormal tone, impaired balance reactions, and abnormal reflexes. Odding et al.[4] found 100% of people diagnosed with CP have motor impairments, the most common of which is spasticity. The severity of spasticity is variable based on the type of CP, as well as the extent of the insult to the brain. Spasticity alters the individual's functional mobility and ease of performance of activities of daily living (ADLs) including feeding, bathing, dressing, and toileting. Additional consequences of spasticity include pain, contractures, bowel and bladder problems, and sleep deficits. Other impairments related to CP include cognitive deficits (23%-44%), speech and language deficits (42%-81%), vision deficits (62%-71%), hearing deficits (25%), epilepsy (22%-40%), feeding and growth abnormalities, seizures, and behavioral and emotional disorders.[2]

A physician traditionally makes the diagnosis of CP; however, the physical therapist can play a vital role in the diagnostic process. For example, the physical therapist may note critical developmental delays, such as delayed reaching, sitting, rolling, crawling, or walking.[2] If developmental delays are noticed, the physical therapist can initiate a follow-up visit with a physician so diagnostic imaging can be performed. There is no single specific gold standard for the diagnosis of CP. The physician first evaluates the child's motor skills, observing for the most typical symptoms including abnormal muscle tone, slow development, and atypical posture, as well as positively confirming the child's condition is *not* worsening. Second, neuroimaging (cranial ultrasound [US], computed tomography [CT] scan, or magnetic resonance imaging [MRI]) may be performed to rule out other movement disorders and to determine the site and nature of damage to the brain.

Neuroimaging is currently the primary method of diagnosing CP in children. Most physicians prefer MRI due to the fine level of detail it provides. A 2004 study by Mirmiran et al.[9] found the sensitivity and specificity of MRI for diagnosing CP in children aged 20 months was 71% and 91%, respectively, and 86% and 89% in children aged 31 months. The study also included cranial US as a method for predicting CP, and found sensitivity and specificity of 29% and 86% in children aged 20 months, and 43% and 82% in children aged 31 months. In 2010, Hnatyszyn et al.[10] found the sensitivity for predicting CP in 47 term and preterm infants using MRI was 100%; specificity was also high (75% and 72%, respectively).

The diagnosis of CP is usually classified based on the form of movement disorder involved.[4] There are three specific kinds: spastic, dyskinetic, and ataxic. Spastic CP is characterized by stiff muscles during movement. Spastic CP may involve the arm and hand unilaterally, and is therefore further classified as spastic hemiplegia or hemiparesis. Spastic hemiplegia/hemiparesis can also affect the leg. Walking is often delayed, and children frequently walk on their toes secondary to tight heel cords. Speech is also frequently delayed with spastic CP, although intelligence is typically normal. In spastic diplegia and diparesis, spasticity is primarily in both legs. The arms and hands may be affected, though with much less severity. The most severe form of CP is spastic quadriplegia/quadriparesis. It is frequently associated with mental retardation.[6] Speaking capability as well as comprehension of the spoken word is minimal. Those affected generally have hypotonicity of the cervical muscles and significant spasticity in their limbs, making ambulation nearly impossible. Dyskinetic CP (also called athetoid, choreoathetoid, and dystonic) is characterized by a combination of hypertonia and hypotonia and may include slow, uncontrolled writhing movements of the hands, feet, arms, or legs.[4] Mixed tone leads to difficulty maintaining upright positions and poor fine motor control. The muscle coordination necessary for speaking may be impaired and hyperactive tongue and facial muscles may cause grimacing and/or drooling. Ataxic CP is rare; it affects the cerebellum and can cause tremors and hypotonia. Coordination deficits are noticeable. Children with ataxic CP have difficulty with rapid or precise movements, and may also demonstrate an intention tremor. Ambulation is impaired, characterized by unsteadiness and an unusually large base of support. It is common for some children to have symptoms of CP that are not consistent with one particular kind of CP (e.g., excessive spasticity in some muscles and hypotonicity in others). In cases where no specific categorization is apparent, the diagnosis becomes known as "mixed type" CP.

Children with CP are also classified according to their level of motor functioning consistent with current concepts of disability, functional limitations, and ability to participate in age-related activities. The **Gross Motor Function Classification System** (GMFCS) was developed by researchers at the CanChild Centre for Childhood Disability at McMaster University in Canada in 1997. The GMFCS classifies individuals with CP into five levels according to functional ability, impairment limitation, mobility, and self-sufficiency (Table 28-1).[11]

Over a 4-year period, Rosenbaum et al.[12] studied 657 children to determine the stability of the GMFCS and they were able to create motor development curves for each level. This allows the physical therapist and physician to predict when the majority of children might reach 90% of their motor function potential. For example, if a child is initially classified as GMFCS Level II, according to the motor development curves, 50% of children in that category reach their highest level of motor function and plateau at age 4.5 years. This prediction assists the therapist in planning the type of therapy interventions and goals by age and classification. Another study has correlated the GMFCS level and the performance by children

Table 28-1 GROSS MOTOR FUNCTION CLASSIFICATION SYSTEM LEVELS FOR CHILDREN WITH CEREBRAL PALSY	
Level I	Walks without restrictions, limitations in more advanced gross motor skills
Level II	Walks without assistive devices; limitations walking outdoors and in the community
Level III	Walks with assistive mobility devices; limitations walking outdoors and in the community, can sit on his own, or with limited support
Level IV	Self-mobility with limitations; children are transported or use power mobility outdoors and in the community, needs support when sitting
Level V	Self-mobility is severely limited even with the use of assistive technology, lacks head and trunk control

using the Gross Motor Function Measure, justifying the use of the GMFCS as a classification level for clinical outcomes.[13]

Physical Therapy Patient/Client Management

Children with CP have a decreased ability to walk efficiently and participate in play and sports activities, which leads to an inability to maintain sufficient strength and cardiorespiratory fitness.[14] It is estimated that 75% of children with CP are ambulatory (and function at a GMFCS Level III or higher).[15] Children with an inability to walk, or who walk with restrictions participate less in social activities with friends compared to those who walk without restrictions.[16] Researchers asked 585 parents of children with CP to identify family priorities for activity and participation. Sixty-one percent identified mobility as a priority (second to self-care).[17] It is critical for physical therapists and the IEP team to identify what the optimal interventions are to improve mobility and function in order to maintain sufficient strength for ADLs, increase cardiorespiratory fitness, and improve the child's overall quality of life related to improving her ability to participate in school and social activities. According to the Individuals with Disabilities Education Act, children are entitled to physical therapy services to maximize their ability to obtain their education.[1] Under this law, children with eligible conditions are evaluated for physical therapy services and in conjunction with the family and educational team, goals for the school year are determined, and the physical therapist provides direct and consultation services in order to meet their educational goals.

Examination, Evaluation, and Diagnosis

The physical therapist needs to acquire information from the medical record and thorough interviews with the parents or caregiver(s). Relevant information to obtain includes the child's birth history, motor milestones, any diagnostic testing, parental concerns, and the child's current level of development. It is also essential to determine the child's and family's priorities based on the child's age and cognitive abilities. According to the *Guide to Physical Therapist Practice*[18] and recent clinical management recommendations for children with CP-Spastic Diplegia[19] to achieve functional mobility outcomes, the examination should start with questions about the child's level of functional mobility at home and school. The examination also includes a systems review and use of specific tests and measures to determine the impairments, functional limitations, and limitations in activity and participation for a same-aged child. In addition to determination of GMFCS level, the therapist can assess the child's motor function using the **Gross Motor Function Measure (GMFM)**. The GMFM measures change in five dimensions including lying and rolling, sitting, crawling and kneeling, standing, and walking, running, jumping. The GMFM is a standardized, reliable, and valid instrument used to detect change in motor skills of children with CP.[20] To assist in identifying the child's current functional level, the physical therapist can use the Pediatric Evaluation of Disability Inventory (PEDI).[21] The PEDI is a standardized assessment tool that measures functional performance

Table 28-2   SAMPLE QUESTIONS FOR ASSESSMENT OF STUDENT IN SCHOOL SETTING
Can the child get on and off the bus independently?
Can the child use the toilet independently in the school setting?
Is the child independent up and down steps or stairs?
Can the child negotiate heavy doors to access the classroom and outdoors?
Are the teachers and aides able to facilitate and assist the child in his/her functional skills?
What kind of training and support in the classroom is required to maximize the student's motor performance?
How long can the child sit in a regular classroom chair to attend to desk and cognitive activities and does the child need modifications to participate in classroom activities?
Does the child have access to the playground and what modifications are needed to improve activity and participation during recess?

and caregiver assistance in the domains of self-care, mobility, and social function in the home and community setting, and is valid for children with disabilities aged 6 months to 7 years.[21] To help set goals for program planning, the physical therapist can use the **School Function Assessment (SFA)**. The SFA is a similar assessment tool, but is valid for children with disabilities from kindergarten to sixth grade and consists of three sections that include all mobility in the school setting: participation, task supports, and activity performance.[22] In order to assess functional limitations and participation, the physical therapist should observe the child's daily mobility routines, including those at home and in the school setting. The physical therapist should also identify how assistive/adaptive devices and orthoses influence mobility. Examples of tasks that must be assessed are listed in Table 28-2.

Plan of Care and Interventions

Specific physical therapy goals are set after the evaluation and should conform to the overarching educational goals of the IEP team. Goals should be attainable and measurable within the school year and include considerations for the child's age and context. This requires identification of primary impairments, dysfunction, and functional limitations such as limitations in walking speed, transitions from walking to sitting, and sitting endurance and posture as well as limitations in activity and participation compared to age-equivalent children. The physical therapist should monitor areas of risk for secondary impairments such as loss of ROM and muscle contractures in spastic muscles, and postural impairments of scoliosis and bony deformities of the lower extremities. Physical therapy interventions most commonly used for treating children with spastic diplegic CP include **strengthening through a functional exercise program**,[23,24] electrical stimulation,[25] bicycling, aquatics, and hippotherapy.[26-28] Improved strength is correlated to improved posture and balance in children with CP.[29] Other treatment interventions include positioning and stretching activities to improve biomechanical alignment, balance and postural activities using neurodevelopmental therapy techniques, activities on an exercise ball, or practice of mobility on uneven or rough surfaces.[30] Partial weightbearing **treadmill training** has also been shown to improve gait parameters and improve overall cardiovascular endurance in children with CP.[31,32]

Evidence-Based Clinical Recommendations

SORT: Strength of Recommendation Taxonomy

A: Consistent, good-quality patient-oriented evidence
B: Inconsistent or limited-quality patient-oriented evidence
C: Consensus, disease-oriented evidence, usual practice, expert opinion, or case series

1. Children with cerebral palsy can be classified according to their functional mobility level using the Gross Motor Functional Classification Scale. **Grade A**

2. Physical therapists can use the Gross Motor Function Measure to measure incremental changes in motor function over time for children with CP. **Grade A**

3. Physical therapists can use the School Function Assessment to identify functional mobility in the school setting, assistance needed from adults, and adaptations and modifications to the environment for optimal functioning. **Grade B**

4. Strengthening, functional mobility training, and treadmill training improve gait and endurance in children with CP. **Grade B**

COMPREHENSION QUESTIONS

28.1 Cerebral palsy is usually diagnosed in the first few years of life and can be categorized in several ways. A child who is demonstrating abnormal postural responses, limitations in selective motor control, and stiff or rigid muscles primarily in the lower extremities would *most* likely be diagnosed based on these clinical signs and symptoms with which of the following types of CP?

    A. Ataxic

    B. Dyskinetic

    C. Quadriplegic

    D. Spastic diplegic

28.2 A physical therapist that is working with a child in the school setting with a diagnosis of CP spastic diplegia must also be concerned with secondary impairments. Typical concerns as a child grows include which of the following?

    A. Obesity and diabetes

    B. Pressure sores and muscle hypertrophy

    C. Muscle contractures, scoliosis, bony deformities

    D. Swallowing disorders, dysphagia

ANSWERS

28.1 **D.** Children with stiff muscles display spasticity in their muscles when they try to move. While their muscles are stiff due to spasticity, they are generally weak and demonstrate more weakness on one side of the body. Children who demonstrate more weakness and spasticity in their legs than their upper extremities are categorized as CP spastic diplegia. Their primary movement disorder is a paucity of movement.

28.2 **C.** Children with CP are at risk for secondary impairments due to the chronic effects of spasticity and postural weakness. As children age, they may develop muscle contractures in their heel cords and hamstrings as well as scoliosis due to trunk and postural weakness. Physical therapists should develop a preventive home stretching and strengthening program and continue to monitor areas of possible secondary impairments.

REFERENCES

1. McEwen I. *Providing Physical Therapy Services under Parts B & C of the Individuals with Disabilities Education Act (IDEA)*. Alexandria, VA: Section on Pediatrics, American Physical Therapy Association; 2009.

2. Rosenbaum P, Paneth N, Leviton A, et al. A report: the definition and classification of cerebral palsy April 2006. *Dev Med Child Neurol Suppl*. 2007;109:8-14.

3. Torpy JM, Lynm C, Glass RM. JAMA patient page. Cerebral palsy. *JAMA*. 2010;304:1028.

4. Odding E, Roebroeck ME, Stam HJ. The epidemiology of cerebral palsy: incidence, impairments and risk factors. *Disabil Rehabil*. 2006;28:183-191.

5. Pharoah P, Cooke T. Cerebral palsy and multiple births. *Arch Dis Child Fetal Neonatal Ed*. 1996;75:174-177.

6. Department of Health and Human Services, National Institute of Neurological Disorders and Stroke (NINDS). Cerebral palsy: hope through research. http://www.ninds.nih.gov/disorders/cerebral_palsy/detail_cerebral_palsy.htm#179323104. Accessed February 14, 2013.

7. Strauss D, Brooks J, Rosenbloom L, Shavelle R. Life expectancy in cerebral palsy: an update. *Dev Med Child Neurol*. 2008;50:487-493.

8. Rosen MG, Dickinson JC. The incidence of cerebral palsy. *Am J Obstet Gynecol*. 1992;167:417-423.

9. Mirmiran M, Barnes DP, Keller K, et al. Neonatal brain magnetic resonance imaging before discharge is better than serial cranial ultrasound in predicting cerebral palsy in very low birthweight preterm infants. *Pediatrics*. 2004;114:992-998.

10. Hnatyszyn G, Cyrylowski L, Czeszynska MB, et al. The role of magnetic resonance imaging in early prediction of cerebral palsy. *Turk J Pediatr*. 2010;52:278-284.

11. Palisano R, Rosenbaum P, Walter S, Russell D, Wood E, Galuppi B. Development and reliability of a system to classify gross motor function in children with cerebral palsy. *Dev Med Child Neurol*. 1997;39:214-223.

12. Rosenbaum PL, Walter SD, Hanna SE, et al. Prognosis for gross motor function in cerebral palsy: creation of motor development curves. *JAMA*. 2002;288:1357-1363.

13. Oeffinger DJ, Tylkowski CM, Rayens MK, et al. Gross motor function classification system and outcome tools for assessing ambulatory cerebral palsy: a multicenter study. *Dev Med Child Neurol*. 2004;46:311-319.

14. Kang LJ, Palisano RJ, Orlin MN, et al. Determinants of social participation-with friends and others who are not family members—for youth with cerebral palsy. *Phys Ther.* 2010;90:1743-1757.

15. Hutton JL, Colver AF, Mackie PC. Effects of severity of disability on survival in north east England cerebral palsy cohort. *Arch Dis Child.* 2000;83:468-474.

16. Chiarello L, Palisano RJ, Maggs JM, et al. Family priorities for activity and participation of children and youth with cerebral palsy. *Phys Ther.* 2010;90:1254-1264.

17. Russell DJ, Avery LM, Rosenbaum PL, et al. Improved scaling of the gross motor function measure for children with cerebral palsy: evidence of reliability and validity. *Phys Ther.* 2000;80:873-885.

18. American Physical Therapy Association. *Guide to Physical Therapist Practice.* 2nd ed. *Phys Ther.* 2001;81:S19-S28.

19. O'Neal ME, Fragala-Pinkham MA, Westcott SL, et al. Physical therapy clinical management recommendations for children with cerebral palsy-spastic diplegia: achieving functional mobility outcomes. *Pediatr Phys Ther.* 2006;18:49-72.

20. Lundkvist Josenby A, Jarnlo GB, Gummesson C, Nordmark E. Longitudinal construct validity of the GMFM-88 total score and goal total score and the GMFM-66 score in a 5-year follow-up study. *Phys Ther.* 2009;89:342-352.

21. Nichols DS, Case-Smith J. Reliability and validity of the Pediatric Evaluation of Disability Inventory. *Pediatr Phys Ther.* 1996;8:15-24.

22. Davies PL, Soon PL, Young M, Clausen-Yamaki A. Validity and reliability of the school function assessment in elementary school students with disabilities. *Phys Occup Ther Pediatr.* 2004;24:23-43.

23. Damiano DL, Abel MF. Functional outcomes of strength training in spastic cerebral palsy. *Arch Phys Med Rehabil.* 1998;79:119-125.

24. Dodd KJ, Taylor NF, Damiano DL. A systematic review of the effectiveness of strength-training programs for people with cerebral palsy. *Arch Phys Med Rehabil.* 2002;83:1157-1164.

25. Kerr C, McDowell B, McDonough S. Electrical stimulation in cerebral palsy: a review of effects on strength and motor function. *Dev Med Child Neurol.* 2004;46:205-213.

26. King EM, Gooch JL, Howell GH, et al. Evaluation of the hip-extensor tricycle in improving gait in children with cerebral palsy. *Dev Med Child Neurol.* 1993;35:1048-1054.

27. Thorpe D, Reilly M. The effect of an aquatic resistive exercise program on lower extremity strength, energy expenditure, functional mobility, balance and self-perception in an adult with cerebral palsy: a retrospective case report. *J Aquatic Phys Ther.* 2000;8:1-24.

28. Sterba JA, Rogers BT, France AP, Vokes DA. Horseback riding in children with cerebral palsy: effect on gross motor function. *Dev Med Child Neurol.* 2002;44:301-308.

29. Shumway-Cook A, Hutchinson S, Kartin D, et al. Effect of balance training on recovery of stability in children with cerebral palsy. *Dev Med Child Neurol.* 2003;45:591-602.

30. Butler C, Darrah J. Effects of neurodevelopmental treatment (NDT) for cerebral palsy: an AACPDM evidence report. *Dev Med Child Neurol.* 2001;43:778-790.

31. Mattern-Baxter K. Effects of partial body weight supported treadmill training on children with cerebral palsy. *Pediatr Phys Ther.* 2009;21:12-22.

32. Van den Berg-Emons RJ, Van Baak MA, Speth L, Saris WH. Physical training of school children with spastic cerebral palsy: effects on daily activity, fat mass and fitness. *Int J Rehail Res.* 1998;21:179-194.

Spina Bifida

Sheryl A. Low

CASE 29

An 11-year-old girl with L4/L5 spina bifida (myelomeningocele) is enrolled in a regular sixth grade class at the local elementary school and uses a manual wheelchair for school and community ambulation. She has always been quite social and verbal and has many friends at school. Immediately after birth, she had surgery to close the myelomeningocele in her lower back and she had a ventriculoperitoneal cerebrospinal fluid (CSF) shunt placed to prevent hydrocephalus. Since then, she has had two shunt revisions due to infection and she also has frequent urinary tract infections. She rolled at 8 months and sat independently at 11 months. She belly crawled at 16 months, and has been using a manual wheelchair since she was 3 years old. She has received physical therapy services regularly since she was a baby. She is now independent in intermittent catheterization during her school day. The school physical therapist has been working with her to maximize her endurance with a walking program using her long leg braces. However, she is only able to ambulate up to 30 ft with her crutches at home and in the classroom, and she is much slower than her peers. She will be going to junior high school next year, which is on a larger campus with hilly terrain, and she will need to change classrooms throughout the day. She is also starting to mature and has gained weight, which has made walking and pushing her wheelchair more difficult. The physical therapist is consulting with the school district and her family to make recommendations for her transfer to junior high and to help establish goals for adaptive physical education.

- ► What are the examination priorities?
- ► What are the most appropriate examination tests?
- ► How would this child's contextual factors influence or change your patient/client management?
- ► Identify her functional limitations and assets.

KEY DEFINITIONS

INDIVIDUALIZED EDUCATION PLAN (IEP): Plan mandated under federal law called the Individuals with Disabilities Education Act (IDEA) and developed annually by the family, school personnel, and occupational, physical, and speech therapists, as indicated by the child's level of functioning; plan may include provision of physical therapy in the school setting, if the team determines it is needed to help the child achieve his/her educational goals[1]

Objectives

1. Describe the primary and secondary impairments and the functional and activity limitations affecting children with spina bifida.
2. Identify key questions to determine the priorities of the child and family in the physical therapy plan of care.
3. Identify reliable and valid outcome tools to measure a child's mobility and level of functioning in school.
4. Discuss appropriate components of the examination.
5. Discuss assistive/adaptive devices and equipment recommendations for a child with spina bifida.
6. Describe attainable age-appropriate goals for a preteen with spina bifida.

Physical Therapy Considerations

PT considerations during management of the child with mobility, activity, and participation limitations in the school setting due to spina bifida at a specific time of transition in the child's life:

▶ **General physical therapy plan of care/goals:** Assess gait and mobility in the school setting including transitions to and from classroom seating, bathroom/toileting, and meal/snack times; assessment of equipment and adaptations needed in school setting; maximization of child's ability to participate in school-related activities with functional independence and safety while minimizing secondary impairments

▶ **Physical therapy interventions:** Patient/teacher/family education on level of assistance required for safe execution of tasks; strengthening; home stretching program; balance and postural control activities; functional mobility training; adapted cardiovascular training program for endurance; coordination and communication with IEP team

▶ **Precautions during physical therapy:** Daily visual inspection for pressure ulcers; close guarding due to osteoporosis and increased risk of fractures with falls

▶ **Complications interfering with physical therapy:** Frequent urinary tract infections, shunt malfunctions, decreased cardiovascular endurance, scoliosis, obesity, improper fit of equipment or orthotics

Understanding the Health Condition

Spina bifida is the term commonly used to describe various forms of myelodysplasia, which is a defective closure of the vertebrae in fetal development. Spina bifida lesions can be classified into *aperta* (visible open lesions) or *occulta* (hidden or not visible). Open lesions leave the meninges and spinal cord protruding in the newborn, which puts the infant at increased risk for damage to the nerves and spinal cord during the birthing process. There is usually sensory and motor loss at or below the level of the lesion causing primary neurologic impairments such as paralysis, club feet, neurogenic bowel and bladder, and hydrocephalus.[2] Spina bifida is a disabling congenital condition that lasts throughout the lifespan. Myelomeningocele (MM) is the most severe form of spina bifida in which defective closure of the vertebrae leaves the meninges and spinal cord protruding dorsally in the newborn.[3] As early as 8 weeks of gestation, the neural tissue folds in on itself to form the neural tube. Later, the neural tube transforms into structures that develop into the central nervous system. Failure of this neuralation process over a specific segment of the spinal column is responsible for the open defect.[3] Neural defects such as MM are thought to be caused by genetic malformations, exposure to alcohol or valproic acid during pregnancy, or lack of folic acid in the maternal diet.[4]

Maternal alpha-fetoprotein screening and better ultrasound technology allow earlier identification of neural tube defects.[5] In utero repair has decreased the occurrence of hydrocephalus (accumulation of CSF in the lateral ventricles) and Arnold-Chiari Type II malformations, which is the caudal displacement of the hindbrain through the foramen magnum.[6] A recent multicenter randomized clinical trial compared prenatal surgical repair with postnatal repair of MM in 158 babies.[7] Only 40% of the prenatal repair group required shunting, whereas 82% of the postnatal repair group required shunting. This promising procedure is still practiced only in a few major centers, but may become more widespread as more surgeons learn the techniques. While the incidence of MM in the United States is lower than before mandatory folic acid fortification to grain products, incidence ranges from 0.17 to 6.39 per 1000 live births.[8] More girls are affected by MM than boys and the prevalence is higher in the eastern and southern United States compared to the West.[9]

MM is easily identifiable at birth when the baby is born with bulging meninges at the area of the defect. Typically, the disorder is managed by postnatal surgery to close the defect.[5] The baby is also screened for hydrocephalus, kidney and urologic defects, and other malformations of the central nervous system.[4] Twenty-five percent of children born with MM present with hydrocephalus, and a further 60% develop it soon after surgical closure of the lesion.[10] If hydrocephalus is present, a ventriculoperitoneal shunt is placed to transfer excess CSF from the brain to the lymph system for reabsorption.[7] Children with shunts are at continued risk for shunt malfunction, which requires immediate surgical correction.[9] Signs of shunt malfunction include edema, vomiting, irritability, lethargy, seizures, new strabismus or squint, headache, redness along shunt track, personality changes, memory changes, handwriting changes, and decreased performance in play or at school.[2]

If the baby has clubfoot deformities, serial casting or splinting is done to achieve a more neutral ankle position to prepare for weightbearing at a later age.[4,11] If serial casting is unsuccessful, children may need surgical intervention to correct foot deformities.[12] Children with MM are referred immediately for physical therapy services in the hospital or to early intervention services.

In MM, primary impairments are evident at birth and are the direct result of the open defect of the neural tube and resulting damage to the central and peripheral nervous systems.[5] Babies often demonstrate flaccid paralysis at or below the level of the primary lesion. The sensory and motor loss may be patchy and asymmetrical and the baby's position in utero can cause range of motion (ROM) deficits and underdevelopment of the lower extremities. Motor levels are assigned to the lowest *intact* dermatome or myotome. There are conflicting systems to classify the level of impairment. The commonly used method of Hoffer et al.[13,14] classifies children with MM according to ambulation status. Hoffer et al.[14] studied 56 individuals with MM between the ages of 5 and 42 years and found such wide variations in function across dermatome and innervation levels that he developed a **functional method to determine ambulation**. Hoffer et al. classified four types of ambulators: nonambulators, nonfunctional ambulators, household ambulators, and community ambulators. Nonambulators are those individuals who are mobile only via a wheelchair but can usually transfer from chair to bed. Nonfunctional ambulators can walk during therapy sessions, at home, in school, or in the hospital, but use a wheelchair for all other transportation. Household ambulators walk only indoors and with orthoses. They are able to get in and out of chairs and bed with little, if any, assistance. They may use a wheelchair for some indoor activities at home and school, but use a wheelchair for all activities in the community. Community ambulators walk indoors and outdoors for most activities and may need crutches, braces, or both. Community ambulators use a wheelchair only for long trips out of the community.

Over time, **secondary impairments** can develop in children with MM. These include scoliosis, obesity, spasticity, decreased cardiac endurance, cognitive dysfunction, upper limb dyscoordination, skin breakdown, muscle contractures, cranial palsies, language dysfunction, chronic urinary tract infections, visual-perceptual deficits, latex allergies, and tethered cord syndrome.[2,4,15-19] Since these children have bowel and bladder dysfunction, they develop frequent urinary tract infections and are often hospitalized with this condition.[2] Secondary impairments can also limit life expectancy for MM.[20,21] In a 25-year follow-up study of individuals with MM, Bowman and colleagues[10] found that 75% of individuals survive into adulthood, and of those, most attended high school or college. Most individuals live with their parents, and 50% have problems with scoliosis, one-third have latex allergies, and others have shunt malfunctions and problems with tethered cord syndrome.

Recent changes in the models of disablement propose that physical therapists change their focus of treatment from an emphasis on the skills a child would need (e.g., walking) to a lifespan enablement approach with an emphasis on independence and participation in society as an adult.[22] The International Classification of Function, Disability and Health (ICF) is a model of classifying individuals with disabilities that is used to help therapists focus their treatment plans on a lifespan approach.[22] There are three domains of this model: body function and structures, activity, and participation. The model relates health to function and starts with the disease process or pathology that causes the impairments which alter structure and function. This leads to restrictions in activity and eventually in participation in age-related activities.

Physical Therapy Patient/Client Management

As this child with MM grows, she receives physical therapy regularly in the school setting or outpatient clinic to help her achieve the highest level of functioning possible. IDEA specifies that physical therapy is part of the Individualized Education Plan (IEP) team that includes the parents, teachers, and educational staff.[1] A child in sixth grade would most likely receive physical therapy services under IDEA through the school district.[1] At 11 years old, this patient is in an important transitional period requiring a comprehensive physical therapy examination and assessment to determine her capabilities in the new larger environment. In junior high school, the role of the physical therapist continues to focus on decreasing the disabling process and helping the adolescent with MM transition to life as an independent adult. Transitional issues include vocational training or planning for college, issues of accessibility on a larger campus or in the community, and training of additional support personnel.[1] Caregiving for a disabled adult is also very stressful on the family and suggests that pediatricians and allied health personnel take a supportive role in assisting families in the transition to adulthood. Mothers often carry the burden of physical care, which can be quite extensive for young adults with MM.[23] In a cross-sectional study of young adults with MM, Bartonek and Saraste[24] found a correlation between neurologic degeneration and shunt revisions with balance problems and functional losses. According to Hirst,[25] functional loss and dependence on others contributes to a social handicap. Other outcome studies have shown that most disabled young adults are unemployed, unmarried, and socially isolated.[10,26] The physical therapist plays a crucial role during this time of transition in assisting the child to achieve increased independence while decreasing caregiver burden on the family.

Examination, Evaluation, and Diagnosis

Given the current goal of preparing the child for the transition to junior high school, the physical therapist should perform a thorough re-examination and evaluation. Standardized tests should be used to assess the child's mobility and functional activities of daily living. The Physical Evaluation of Disability Inventory (PEDI) is a useful tool to determine self-care and level of assistance required for daily activities. This tool that measures self-care and mobility capabilities and performance in home and community environments includes the three domains of self-care, mobility, and social function.[27] The **School Function Assessment (SFA)** can be used to determine the child's functional level in the school setting. The SFA is a reliable criterion referenced tool to assess function and guide program planning for students with disabilities within the educational environment.[28] The areas assessed are participation, task supports, activity performance, including all mobility in the school setting. The child should also be examined in all areas for primary and secondary impairments according to the *Guide to Physical Therapist Practice*.[29] Specific areas that should be assessed for an 11-year-old child with MM include changes in paralysis or sensation, ROM, and changes in postural alignment in sitting and lying. Secondary impairments to assess include cardiovascular endurance and perceived exertion during wheelchair propulsion or walking with assistive equipment. Pulmonary function tests are also indicated if the child has postural changes impacting lung capacity.[29] The physical therapist should also assess the child's activity and participation according to the **ICF model of enablement**.[22] Indeed, Goldstein et al.[30] have proposed focusing on what the child *can* do instead of the child's limitations. This focus requires that the physical therapist investigate options and adaptations available for the child to enable her to participate in activities with her peers. Considerations at this transition from childhood to preteen include appropriate independence for bowel and bladder care, ability to keep up with peers on a larger school campus, independence in transfers, alternate methods of maintaining cardiovascular endurance and preventing obesity, pressure relief and skin care, and prevention of muscle contractures.[4]

Over time, children with MM gain weight and find it more difficult to maintain their ability to ambulate, even with orthotics.[31] The increased energy expenditure spent ambulating with assistive devices can make school performance on cognitive tasks more difficult compared to performance when students with MM use a wheelchair for mobility.[32] Therefore, the physical therapist must assess the endurance, efficiency, safety, and effectiveness of the child's gait. The overall goal for this emerging teenager is to keep up with her peers in an integrated setting in the most energy-efficient manner possible. Ideally, the therapist would assess the child's ability to manually propel her wheelchair across campus and from class to class within the allotted time allowed between classes. Meiser et al.[33] compared energy expenditure and perceived exertion during a 2-minute propulsion test for two children with spina bifida when using a lightweight wheelchair (weighing an average of 45 lb) versus an ultralight wheelchair (weighing an average of 32 lb) and found increased exertion and fatigue using the lightweight wheelchair. If it is not possible for the therapist to accompany the child to the new campus, the therapist could estimate the distances needed to be traveled and perform a timed wheelchair propulsion test while measuring the child's perceived exertion during this task. Perceived exertion in children can be measured using the **Children's OMNI Perceived Exertion Scale**, a 10-point scale with four activity pictures to rate perceived exertion. This scale has been validated over a wide metabolic intensity range in healthy boys and girls of different ethnicities and has also been used in children with post-traumatic brain injury and spina bifida.[34,35] Energy expenditure can also be calculated using the **Energy Expenditure Index (EEI)**, which is calculated by subtracting the resting heart rate (HR) from the propulsion HR divided by the speed.[33] Another method to determine the child's functional performance is to time her ability to propel her manual wheelchair over a 50-ft distance and **compare the wheelchair propulsion speed to walking speeds of**

Table 29-1 POTENTIAL EXAMINATION QUESTIONS FOR A PRETEEN WITH MYELOMENINGOCELE
What is the new campus like? (hilly or flat; distances between classes, etc.)
Is the child fast enough in the manual wheelchair to move around campus during the allotted classroom breaks?
Is the child going to sit in the wheelchair all day or transfer to a desk in classes?
Is the child independent in all transfers?
Is the child capable of performing pressure relief during the day?
Is the child able to perform intermittent catheterization independently? Where will the child do this?
What is the school proposing for participation during physical education?
What sports or leisure activities is the child interested in?
Will the child be participating in extracurricular groups or activities?
Does the home program need to be modified?
Will the child continue a walking or standing program at home?
Is there an activity to keep the child's cardiovascular system healthy?
What could be modified to allow the child more participation in peer-related activities?
What postural and structural concerns need to be addressed (*e.g.*, spine, legs)?

peers for the same distance. David and Sullivan[36] studied the walking speeds of 370 children in the school setting for a 50-ft distance and determined the mean walking speed for sixth graders to be 10.6 seconds. If the child does not have sufficient endurance and speed in her manual wheelchair, a power wheelchair may be indicated.[2] Documentation supporting justification for a power wheelchair can be provided by her exertion rating on the Children's OMNI Perceived Exertion Scale and her EEI during a timed wheelchair propulsion test, as well as her ability to cover required distances in a specific timeframe and comparison to walking speeds of her peers.

As a consultant to the Local Education Agency (LEA), the physical therapist recommends changes to the environment that are needed for accessibility. The physical therapist also trains the teacher(s) or staff regarding the mobility and/or standing program for the child and use of any adaptive equipment. A child with MM may also need accommodations for intermittent catheterization and adaptive physical education.[1,2] Questions to consider during the examination process are listed in Table 29-1.

Plan of Care and Interventions

Applying the ICF enablement model assists the physical therapist in determining the intervention plan. As the child grows, the role of the physical therapist begins to focus more on helping the family and child prepare for adulthood, so it is not unusual for the frequency of therapy services to decrease, become episodic, and focus on more specific objectives. Initially, the therapist may work with the teachers, school staff, and nursing personnel to train them in transfers, equipment needs, and adaptations needed for the child's daily classroom program. A typical daily classroom program might include skin checks, intermittent catheterizations, pressure relief, and perhaps a special program for adapted physical education. In order to facilitate the child moving from classroom to classroom, special desks may be required that can accommodate a power or manual wheelchair, and two sets of textbooks may be needed—one for school and another for home. The physical therapist should also monitor that the program is being carried out correctly and modify it if any changes are required.[1]

The therapist also works with the family to prevent secondary impairments.[4] A child in a rapid growth spurt may develop contractures when bones grow faster than muscles.[37] Children with MM have an increased risk for contractures due to spending longer periods of time sitting in wheelchairs. The physical therapist should closely monitor the child's ROM and continue to focus on interventions such as a home stretching and standing program to prevent contracture development.[38]

Since the child may be busier with school and social activities, leisure activities may take the place of therapy. Activities that can help maintain cardiovascular fitness could include swimming, an adapted cycling program or a hand bike, or adapted sports activities such as therapeutic horseback riding, skiing, kayaking, sailing, camping, and yoga.[2,30] The role of the physical therapist is to consult and teach the child to maintain proper conditioning, warm-up, and cool down as she participates in sports and recreational activities. Upper extremity strength training can assist the child with MM in improving function and metabolism.[39] Involvement in sports activities also encourages social involvement and lessens disability and isolation. Figure 29-1 applies the ICF model to the child with MM.

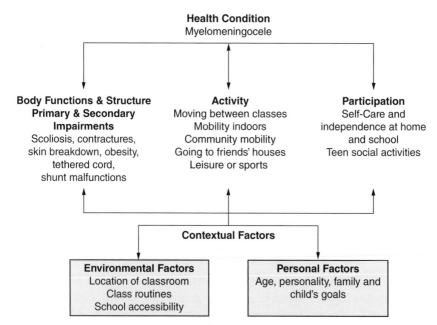

Figure 29-1. International Classification of Functioning (ICF) enablement model applied to the child with myelomeningocele. (Modified with permission from World Health Organization. International Classification of Functioning, Disability and Health [ICF]; 2001. http://www.who.int/classifications/icf/en/. Accessed June 25, 2012.)

Last, the physical therapist's role is to continue assisting the individual and family in the transition to adulthood focusing on a lifelong plan for maintaining the highest functional level.[26] The goal of physical therapy for children with disabilities is to assist in the development of a useful, productive adult who can participate and function in society.

Evidence-Based Clinical Recommendations

SORT: Strength of Recommendation Taxonomy

A: Consistent, good-quality patient-oriented evidence
B: Inconsistent or limited-quality patient-oriented evidence
C: Consensus, disease-oriented evidence, usual practice, expert opinion, or case series

1. Classification of intact motor level is less important than documenting the functional ambulation level for children with myelomeningocele. **Grade B**

2. Secondary impairments such as pressure ulcers, progressive neurological loss, osteoporosis, shunt malfunctions, and urological infections are common problems for teenagers and young adults with MM. **Grade A**

3. Physical therapists can use the School Function Assessment (SFA) to identify functional mobility in the school setting, assistance needed from adults, and adaptations and modifications to the environment needed for optimal functioning. **Grade B**

4. As children with MM mature, focus on a lifespan approach by the physical therapist increases activity and participation. **Grade C**

5. Functional mobility of the child with MM should include a comparison of the child's gait (or wheelchair propulsion) speed to their peers, assessment of perceived exertion using the Children's OMNI Perceived Exertion Scale, and estimated energy expenditure. **Grade B**

COMPREHENSION QUESTIONS

29.1 Children born with myelomeningocele are likely to develop which of the following secondary impairments?
   A. Scoliosis
   B. Tethered cord
   C. Obesity
   D. All of the above

29.2 A focus of the physical therapy examination for a child transferring to junior high school should emphasize which of the following?

A. Maintenance of her walking ability

B. Wheelchair endurance program

C. Increasing participation with peers at school

D. Home stretching program

ANSWERS

29.1 **D.** Children with myelomeningocele are at high risk for developing scoliosis due to the asymmetrical nature of their muscle weakness and structural spinal deformities from birth. Scarring from the surgical repair or a congenital anomaly may result in a tethered spinal cord as the child grows. Since children with myelomeningocele often use a wheelchair for mobility, their energy expenditure is much lower, making them prone to obesity as teenagers.

29.2 **C.** During the crucial transition from grade school to junior high school, the focus would change from direct therapeutic interventions to increasing participation with peers in school. Children with myelomeningocele often decrease their ability to maintain their ambulation status as they grow and move into a larger and more complex school environment. A stretching program is important (option D) and should be monitored as a home program, but it is no longer the focus of therapy. The goal is to increase the child's independence and ability to keep up with peers in the school setting.

REFERENCES

1. McEwen I. *Providing Physical Therapy Services under Parts B & C of the Individuals With Disabilities Education Act (IDEA)*. Alexandria, VA: Section on Pediatrics, American Physical Therapy Association; 2009.

2. Hinderer KA, Hinderer SR, Shurtleff DB. Myelodysplasia. In: Campbell SK, ed. *Physical Therapy for Children*. Philadelphia, PA: WB Saunders; 2012:703-755.

3. Adzick NS, Walsh DS. Myelomeningocele: prenatal diagnosis, pathophysiology and management. *Semin Pediatr Surg*. 2003;12:168-174.

4. Elias ER, Hobbs N. Spina bifida: sorting out the complexities of care. *Contemp Pediatr*. 1998:15;156-171.

5. Bowman RM, McLone DG. Neurosurgical management of spina bifida: research issues. *Dev Disabil Res Rev*. 2010:16;82-87.

6. Bruner JP, Tulipan N, Paschall RL, et al. Fetal surgery for myelomeningocele and the incidence of shunt-dependent hydrocephalus. *JAMA*. 1999:282;1819-1825.

7. Adzick NS, Thom EA, Spong CY, et al. A randomized trial of prenatal versus postnatal repair of myelomeningocele. *N Engl J Med*. 2011;364:993-1004.

8. Williams LJ, Mai CT, Edmonds LD, et al. Prevalence of spina bifida and anencephaly during the transition to mandatory folic acid fortifications in the United states. *Teratology*. 2002;66:33-39.

9. Bowman RM, Boshnjaku V, McLone DG. The changing incidence of myelomeningocele and its impact on pediatric neurosurgery: a review from the Children's Memorial Hospital. *Childs Nerv Syst*. 2009;25.7:801-806.

10. Bowman RM, McLone DG, Grant JA, Tomita T, Ito JA. Spina bifida outcome: a 25-year prospective. *Pediatr Neurosurg*. 2001;34:114-120.

11. Brown JP. Orthopedic care of children with spina bifida: you've come a long way, baby! *Orthop Nurs.* 2001;20:51-58.

12. Staheli LT. *Practice of Pediatric Orthopedics.* Philadelphia, PA: Lippincott Williams & Wilkins; 2001.

13. Bartonek A, Saraste H, Knutson LM. Comparison of different systems to classify the neurological level of lesion in patients with myelomeningocele. *Dev Med Child Neurol.* 1999;41:796-805.

14. Hoffer M, Feiwell E, Perry J, Bonnett C. Functional ambulation in patients with myelomeningocele. *J Bone Joint Surg Am.*1973;55:137-148.

15. Golge M, Schutz C, Dreesmann M, et al. Grip force parameters in precision grip of individuals with myelomeningocele. *Dev Med Child Neurol.* 2003;45:249-256.

16. Burmeister R, Hannay HJ, Copeland K, Fletcher JM, Boudousquie A, Dennis M. Attention problems and executive functions in children with spina bifida and hydrocephalus. *Child Neuropsychol.* 2005;11:265-283.

17. Lapsiwala SB, Iskandar BJ. The tethered cord syndrome in adults with spina bifida occulta. *Neurol Res.* 2004;26:735-740.

18. Majed M, Nejat F, Khashab ME, et al. Risk factors for latex sensitization in young children with myelomeningocele. Clinical article. *J Neurosurg Pediatr.* 2009;4:285-288.

19. Shurtleff DB, Walker WO, Duguay S, Peterson D, Cardenas D. Obesity and myelomeningocele: anthropometric measures. *J Spinal Cord Med.* 2010;33:410-419.

20. Dillon CM, Davis BE, Duguay S, Seidel KD, Shurtleff DB. Longevity of patients born with myelomeningocele. *Eur J Pediatr Surg.* 2000;10(suppl 1):33-34.

21. Davis BE, Daley CM, Shurtleff DB, et al. Long-term survival of individuals with myelomeningocele. *Pediatr Neurosurg.* 2005;41:186-191.

22. World Health Organization. International Classification of Functioning, Disability and Health (ICF); 2001. http://www.who.int/classifications/icf/en/. Accessed June 25, 2012.

23. Lie HR, Borjeson MC, Lagerkvist B, Rasmussen F, Hagelsteen JH, Lagergren J. Children with myelomeningocele: the impact of disability on family dynamics and social conditions. A Nordic study. *Dev Med Child Neurol.* 1994;36:1000-1009.

24. Bartonek A, Saraste H. Factors influencing ambulation in myelomeningocele: a cross-sectional study. *Dev Med Child Neurol.* 2001;43:253-260.

25. Hirst M. Patterns of impairment and disability related to social handicap with cerebral palsy and spina bifida. *J Biosoc Sci.* 1989;21:1-12.

26. Bottos M, Feliciangeli A, Scuito L, Gericke C, Vianello A. Functional status of adults with cerebral palsy and implications for treatment of children. *Dev Med Child Neurol.* 2001;43:516-528.

27. Nichols DS, Case-Smith J. Reliability and validity of the pediatric evaluation of disability inventory. *Pediatr Phys Ther.* 1996;8:15-24.

28. Davies PL, Soon PL, Young M, Clausen-Yamaki A. Validity and reliability of the school function assessment in elementary school students with disabilities. *Phys Occup Ther Pediatr.* 2004;24:23-43.

29. American Physical Therapy Association. *Guide to Physical Therapist Practice.* 2nd ed. *Phys Ther.* 2001;81:S19-S28.

30. Goldstein DN, Cohn E, Coster W. Enhancing participation for children with disabilities: application of the ICF enablement framework to pediatric physical therapist practice. *Pediatr Phys Ther.* 2004;16:114-120.

31. Bare A, Vankoski SJ, Dias L, Danduran M, Boas S. Independent ambulators with high sacral myelomeningocele: the relation between walking kinematics and energy consumption. *Dev Med Child Neurol.* 2001;43:16-21.

32. Franks CA, Palisano RJ, Darbee JC. The effect of walking with an assistive device and using a wheelchair on school performance in students with myelomeningocele. *Phys Ther.*1991;71:570-579.

33. Meiser JM, McEwen IR. Lightweight and ultralight wheelchairs: propulsion and preferences of two young children with spina bifida. *Pediatr Phys Ther.* 2007;19:245-253.

34. Robertson RJ, Goss FL, Boer NF, et al. Children's OMNI scale of perceived exertion: mixed gender and race validation. *Med Sci Sports Exerc.* 2000;32:452-458.

35. Katz-Leurer M, Rotem H, Keren O, Meyer S. The relationship between step variability, muscle strength and functional walking performance in children with post-traumatic brain injury. *Gait Posture.* 2009;29:154-157.

36. David KS, Sullivan M. Expectations for walking speeds: standards for students in elementary schools. *Pediatr Phys Ther.* 2005;17:120-127.

37. Tardieu C, Lespargot C, Tabary C, Bret MD. For how long must the soleus muscle be stretched each day to prevent contracture? *Dev Med Child Neurol.* 1988:30;3-10.

38. StubergWA. Consideration related to weight-bearing programs in children with developmental disabilities. *Phys Ther.* 1992;72:35-40.

39. Hurd WJ, Morrow MM, Kaufman KR, An KN. Wheelchair propulsion demands during outdoor community ambulation. *J Electromyogr Kinesiol.* 2009;19:942-947.

Down Syndrome

Cornelia Lieb-Lundell

CASE 30

A 7-year-old girl with a diagnosis of Down syndrome was referred to outpatient physical therapy for an evaluation to address the child's deteriorating gait and obtain recommendations for orthotic devices. The mother reports that the child had bilateral bunionectomies (performed by a podiatrist) 6 months earlier and an improvement in her gait was noted briefly after the surgery. However, in the last 3 months her gait appears to have regressed and is now at the level that it was before the surgery. The child's previous history was gathered from the details provided by the parent and from available medical records. She was born at term (weighing 6 lb 2 oz) and had Apgar scores of 6 and 8 (at 1 and 5 minutes, respectively) and was diagnosed at birth to have Down syndrome. Subsequent genetic testing confirmed the diagnosis of Trisomy 21. No other medical complications were identified and she passed the newborn hearing screen. She was discharged with her mother 48 hours after birth. The mother describes the child's development as slower than her brother who is 18 months older. However, she sat independently at her first birthday and began taking first steps at age of 22 months. Around that time, the mother noticed that the child's knees intermittently tended to be red and slightly inflamed and she occasionally gave her ibuprofen. The mother thought these signs were related to the child transitioning from creeping to walking with support and because she sometimes let go of her support and fell on her knees. The knee swelling episodes continued intermittently for about a year. The mother took her to the pediatrician, but the problem had usually subsided by the time of the appointments. When the child was 4 years old, the pediatrician referred her for an orthopaedic evaluation. The report indicated that there were no significant findings other than usual problems consistent with the diagnosis of Down syndrome. Between the ages of 4 and 6 years, she was screened for thyroid dysfunction and the results were described as normal for age. During that period, the mother noted that her daughter seemed to be developing a slightly "shuffling" gait. She became concerned that her daughter may need orthoses because she was also developing noticeable bilateral bunions at the first metatarsal joints.

Review of school records revealed that between the ages of 5 and 7 years, the child demonstrated no progress in Adaptive Physical Education (APE) so the goals written at age 5 were carried over yearly for 2 more years. To address concerns about the child's walking, the mother took the child to a podiatrist. The podiatrist recommended and scheduled bilateral bunionectomies, which were completed without complications. She received routine postsurgical care and remained hospitalized for 5 days. The mother noted that the child walked with decreased stiffness by the end of her hospital stay. This improvement continued for about 3 months when the mother noted increased stiffness again and sought out a physical therapist to explore management options. The therapist noted that the child took a full 15 minutes to cross a 50-ft distance from the parked car to the front door of the clinic.

- ► What examination signs may be associated with this diagnosis?
- ► Based on the patient's health condition, what do you anticipate will be the contributors to activity limitations?
- ► What are the physical therapy examination priorities?
- ► Identify referrals to other medical team members.
- ► What are the most appropriate physical therapy interventions?

KEY DEFINITIONS

ADAPTIVE PHYSICAL EDUCATION (APE): Program designed for children with disability by modifying physical education activities to make the program accessible for this special population; APE is a federally mandated component of special education services[1]

BUNIONECTOMY: Surgical removal of protruding bony prominence of the first metatarsal joint of either foot

Objectives

1. Describe typical development for children with Down syndrome.
2. Define common orthopaedic problems associated with Down syndrome.
3. Define key questions needed to establish a physical therapy diagnosis.
4. Identify tests and outcome measures appropriate for children with Down syndrome to assess developmental and/or functional level, range of motion, strength, and gait dysfunction.
5. Define relevant components of the physical therapy evaluation.

Physical Therapy Considerations

PT considerations during management of the child with Down syndrome presenting with deteriorating gait and poor lower extremity strength and mobility:

▶ **General physical therapy plan of care/goals:** Reflex testing, developmental testing such as the Peabody or Bruininks-Oseretsky Test of Motor Proficiency (BOT-2); assessment of range of motion (ROM), strength, posture, balance, pain, endurance, and gait

▶ **Physical therapy interventions:** Strength training to improve core strength, pelvic stability and lower extremity weight shifting; orthotic fitting and fabrication; gait training including treadmill training to increase cadence, step length, and base of support

▶ **Precautions during physical therapy:** Pain, limited aerobic endurance, fear of falling

▶ **Complications interfering with physical therapy:** Fatigue, falls, pain

Understanding the Health Condition

Down syndrome is the most common autosomal chromosome condition linked with decreased intellectual function and is usually diagnosed at birth.[2] Most often, it is a spontaneously occurring duplication of the 21st chromosome yielding one additional chromosome (*i.e.*, Trisomy 21), although about 4% of cases are inherited. Infants born with Down syndrome have a pattern of distinct features that includes an index of eight physical features developed by Rex and Preus[3] as well as central hypotonia (low muscle tone) and ligamentous laxity. Children with Down syndrome may have additional medical problems such as congenital heart disease (40%-50%),[4] gastro-intestinal problems, hypothyroidism, and atlantoaxial instability due to significant ligamentous laxity.[2,5]

Physical development is typically delayed and children with Down syndrome are at high risk for developing secondary musculoskeletal disorders such as general joint hypermobility, excessive foot pronation, and patellar instability. Signs and symptoms of a subluxation at the level of C1/C2 vertebrae can include fatigue, altered ambulatory pattern, neck pain with limited mobility, torticollis, change in bowel and bladder function, and/or sensory impairments.[4] Because of the increased prevalence of **juvenile idiopathic arthritis (JIA)** in this population (more than six times higher than in the general population), JIA should be considered as a potential comorbidity in individuals who present with a constellation of symptoms that may include intermittent joint pain and swelling, general stiffness, antalgic gait pattern, and decreased ROM of major joints over time.[6] JIA is the most common form of arthritis in children and is usually an autoimmune disorder. The condition typically affects children under 16 years of age and may be diagnosed when joint inflammation occurs and persists for 6 or more weeks.[2]

Persons with Down syndrome are also at increased risk for medical complications of multiple organ systems at birth and throughout the lifespan. They are thought to be at risk for developing early Alzheimer's disease[7] and are at risk for early deterioration of hearing and vision.[5] The most common developmental motor profile for persons with Down syndrome includes delayed gross motor skills with independent walking usually achieved at 18 to 21 months of age, but for some children, walking may not be achieved until up to age 3 years.[8] Over time, children with Down syndrome generally can learn to walk, run, ride a bicycle, and participate in sports.[9] Language development is often delayed and receptive language skills are generally better than expressive skills. Children typically receive speech therapy to improve speech intelligibility. Further, they need the support of a special education environment in order to optimize learning potential.

Physical Therapy Patient/Client Management

Intervention for infants with Down syndrome typically begins when the family participates in a home-based early intervention program in which an educational program and physical, occupational, and speech therapy services are provided for infants (from birth) to 3 years of age to address feeding issues, motor delays, and speech delays. Children with identified motor delays may also receive individual physical therapy episodes to address these delays. Many families also participate in a range of complementary or alternative therapies (*e.g.*, vitamin therapy, stem cell therapy, cognitive enhancement treatments) that are widely available, but often are not based on or supported by patient-based outcome data. When viewing the life-course challenges that are associated with a diagnosis of Down syndrome, the physical therapist is well positioned to provide primary intervention in the assessment and management of musculoskeletal issues, ongoing assessment of neurological stability, promotion of gross motor development, assistance in needed environmental adaptations, and parent and caregiver education. The physical therapist may make referrals to rheumatologists to address joint and/or muscle inflammation, work with orthotists to address foot function and occupational therapists to address activities of daily living function, and consult with the education team to reassess school progress.

Examination, Evaluation, and Diagnosis

The child with Down syndrome typically presents with generalized hypotonia with joint hypermobility, gross motor delay as part of developmental delay, and a limited repertoire of postural control strategies. At age 7 years, the child should have developed a mature gait pattern with bilateral arm swing, the ability to run, and the ability to maintain her posture on variable surfaces. When the patient does not fit this profile, as is the case with this child, the physical therapist must apply diagnostic skills and choose appropriate outcome measures to determine if the patient's delays are based on general developmental delay or dysfunctions in the area of musculoskeletal, neuromuscular, cardiovascular/pulmonary, and/or integumentary systems.[10]

With young children, the parent(s) are the primary source for obtaining a summary of the current problem and also relating the child's history. In addition to reviewing the birth history, the therapist asks about past illnesses, injuries, hospitalizations, medications the child currently takes or was recently taking, and any other relevant medical information such as imaging or laboratory tests. Examination includes observation of posture and alignment and assessment of deep tendon and postural reflexes, strength, ROM, balance, and functional status. Motor development and proficiency can be comprehensively examined using the Bruininks-Oseretsky Test of Motor Proficiency (BOT-2).

Typical posture for a 7-year-old with Down syndrome is a slightly wide-based stance with mild to moderate ankle pronation and flat-foot contact, knee hyperextension, mild hip flexion, excessive lumbar lordosis with a protruding abdomen, and poor shoulder stability. Overall strength can be expected to be better than 3/5 on a manual muscle test, but is often slightly below normal for age.[11,12] Use of a handheld dynamometer is a valid and reliable evaluation approach for this population.[13] Joint hypermobility of the foot and ankle, knees, hips, shoulders, elbows, and fingers is typical for this diagnosis and deviations from normal should be documented.

Acquiring stable motor skills and developing a range of functional postural control mechanisms are central themes for persons with Down syndrome. After the therapist has established a child's motor developmental level by applying a standardized test, the level of postural stability and/or mobility should be assessed. In contrast to the variety of postural control tests available for adults, fewer tests are available for children and those available largely lack sound validation. The therapist may start with tests such as the Pediatric Berg Balance Scale[14] and the Observational Gait Scale.[15]

Assessment of motor skills needs to be repeated over time and the **Bruininks-Oseretsky Test of Motor Proficiency (BOT-2)** is an appropriate tool for this task. This test has been widely used for assessing motor skills in children and takes approximately 45 to 60 minutes to administer. The BOT-2 measures gross and fine motor skills of individuals 4 to 21 years of age. It was specifically designed to measure body coordination, fine manual control and coordination, strength, and agility.[16] The BOT-2 has been validated for use with children diagnosed with Down syndrome and other diagnoses associated with mild to moderate developmental delay.[17]

Serial assessment of motor skills of a child with Down syndrome should provide a picture of delayed-for-age, but steady longitudinal achievement of motor milestones. After the systems review and examination, the physical therapist identified that the child had shown no progress in gross motor development over 2 years (as documented by her lack of progress in APE) and her composite scores on the BOT-2 were lower than anticipated for her age and primary diagnosis of Down syndrome. After the child's foot surgery, she initially gained stability with walking, but quickly lost stability again. In addition, the physical therapist carefully considered the mother's report that the child's knees intermittently tended to be red and inflamed since the age of approximately 2 years with short-term positive response to nonsteroidal anti-inflammatory drugs (NSAIDs). Upon further questioning, the mother reported that the child has been experiencing a more recent bout of chronic intermittent inflammation of the knees and hips over the past several months. Based on the summary of the examination findings, the therapist concluded that the child's developmental profile was not typical for the sole diagnosis of Down syndrome. Rather, her clinical presentation was consistent with a chronic inflammatory disease such a JIA.

Plan of Care and Interventions

The physical therapist implemented a group of interventions that included both therapeutic exercises and functional training sessions. The therapist initiated a referral to a rheumatologist to evaluate the child and summarized her examination findings to this healthcare provider. The therapist also participated in interdisciplinary planning to focus on communication and service coordination across settings (*e.g.*, home, classroom, APE). The expected outcome of the interventions is that this child will improve her mobility, strength, stability/balance, and overall developmental level, which may lead to increased independence in her home, school, and community.

The structure of the **therapeutic exercise routine** must consider the needs and constraints present with a child that carries dual diagnoses of underlying joint hypermobility (due to Down syndrome) and limited ROM (due to JIA) that is additionally complicated by increased pain. Table 30-1 illustrates specific exercises focusing on advancing development, improving balance, improving efficiency of gait, improving joint ROM using active and active assisted techniques, and increasing endurance. Finally, the focus of the therapist's team participation is family-child and caregiver-child instruction and adding environmental adaptations to increase the child's home, school, and community participation.

Table 30-1	THERAPEUTIC EXERCISE PLANNING
Focus Area	**Example Activities**
Development	• Assess climbing on various structures using alternating directions and hands and feet • Practice walking on various surfaces and stepping up and down curb • Introduce bicycle with training wheels, start propelling with feet on floor and gradually fade training wheels out
Balance	• With child sitting on a Physioball, challenge balance in all directions • Stand on small piece of foam balancing with both legs, then single limb stance; introduce ball catching, bean tossing, etc. • Stair climbing (up and down) with decreasing support • Practice donning and doffing sweater or coat in standing • Practice standing while forward reaching for a toy with a tape measure on the wall to document progress
Gait efficiency	• Provide visual prompts to vary step length • Practice walking on toes, on heels, high steppage gait • Use metronome or music to prompt varying speed • Introduce 3-minute walk, progress to 6 minutes
Range of motion	• Schedule ROM with regard to pain management schedule • Instruct in self-ranging activities • Practice putting shoes and socks on in sitting • Provide active assisted ROM when pain is present
Endurance	• Practice sit to stand and stand to sit to the count of five, six, etc. • Abdominal exercises: sit on ball and encourage rotation with extension • See gait efficiency above

Evidence-Based Clinical Recommendations

SORT: Strength of Recommendation Taxonomy

A: Consistent, good-quality patient-oriented evidence
B: Inconsistent or limited-quality patient-oriented evidence
C: Consensus, disease-oriented evidence, usual practice, expert opinion, or case series

1. Juvenile idiopathic arthritis (JIA) should be considered as a potential comorbidity in young persons with Down syndrome who present with intermittent joint pain and swelling, general stiffness, antalgic gait pattern, and decreased ROM of major joints. **Grade B**

2. The Bruininks-Oseretsky Test of Motor Proficiency (BOT-2) is validated for use with children diagnosed with Down syndrome and other diagnoses associated with mild to moderate developmental delay as an evaluation of gross and fine motor skills of individuals 4 to 21 years of age. **Grade A**

3. A specific therapeutic exercise routine focusing on advancing development, increasing endurance, and improving balance, gait efficiency, and joint ROM improves children's mobility, strength, stability, and overall developmental level. **Grade C**

COMPREHENSION QUESTIONS

30.1 The physical therapist has evaluated a 7-year-old child with Down syndrome who was referred because her gait has deteriorated over the last 2 years. Initially, the therapist will *most* likely be concerned about which of the following test results?

A. Child's inability to climb up a set of three 3-inch steps

B. Generalized loss of strength (≤3/5 MMT, overall)

C. Hyperactive lower extremity deep tendon reflexes

D. Low score on the Pediatric Balance Scale

30.2 The physical therapist has evaluated a 7-year-old child with Down syndrome who was referred because her gait has deteriorated over the last 2 years. The evaluation demonstrated average strength, decreased ROM of major joints, intermittent joint pain, slow and tedious gait with minimal heel strike, no sensory loss, and no change in bowel and bladder habits (by parent report). The therapist should consider requesting a referral to which specialist?

A. Gastroenterologist

B. Neurologist

C. Orthopaedist

D. Rheumatologist

30.3 Which of the following tests would be *most* ideal for assessing the developmental skills of a 7-year-old with Down syndrome?

A. Bruininks-Oseretsky Test of Motor Proficiency (BOT-2)

B. Interviewing parent regarding his/her assessment of the child's development

C. Observational Gait Scale

D. Pediatric Berg Balance Scale

30.4 The features that *best* describe the limitations that are consistent with a diagnosis of Down syndrome are:

A. Cognitive delay, persistent joint pain over 6 or more weeks, joint hypermobility

B. Delayed gross motor development, joint instability, reduced joint discomfort with use of NSAIDs

C. Developmental delay, limited development of postural stability, ligamentous laxity

D. Normal intellectual functioning, excessive instability of major joints, bladder incontinence

ANSWERS

30.1 **C.** The therapist would most likely be ruling out atlantoaxial (C1/C2) subluxation because this occurs in approximately 14% of children with Down syndrome.[5] Options A and B could be explained simply by disuse atrophy. Option D is not the best choice because although the test is a reliable measure of functional balance for school-aged children, it is specifically appropriate to use with individuals with mild to moderate motor impairment.[14]

30.2 **D.** The clinical presentation suggests a systemic disease versus an orthopaedic (*e.g.*, atlantoaxial subluxation) or neurological disorder since the child had no change in bowel and bladder function and no sensory loss.

30.3 **A.** The BOT-2 is considered a reliable and valid test of gross and fine motor skills for children ages 4 to 9 years without and with disabilities. Parent interview is an important component of the evaluation process, but is not an objective measure of motor development (option B). While both the Observational Gait Scale and the Pediatric Berg Balance Scale provide a functional level assessment of gait and balance, neither is appropriate as a tool for the assessment of motor performance (options C and D).

30.4 **C.** Developmental delay, limited development of postural stability, and ligamentous laxity provides a typical portrait of a child with Down syndrome. Persistent joint pain is not typical for children with Down syndrome (option A), who may have a problem recognizing pain and may lack the ability to express feeling pain. Delayed gross motor development and joint instability are consistent with Down syndrome, but there is no evidence to indicate that NSAIDs specifically address pain better than other analgesic medications (option B). Option D describes one major problem of children with low tone (excessive instability of major joints) related to a diagnosis of Down syndrome; however, normal intellectual functioning is not consistent with a diagnosis of Down syndrome and bladder incontinence would more appropriately apply specifically if C1/C2 instability is present.

REFERENCES

1. U.S. Government. USCA. 1402(25). http://idea.ed.gov/. Accessed September 01, 2012.

2. Drnach M. *The Clinical Practice of Pediatric Physical Therapy*. Philadelphia, PA: Wolters Kluwer; 2008:87-88.

3. Rex AP, Preus M. A diagnostic index for Down syndrome. *J Pediatr*. 1982;100:903-906.

4. NICHCY. Down syndrome disability fact sheet #4 June 2010. http://nichcy.org/disability/specific/downsyndrome. Accessed August 03, 2012.

5. Smith DS. Health care management of adults with Down syndrome. *Am Fam Physician*. 2001;64:1031-1038.

6. Juj H, Emery H. The arthropathy of Down syndrome: an underdiagnosed and underrecognized condition. *J Pediatr*. 2009;154:234-238.

7. Roizen N. Down syndrome. In: Batshaw ML, Pellegrino L, Roizen NJ, eds. *Children with Disabilities*. Baltimore, MD: Brookes Publishing Co.; 2007:263-273.

8. Looper J, Benjamin D, Nolan M, Schumm L. What to measure when determining orthotic needs in children with Down syndrome: a pilot study. *Pediatr Phys Ther.* 2012;24:313-319.

9. Sacks B, Buckley SJ. Motor development for individuals with Down syndrome: an overview. *Down Syndrome Issues and Information.* 2003. http://www.down-syndrome.org/information/motor/overview/. Accessed July 01, 2012.

10. Harris SR, Heriza CB. Measuring infant movement: clinical and technological assessment techniques. *Phys Ther.*1987;67:1877-1880.

11. Wu J, Looper J, Ulrich BD, Ulrich DA, Angulo-Barroso RM. Exploring effects of differential treadmill interventions on walking onset and gait patterns in infants with Down syndrome. *Dev Med Child Neurol.* 2007;49:839-845.

12. NCHPAD. Down syndrome and exercise. 2012-09. http://www.ncpad.org/117/910/Down~Syndrome~and~Exercise. Accessed October 10, 2012.

13. Bergeron K, Dichter C. Case study: Down syndrome. In: Effgen S, ed. *Meeting the Physical Therapy Needs of Children.* Philadelphia, PA: F.A. Davis; 2005:516-538.

14. Franjoine MR, Gunther JS, Taylor MJ. Pediatric balance scale: a modified version of the Berg balance scale for the school-age child with mild to moderate motor impairment. *Pediatr Phys Ther.* 2003;15:114-128.

15. Martin K, Hoover D, Wagoner E, et al. Development and reliability of an observational gait analysis tool for children with Down syndrome. *Pediatr Phys Ther.* 2009;21:261-268.

16. Bruininks R, Bruininks B. Bruininks-Oseretsky test of motor proficiency. 2nd ed. 2005. https://blogs.elon.edu/ptkids/2012/03/16/bruininks-oseretsky-test-of-motor-proficiency/. Accessed June 30, 2012.

17. Wuang YP, Su CY. Reliability and responsiveness of the Bruininks-Oseretsky test of motor proficiency: second addition in children with intellectual disability. *Res Dev Disabil.* 2009;30:847-855.

Lissencephaly

Lisa Marie Luis

CASE 31

A 4.4-year-old boy was referred to outpatient pediatric physical therapy services secondary to global developmental delay. His medical and physical therapy records document a diagnosis of mild lissencephaly or pachygyria. There were no complications during the mother's pregnancy or after delivery, which was a normal vaginal birth at full term. The parents report that he progressed through his motor milestones slowly. He first rolled over at 7 months, sat independently at 12 months, crawled at 18 months, walked at 30 months, and ran at 42 months. He has no other significant medical history, currently takes no medications, and has no reported allergies. He attends a preschool where he is in a special education program and has an Individualized Education Program (IEP; for description of IEP, see Case 29). He is receiving physical, occupational, and speech therapy at his preschool. He wears bilateral articulating ankle foot orthoses (AFOs) during gait and play activities. His parents' primary concern and reason for seeking outpatient physical therapy is that their son frequently trips and falls and requires assistance on stairs.

▶ Based on his health condition, what do you anticipate will be the contributors to activity limitations?
▶ What are the examination priorities?
▶ What is the most appropriate physical therapy outcome measure for functional mobility in children with global developmental delay?
▶ What are possible secondary impairments for a child with mild lissencephaly?

KEY DEFINITIONS

BLOCKED PRACTICE: Practicing one task for a block of trials then moving on to the next task

POSTURAL INSECURITY: Describes when an individual demonstrates extreme caution as a result of decreased postural ability during physical challenges that require postural strength and stability[1]

RANDOM PRACTICE: Practicing a task in random-ordered conditions with multiple skills being practiced within the same session

Objectives

1. Identify key questions to determine the priorities of the child and family in the physical therapy plan of care.

2. Discuss appropriate components of the examination for a child with global developmental delays.

3. Identify the most appropriate physical therapy interventions for a child with global developmental delays.

4. Discuss potential precautions that should be taken during physical therapy examination and/or interventions.

Physical Therapy Considerations

PT considerations during management of the child with mobility, activity, and participation limitations due to mild lissencephaly:

▶ **General physical therapy plan of care/goals:** Assess gait, mobility, functional strength, and equipment needs; enhance the child's ability to participate in play, home, and school activities with functional independence and safety

▶ **Physical therapy interventions:** Blocked and random practice with obstacle courses that provide variable practice of tasks; strengthening; improving balance and postural control; stretching; functional play activities; home exercise program

▶ **Precautions during physical therapy:** Decreased safety awareness and postural insecurity; awareness of potential comorbidities such as seizure disorders, aspiration, pneumonia, and secondary impairments of decreased postural control, below age level transitional and core strength, and poor dynamic standing balance

▶ **Complications interfering with physical therapy:** Cognitive level of the child and motivation for participation; frequent checking for proper equipment fit because natural maturation may interfere with joint range of motion and muscle length; decreased family involvement in care; decreased functional skills due to seizures

Understanding the Health Condition

Lissencephaly literally means "smooth brain." It is a congenital disorder in which the normal sulcal and gyral patterns of the brain are replaced by a reduced number of shallow sulci with fewer and thicker gyri (pachygyria) or a complete loss of gyri (agyria), giving the brain a smooth appearance.[2,3] Children with classic lissencephaly present with mental retardation and mixed hypotonia that is seen early and persists, spasticity that appears later, opisthotonus, poor feeding, poor control of secretions, motor delay, and seizures.[4] There may be a history of excessive accumulation of amniotic fluid (polyhydramnios) during pregnancy that is often caused by a birth defect that affects the gastrointestinal tract or central nervous system of the fetus.[3,5] Children with lissencephaly tend to be small for their gestational age and may fail to thrive—experiencing frequent episodes of aspiration and gastroesophageal reflux. Feeding problems are present within the first few months of life but usually resolve within weeks to months. Aspiration often becomes worse as spasticity increases, and infantile spasms usually occur from the 3rd to the 12th month. It is uncommon for children with lissencephaly to not experience seizures. Multiple seizure types are common, including atypical absence, myoclonic, tonic, and tonic-clonic seizures that are often intractable. Characteristic craniofacial features of a child with lissencephaly include prominent forehead, bitemporal hollowing, short nose with upturned nostrils, flat midface, protuberant upper lip, thin vermilion border of the upper lip, and small jaw.[4] A shortened life span is likely expected and related to the severity of the condition. In a study to determine survival of patients with classic lissencephaly, de Wit et al.[6] noted that approximately 50% of 24 patients with severe forms of lissencephaly were alive at 14 years, and all were severely disabled and needed complete care. They also concluded that life expectancy was related to the severity of the lissencephaly observed on neuroimaging. Table 31-1 shows the six grades of lissencephaly, which is a patterning scale used to determine the severity of brain malformation based on neuroimaging.[4] A low grade on neuroimaging is indicative of more severe forms of lissencephaly and survival rates are expected to be low. Children with a lissencephaly grade of 1 or 2 demonstrate severe psychomotor impairment and intractable epilepsy. Milder phenotypes may only present with epilepsy and have normal cognitive development.[3,4,6]

Lissencephaly is a relatively rare disorder. It is estimated to occur in at least 1 in 100,000 live births, although some sources believe this may be an underestimate.[3,4,6] In 80% of the cases, there is a distinct genetic abnormality and the remaining 20%

Table 31-1	GRADES OF LISSENCEPHALY
Grade 1	Complete agyria
Grade 2	Diffuse agyria with frontal or occipital undulations
Grade 3	Posterior agyria and anterior pachygyria
Grade 4	Anterior or posterior preponderance with either mixed or diffuse pachygyria
Grade 5	Anterior to gradient of pachygyria with subcortical band heterotopias
Grade 6	Subcortical band heterotopia only

are considered familial in origin. There are several genes that are involved in the pathogenesis of lissencephaly. *Lissencephaly 1 (LIS1)*, *Doulecortin (DCX or XLIS)*, *Reelin (RELN)*, and *Aristlass-Related Homeobox (ARX)* are the main genes that are affected. Lissencephaly is associated with deletions on the 17th chromosome and always includes the *LIS1* gene.

All patients with severe lissencephaly have profound mental retardation. Approximately half of all children with lissencephaly will be able to roll, move short distances when placed on the floor, reach for objects, and sit. The incidence of purposeful movement is higher when seizures are better managed. The most common complications are seizures, poor feeding, and pneumonia. de Wit et al.[6] found that children with severe grades of type 1 lissencephaly had severe intellectual and motor disability and epilepsy was intractable in all cases. They found that treatment of epilepsy was important because seizures may lead to loss of skills and death. Life expectancy was found to be limited in this cohort; however, with care that was focused on infection and scoliosis prevention, many of the children reached adulthood. A limitation of this study was that it did not include children with milder phenotypes of lissencephaly because these individuals were not diagnosed with the disorder prior to 1990 due to limitations in neuroimaging.

Physical Therapy Patient/Client Management

The child with lissencephaly presents with a complex medical history and requires multidisciplinary care. Clinical manifestations may include mental retardation, mixed hypotonia, spasticity, poor feeding, and poor control of secretions that predispose them to pneumonia and seizures. These children may also have various comorbidities. Medical management of seizures is of utmost importance secondary to regression of skills or even death. Feeding issues, dysphagia, control of secretions, speech delays, and pneumonia prevention may be best managed under the care of a speech language pathologist. Evaluation and treatment from an occupational therapist may be necessary for psychomotor disability and sensory integration difficulties. An occupational therapist also plays an important role for children with lissencephaly that present with postural and gravitational insecurity as well as movement intolerance.[1] Due to global gross motor delay, mild spasticity, and mixed hypotonia, these children are prone to the development of scoliosis and benefit from the care and treatment of a physical therapist. Since there is a significant range of psychomotor disability based on the grades and severity of lissencephaly, these children may or may not be mainstreamed into a typical school setting. Survival rate in this population may also depend on quality of care received. In the study by de Wit et al.,[6] many of the patients died before the era of routine gastrostomy (surgical opening into the stomach for nutritional support).

It is unknown if neural plastic changes occur in children with lissencephaly over time. Disruption of the *RELN (Reelin)* gene in humans is linked to lissencephaly. *RELN* is a large extracellular matrix protein that is secreted by specialized neurons (called Cajal-Retzius cells) located in the marginal zone. *RELN* serves as a molecular guiding cue for the subventricular migrating neurons during embryonic development of the central nervous system. Banko et al.[7] investigated the importance of *RELN* expression in mice. *RELN* is mutated in the naturally occurring mutant reeler mice. Reeler mice have similar characteristics to those of children with lissencephaly. They demonstrate a reeling gait pattern (staggering or drunken gait), impaired learning and memory, and abnormal cerebral layering in the neocortex, cerebellum, and hippocampus. Mice exposed to *Reelin* via bilateral ventricle cannulation exhibit enhanced spatial and associative learning. This suggests that alterations in adult *RELN* signaling could affect hippocampal plasticity and cognitive ability. While there is currently no treatment for lissencephaly, this study identified that humans with deficiencies in *RELN* signaling share several phenotypic features of reeler mice. This signaling defect demonstrates a need for further investigation into the potentially important role *RELN* has on the adult and developing brain.[7]

Examination, Evaluation, and Diagnosis

The physical therapist obtains information from medical records and interviews with the parents to determine the child's birth history, previous diagnostic testing, motor milestones, and concerns that the parents have for the child. Additional relevant questions include: "Can the child walk and how far can he walk?" and "Can he participate in play with siblings or age-matched peers?" If the child cannot ambulate long distances, the therapist should consider whether an adaptive stroller would be an option to support the parents. The examination should include tests and measures and a systems review to determine the primary and secondary impairments, functional limitations, and participation restrictions.

Since the parents are concerned about their son's frequent falling and needed assistance on the stairs, the therapist should consider what adaptive/assistive devices or orthoses could assist in the child's safe functional mobility. The therapist performs a functional assessment to determine whether the child can demonstrate sufficient functional strength to transition from one position to another. In starting out the evaluation, some questions are directed at the child. How and whether the child answers the questions helps the therapist understand his cognitive ability. If the child appears not to understand verbal directions, then the therapist can demonstrate a requested task. Observation is a critical skill that the physical therapist must utilize when working with any pediatric client. As the therapist is conducting the interview with the parents, the therapist observes how the child walks and moves, which provides necessary information to determine appropriate adaptive/assistive equipment needs that are best for the child and also to support the parents.

The physical therapist can use the **Peabody Developmental Motor Scales, 2nd edition (PDMS-2)** to help identify the child's level of function as compared to his typical age-matched peers. The PDMS-2 gross motor section contains 151 items equally divided among age levels from 15 days to 71 months. Items are grouped into four skill categories (reflexes, stationary, locomotion, and object manipulation) that represent the clustering of items that place similar demands on the child. Items are scored on a three-point scale (0, 1, and 2). A score of 0 indicates that the criterion has not been met, a score of 1 indicates that the behavior is emerging but that the criterion for successful performance has not been fully met, and a score of 2 indicates that all criteria for the skill have been fully met. The PDMS-2 has high diagnostic accuracy for motor delay with reports that results of the test can correctly diagnose motor delay 98% of the time.[8,9]

Plan of Care and Interventions

Presently, there is no research regarding which physical therapy interventions are most effective for children with mild lissencephaly. Interventions are based on the child's impairments, functional limitations, and participation restrictions. Identification of primary and secondary impairments, functional limitations, and participation restrictions as compared to typical age-matched peers is necessary to construct goals that are pertinent to the child and his parents. Goals should be specific, measureable, attainable, reasonable, and time dependent. Physical therapy interventions that could be used for a child with mild lissencephaly include strengthening exercises, balance training, positioning, stretching, gait, and functional activity training. **Blocked and random practice schedules** can be used during therapy sessions to promote long-term motor learning and transfer of learning. Given that transfer of learning is best accomplished when the practice environment closely matches the processing demands of those in the actual environment,[10] treatment rooms can be set up using ramps, stairs, steps, swings, and variety of toys, and surfaces to mimic school, home, and community environments. For example, the parents stated that the stairs at home are 8 inches in height. The therapist could incorporate a step into a game in which the child would have to climb up a step (beginning with a shorter step of approximately 4 inches) to get to a puzzle or game that is on a raised surface or on the wall. Once the child masters the 4-inch step, the therapist can increase the difficulty by increasing the height and number of stairs the child ascends and descends. This task encourages postural security with the activity and increases lower extremity strength.

Another intervention strategy that provides variable practice of tasks related to impairments and goals is the use of obstacle courses to improve walking, running, squatting, climbing, bilateral and single-leg balance, and coordination activities. Obstacle courses may also be repeated in reverse order to further randomize the practice. The child in this case demonstrates postural insecurity on raised or uneven surfaces, decreased range of motion in bilateral ankles, and decreased functional strength. An example of an obstacle course that would be beneficial for him would be one consisting of transitions from firm to soft surfaces (*e.g.*, hard wood to carpet to foam mat), a ramp that would promote mild heel cord stretching, stairs, and a balance beam for postural control, balance, and strength. Mixed hypotonia is common in children with lissencephaly, and these children have a tendency to "lock" weightbearing joints or assume positions that provide a wide base of support.[11] Special attention should be paid to sitting, standing, walking, and running postures to ensure that weightbearing is equally distributed and alignment is neutral. It is also important to include activities that focus on postural insecurity given that children with hypotonia generally have limited movement experiences and typically do not develop a well-adapted sensory system.[11]

Evidence-Based Clinical Recommendations

SORT: Strength of Recommendation Taxonomy

A: Consistent, good-quality patient-oriented evidence
B: Inconsistent or limited-quality patient-oriented evidence
C: Consensus, disease-oriented evidence, usual practice, expert opinion, or case series

1. Physical therapists can use the Peabody Developmental Motor Scales, 2nd edition (PDMS-2), to identify children with motor disability. **Grade A**

2. Physical therapists can use blocked and random practice schedules to increase long-term motor learning and transfer of learning. **Grade B**

3. Blocked and random practice schedules increase long-term motor learning in children with lissencephaly. **Grade C**

COMPREHENSIVE QUESTIONS

31.1 What conditions should the physical therapist be aware of when evaluating and treating the child with an unknown grade of lissencephaly?

 A. Diabetes, hypertension

 B. Seizures, poor feeding, pneumonia

 C. Cardiac arrhythmias

 D. Scoliosis, breathing difficulty

31.2 Which is the *most* appropriate practice schedule to use when the learner does not understand the dynamics of the task being learned?

 A. Random

 B. Full task

 C. Blocked

 D. Random and blocked

ANSWERS

31.1 **B.** The most common complications with lissencephaly are seizures, poor feeding, and pneumonia. It is uncommon for children with lissencephaly to not experience seizures. Feeding problems are often noticed within the first few months of life and usually resolve within weeks to months. Aspiration, which can cause pneumonia, often becomes worse as spasticity increases.

31.2 **C.** Blocked practice is the most appropriate practice schedule to use until the learner understands the dynamics of the task being learned. Once the learner understands the dynamics of the task, research shows that there is increased motor learning when a random practice schedule is used.[10]

REFERENCES

1. May-Benson T, Koomar JA. Identifying gravitational insecurity in children: a pilot study. *Am J Occup Ther.* 2007;61:142-147.

2. Landrieu P, Husson B, Pariente D, Lacroix C. MRI-neuropathological correlations in type 1 lissencephaly. *Neuroradiology.* 1998;40:173-176.

3. Nasrallah IM, Golden JA. Brain malformations associated with cell migration. *Pediatr Dev Pathol.* 2006;9:89-97.

4. Dobyns WB, Seibert JR, Sarnat HB. Lissencephaly. Medlink Neurology. 2011.

5. Mayo Clinic. Polyhydramnios. http://www.mayoclinic.com/health/polyhydramnios/DS01156. Accessed May 25, 2012.

6. de Wit MC, de Rijk-van Andel J, Halley DJ, et al. Long-term follow-up of type 1 lissencephaly: survival is related to neuroimaging abnormalities. *Dev Med Child Neurol.* 2011;53:417-421.

7. Banko JL, Trotter J, Weber EJ. Insights into synaptic function from mouse models of human cognitive disorders. *Future Neurol.* 2011;6:113-125.

8. Palisano RJ, Kolobe TH, Haley SM, Lowes LP, Jones SL. Validity of the Peabody Development Gross Motor Scale as an evaluative measure of infants receiving physical therapy. *Phys Ther.* 1995;75: 939-948.

9. Wang HH, Liao HF, Hsieh CL. Reliability, sensitivity to change, responsiveness of the Peabody developmental motor scales second edition for children with cerebral palsy. *Phys Ther.* 2006;86: 1351-1359.

10. Shumway-Cook A, Woollacott M. *Motor Control: Theory and Practical Applications.* 3rd ed. Baltimore, MD: Lippincott Williams and Wilkins; 2007.

11. Umphred DA. *Neurologic Rehabilitation.* 5th ed. St. Louis, MO: Mosby; 2007.

Listing of Cases

Listing by Case Number

Listing by Health Condition (Alphabetical)

Listing by Case Number

Listing by Health Condition (Alphabetical)

NOTE: Page numbers followed by *f* or *t* indicate figures or tables, respectively.